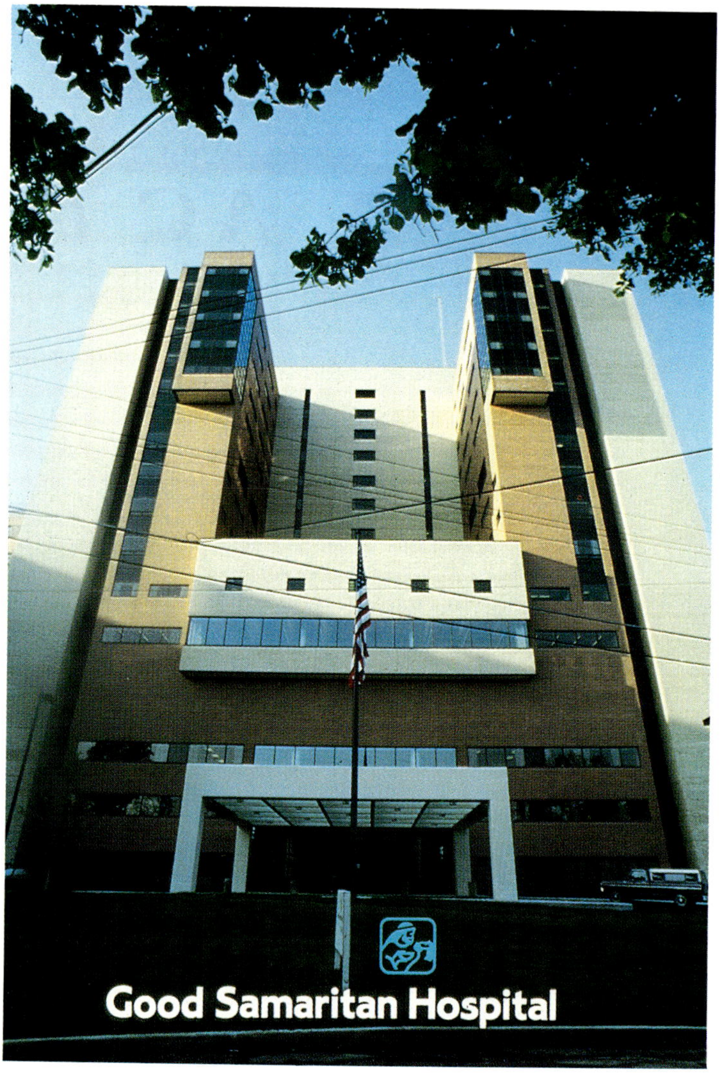
Good Samaritan Hospital

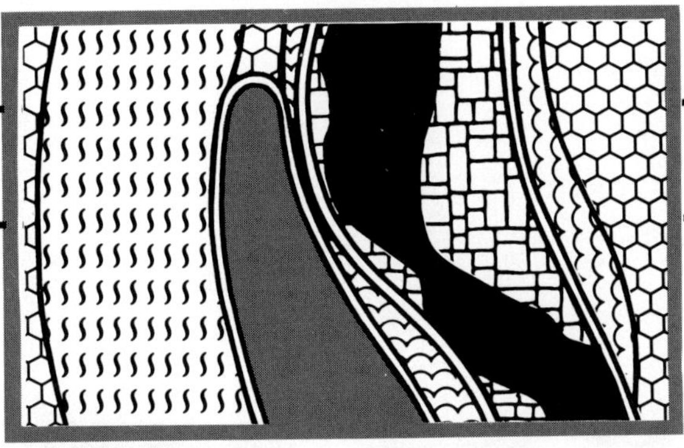

ATLAS OF DUPLEX SCANNING

CAROTID ARTERIES

John J. Cranley, Jr., M.D.
Director Emeritus
Department of Surgery
Director, Vascular Laboratory
Good Samaritan Hospital
Cincinnati, Ohio

William S. Karkow, M.D.
Associate Director
Vascular Laboratory
Good Samaritan Hospital
Cincinnati, Ohio

E. Douglas Baldridge, M.D.
Peripheral Vascular Fellow
Good Samaritan Hospital
Cincinnati, Ohio

1989

W.B. SAUNDERS COMPANY

Harcourt Brace Jovanovich, Inc.

Philadelphia ○ London ○ Toronto ○ Montreal ○ Sydney ○ Tokyo

W. B. SAUNDERS COMPANY
Harcourt Brace Jovanovich, Inc.

The Curtis Center
Independence Square West
Philadelphia, PA 19106

Library of Congress Cataloging-in-Publication Data

Cranley, John J.
Atlas of duplex scanning : carotid arteries / John J. Cranley, William S. Karkow, E. Douglas Baldridge, Jr.
p. cm.
ISBN 0-7216-2303-4
1. Carotid artery—Diseases—Diagnosis—Atlases. 2. Carotid artery—Ultrasonic imaging—Atlases. 3. Duplex ultrasonography—Atlases. I. Karkow, William S. II. Baldridge, E. Douglas. III. Title.
[DNLM: 1. Carotid Arteries—radiography—atlases. 2. Carotid Artery Diseases—diagnosis—atlases. 3. Ultrasonic Diagnosis—atlases. WG 17 C891a]
RC691.6.D87C73 1989
616.1′3—dc19

88–15670

Editor: W. B. Saunders Staff
Designer: Maureen Sweeney
Production Manager: Bob Butler
Manuscript Editor: Mary Anne Folcher
Illustration Coordinator: Walt Verbitski
Indexer: Ann Kassar

Atlas of Duplex Scanning: Carotid Arteries ISBN 0-7216-2303-4

Last digit is the print number: 9 8 7 6 5 4 3 2 1

PREFACE

The development of instrumentation combining B-mode ultrasound and Doppler velocity detection for purposes of studying vascular disease was the work of Strandness and associates. They coined the term duplex scanning. Originally, it was used primarily for the study of the carotid arteries. Ford and Talbot, to our knowledge, were the first to use duplex scanning to study the venous system and recommended the technique to us. While using it in the study of veins of the lower extremities, it soon became apparent that this modality was an excellent one for investigating venous problems, such as venous thrombosis and chronic venous insufficiency, and for vein mapping prior to in situ vein surgery for revascularization of the lower extremity and for coronary grafting. Further, once we started scanning extremities, we realized how extremely useful the technique was for the study of arterial aneurysms, anastomotic aneurysms, and stenoses of grafts. In addition, it proved to be of value in diagnosing cysts, localized hemorrhage, perigraft hematomata and infections, lymphadenopathy, and edema of the extremity.

Our experience with carotid scanning began in 1979 and extremity scanning in 1982. These modalities had an explosive effect on our laboratory, so that today, ultrasound is the single, most used diagnostic method in the laboratory. To date, we have scanned cases involving an excess of 9000 carotid arteries and 7000 extremities.

Along with the growth in our laboratory came requests from physicians and technicians for training in ultrasound. While videotapes are the best way to learn to interpret scans, there is still a need for drawings correlated with actual photographs of the images to help the trainee understand the procedure fully. From this need for instruction, the idea occurred to us to prepare an atlas on scanning, specifically designed for physician and technician trainees.

The atlas has been compiled to accomplish several specific objectives as follows: to permit the student to recognize the appearance of normal tissues in the neck, as viewed from several angles; to differentiate the normal from the abnormal and to be able to identify the nature of the abnormality; to formulate a consistent method of evaluation and degree of the abnormality; and, finally, to recognize artifacts and thereby eliminate errors both in the performance and interpretation of the test, so as to provide a scanning technique in which maximum confidence can be placed.

Duplex scanning is a combination of B-mode imaging and Doppler signals. Since much has already been published on interpretation of Doppler signals, the topic will not be included in this text. We believe the quality of the image is the most important entity in determining whether or not the scan can be interpreted properly. The Doppler signal, while at times very valuable, is of lesser importance. Thus, it is the image that is primarily addressed in this volume. However, in practice one does not need to depend on exclusive use of either modality.

ACKNOWLEDGMENTS

As the first year fellow, at the time we obtained our first duplex scanner, Dr. Anthony Comerota was given the assignment of developing a protocol for the use of ultrasound in our vascular laboratory. Each year thereafter, the following successive fellows have continued our investigations in this field: Drs. Stephen Cook, Peter Sippel, Larry Flanagan, William Karkow, Bruce Ruoff, Douglas Baldridge, and Robert Cranley. Our technologists, mostly premedical students, have been outstanding. The first of them, David Peter, is currently a graduate physician; Larry Hanrahan and Kurt Stedje are in medical school; and Larry Hannan is in dental school. These young men worked intensely, providing us with teaching material for this first volume and for other exhibits and presentations. Daniel Meibers contributed many overtime hours with us in the preparation of this volume.

We acknowledge Strandness and associates for having the wisdom to combine B-mode scanning and Doppler signals. We acknowledge a debt of gratitude to Dr. Clynn Ford and his technologist, Steve Talbot, at the University of Utah for kindling our interest in venous scanning.

Dr. Douglas Baldridge did yeoman's work in the development of this first volume, he not only made valuable contribution to the editing but also personally photographed most of the carotid scans, and has very nearly completed the pictures that will be needed for the second volume on venous scanning.

Dr. William Karkow has single-handedly compiled and organized the vast accumulation of material into its present format. In this volume, his singular genius for three-dimensional analysis of the scanning technique is superbly displayed. With his wife, Louaine Karkow, Dr. Karkow has produced all the drawings, using their own home computer. Louaine also did the typing of the manuscript. Rosamunde M. Preuninger, Ph.D., our research associate since the establishment of our laboratory, proofread all the material.

To Biosound, Inc., of Indianapolis, we express our sincere thanks for their support for almost a decade.

To all those mentioned, and to the other technicians in the vascular laboratory, to the late Charles F. McCurdy, an early and faithful benefactor, and to those in the administration of Good Samaritan Hospital who have supported us so long and so loyally, we are deeply grateful.

Finally, to the Trustees of Kachelmacher Memorial Inc. of Logan, Ohio, I express my profound gratitude for the funding that has permitted us to have a two-year vascular fellowship for the past 18 years. Without the contributions of these brilliant, hard working postgraduate physicians, none of our research would have been possible.

John J. Cranley, M.D.

TO
the late Nils Kachelmacher
and
the trustees of Kachelmacher Memorial, Inc. of
Logan, Ohio.

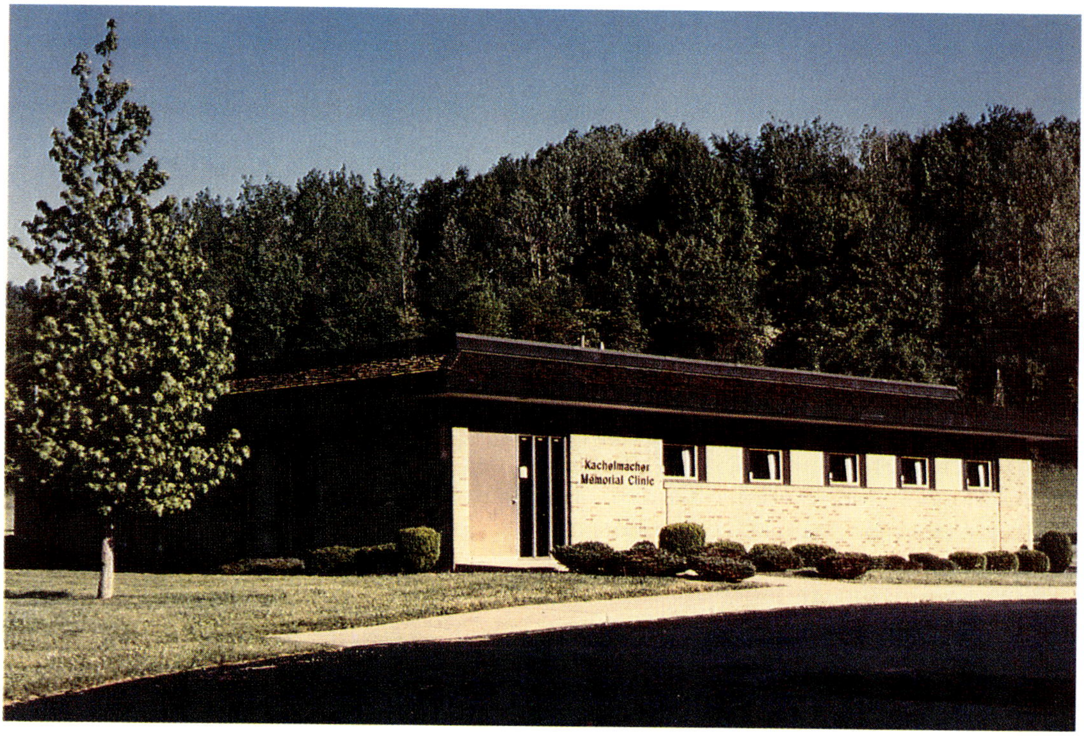

CONTENTS

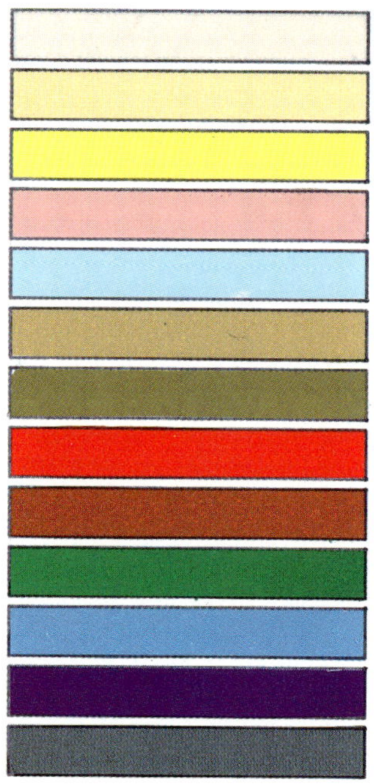

LYMPH NODE, TUMOR
CYST
GEL GAP
ARTERY WALL
VEIN WALL
PLAQUE
DACRON
ARTERIAL BLOOD
THROMBUS
PROBE MEMBRANE
VENOUS BLOOD
ARTIFACT
NERVE

CHAPTER 1

NORMAL ANATOMY

Figure 1. SCAN ORIENTATION

This schematic diagram is included to define terms in all of the ultrasound images that follow. Blood vessels are seen either in transverse (TRANS) or longitudinal (LONG) orientation. The position of the probe is such that the skin surface (SKIN) lies to the left edge of view, and the deep tissues (DEEP) lie to the right. The direction of penetration of the ultrasound beam is represented by the long arrow. The superficial wall (SW) and deep wall (DW) of the vessels are clearly seen in either view. However, only the transverse view demonstrates both top and bottom "back walls" (BW). As the probe is held against the skin, the left corner (LC) of the probe corresponds to the top LC of the image, and the right corner (RC) of the probe corresponds to the bottom LC of the image. It is easiest to imagine holding the probe in the right hand, in which case the top border of the image corresponds to the "thumb side" of the ultrasound beam, and the bottom border corresponds to the "little finger side." In this diagram, the artery in longitudinal view is shaded to indicate the back wall, which is out of the plane of the beam and not seen.

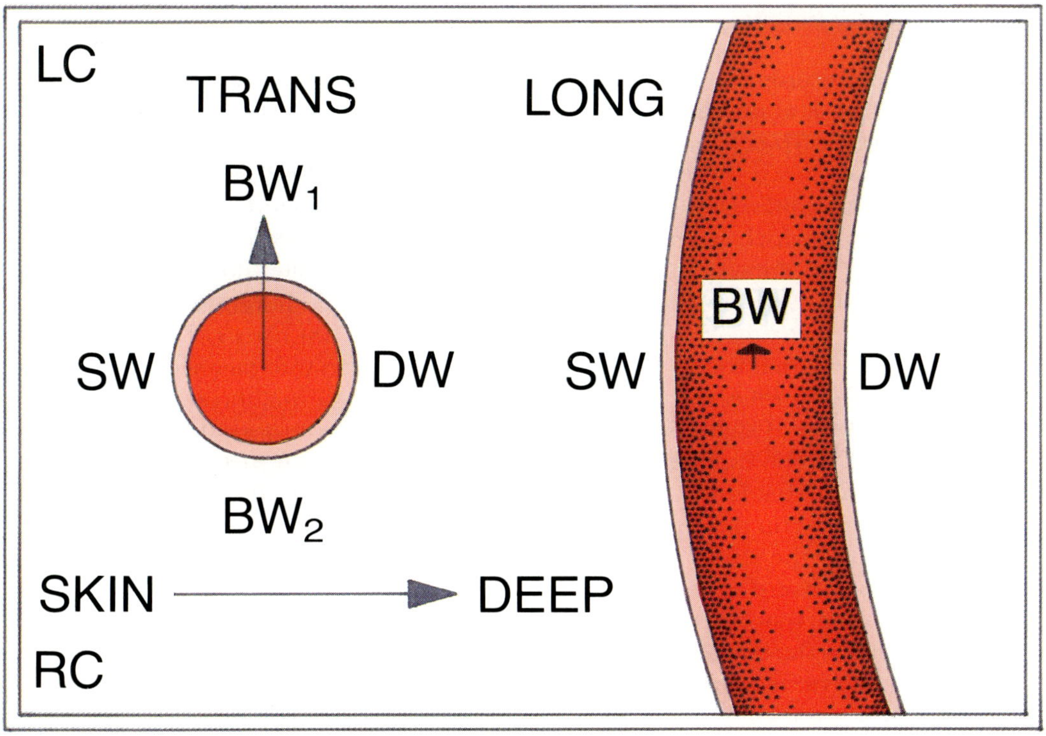
LC
TRANS
LONG
BW1
SW
DW
BW
SW
DW
BW2
SKIN
DEEP
RC

Figure 2. NORMAL COMMON CAROTID ARTERY

This is an example of a normal artery; in this case, the right common carotid artery (CCA) is at mid neck with the head toward the top of the screen as indicated by the arrow. The component parts of the arterial wall are diagrammed in greater detail than shown throughout much of the atlas. As one proceeds outward from the central lumen, shown in red, one first encounters the dark gray zone in the photograph, which is shown as a dotted pink portion (I) in the corresponding diagram. This zone is often referred to as the "intimal stripe"; but, in fact, the true intima is only a few cell layers thick, is measured in microns, and is invisible to existing instruments. The surface echo is bright not because one is actually seeing the intimal tissue, but because this solid/liquid interface with the flowing blood makes a reflective boundary, and one is seeing the abrupt transition between tissues of different densities. The rest of this intimal stripe, in fact, is composed of the inner two thirds of the media or smooth muscle layer of the arterial wall. This is the portion that does not contain vasa vasorum. Notice its similarity in echo density to the sternocleidomastoid muscle (M), which is seen quite well to the left of the artery with its typical longitudinal striations. As one proceeds outward from the intimal stripe, one sees a layer of very bright echoes representing the outer medial and adventitial layers of the arterial wall and presented in the diagram as a clear pink layer A for adventitia. Proceeding outward from this layer is a third layer that is not as brightly echogenic as the adventitial layer but is more brightly echogenic than the surrounding tissue. This third layer is presented in the diagram by the zigzag lines. These correspond to periadventitial tissue, in this case, the carotid sheath.

It is most important to recognize that the intimal stripe is normally present and measures up to 1 mm in thickness and should not be mistaken for smooth plaque. (The Doppler cursor in the center of the picture is equal to 0.9 mm. SQ = subcutaneous tissue (including, in this case, both the deeper layer of the dermis and platysma muscle); F = fascia (including both the investing cervical fascia and the carotid sheath). In this and all subsequent drawings all deeper tissues, in which a definite identification of tissue type cannot be made, are represented by a honeycomb pattern.

To remind the reader in regard to the orientation of the scan, it is understood that the skin is always located to the left with the deeper tissues located to the right. There are no exceptions to this left-to-right direction of penetration into the deeper tissues. In addition, each longitudinal scan, as in this example, has an arrow indicating the direction toward which the head is located. In the case of transverse scans the arrow indicates in which direction the medial aspect of the body is located, because in carotid scans we view the left bifurcation upside down for the sake of ease in positioning the probe. In lower extremity studies the orientation varies occasionally for the same reason.

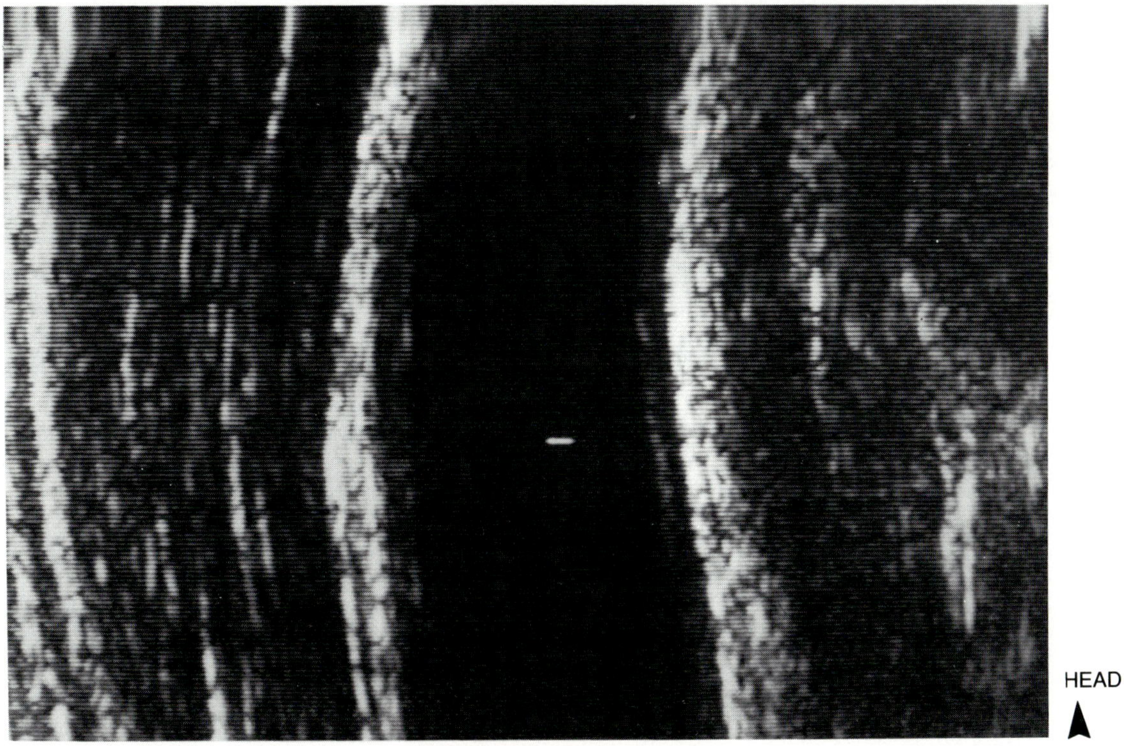
HEAD

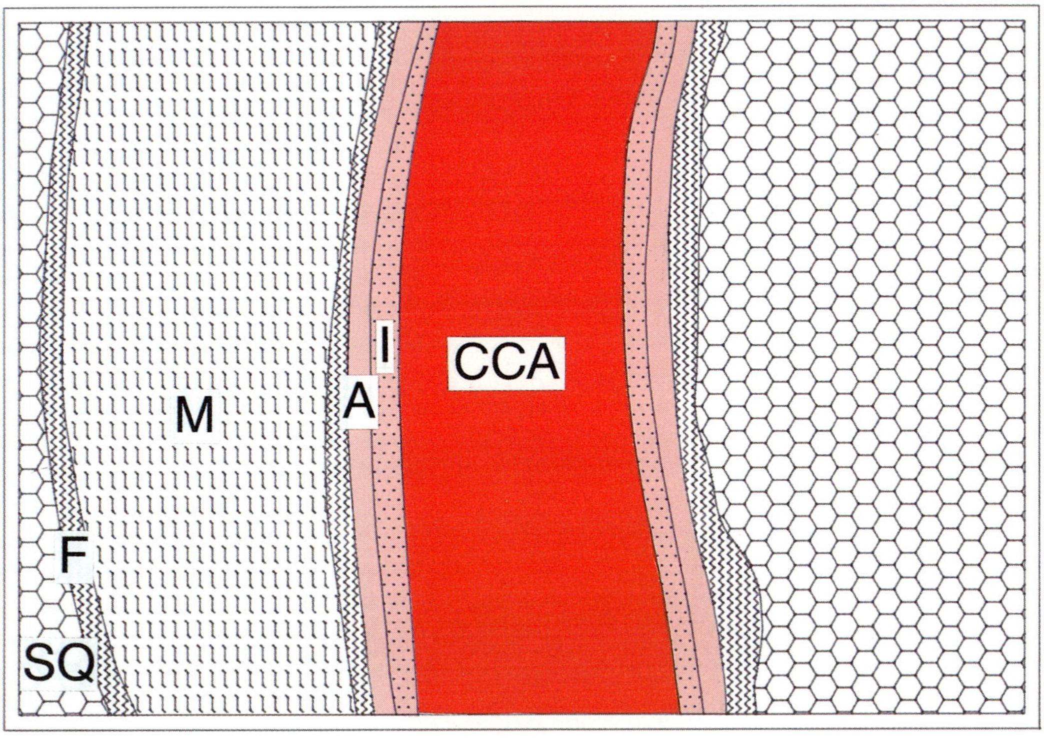
I
CCA
A
M
F
SQ

Figure 3. NORMAL LEFT COMMON CAROTID

This is a longitudinal view of another normal left common carotid artery (CCA) in its mid section. In the center of the photograph at mid neck, is shown the measurement of a residual lumen (RL2), which is slightly larger than the residual lumen (RL1) of the common carotid at the base of the neck; this is typical. These residual lumens are most properly measured with calipers in a perpendicular fashion to the long axis of the artery at that particular level. Note the exact end points of the residual lumens that extend from the inner surface of the normal "intimal stripes" (I), not the brighter adventitial boundaries (A). This photograph and the following two photographs are of the same carotid system and are shown to give the reader an overall view of the approximately 12 cm of carotid arteries that can be visualized in the normal adult neck. G = gel, S = skin, PM = platysma muscle, F = fascia, SCM = sternocleidomastoid muscle, DIST = distal common carotid, ? = tissue of uncertain composition.

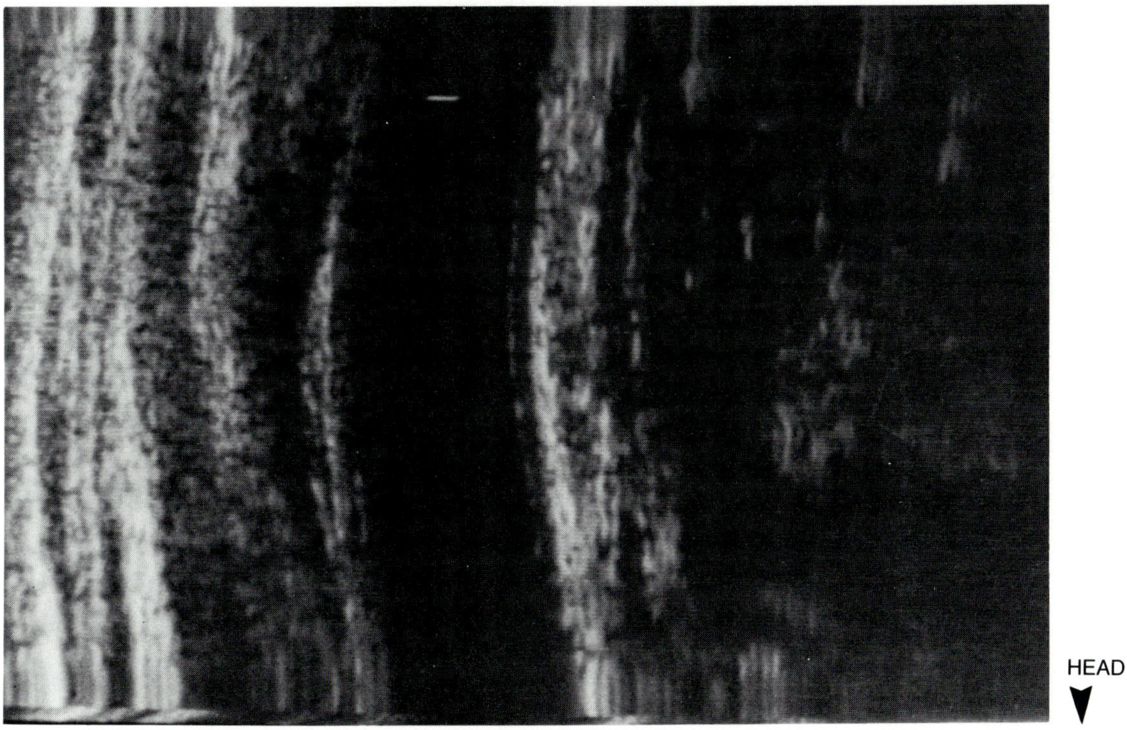
HEAD

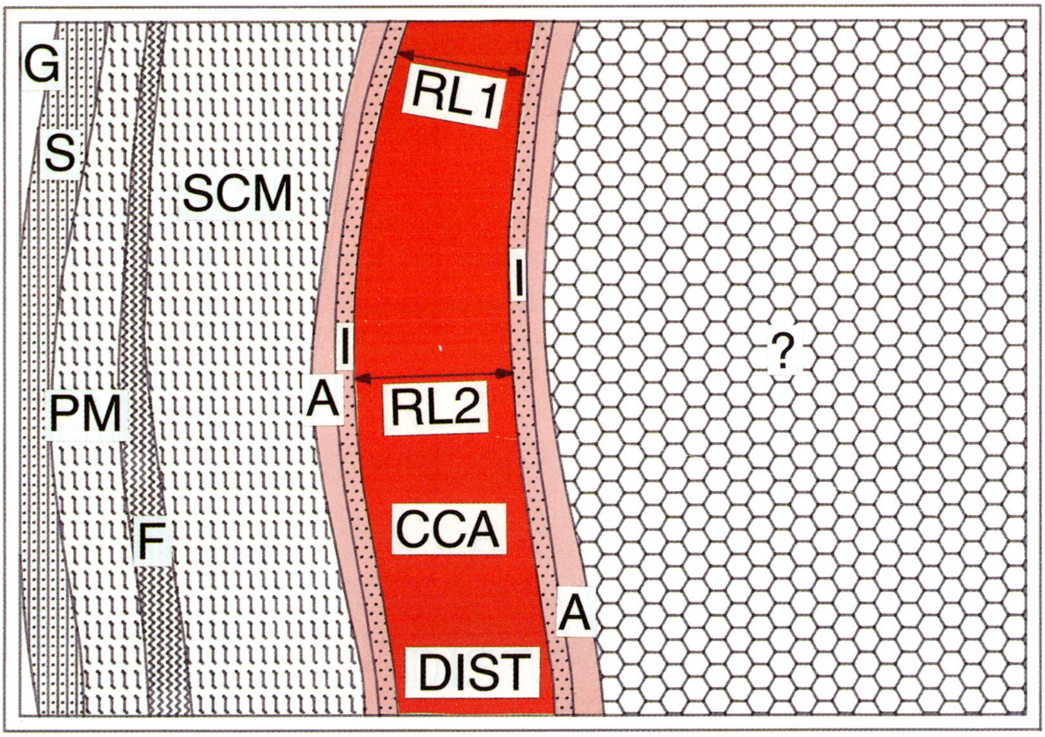
G
S
SCM
PM
F
RL1
I
I
A
RL2
CCA
A
DIST
?

Figure 4. NORMAL LEFT CAROTID BIFURCATION

In this view the same common carotid artery (CCA) is followed up to the bifurcation, which is in the center of this photograph. Note the larger size of the bulb of the internal carotid artery (ICA) represented by the residual lumen (RL3) in comparison with the residual lumen (RL4) of the distal artery, which is not well visualized at the bottom of the screen but is better visualized on the next photograph. The external carotid artery is seen deep to the internal carotid in this view of the left bifurcation. This orientation is quite frequent on the left, presumably because of the fashion in which our technicians hold the probe from a somewhat more posterior position on the neck and thus closer to the internal than the external carotid. G = gel, S = skin, M = platysma muscle, F = fascia, SCM = sternocleidomastoid muscle, V = internal jugular vein, I = intimal stripe (not well seen in this photograph), ? = tissue of uncertain composition.

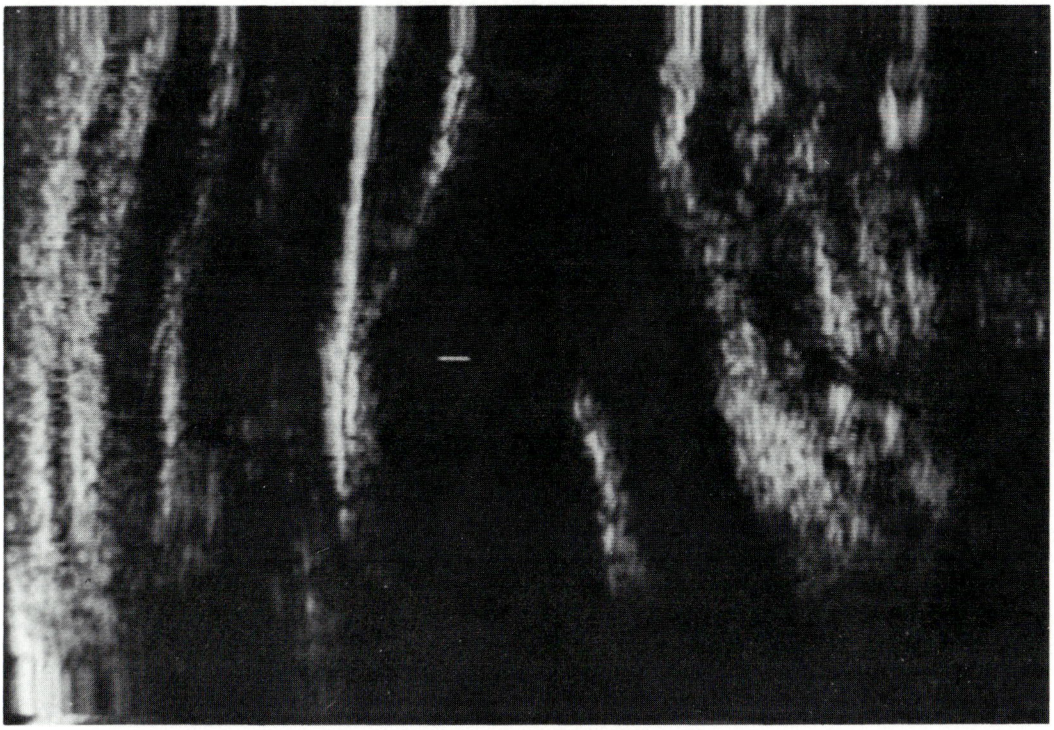

HEAD

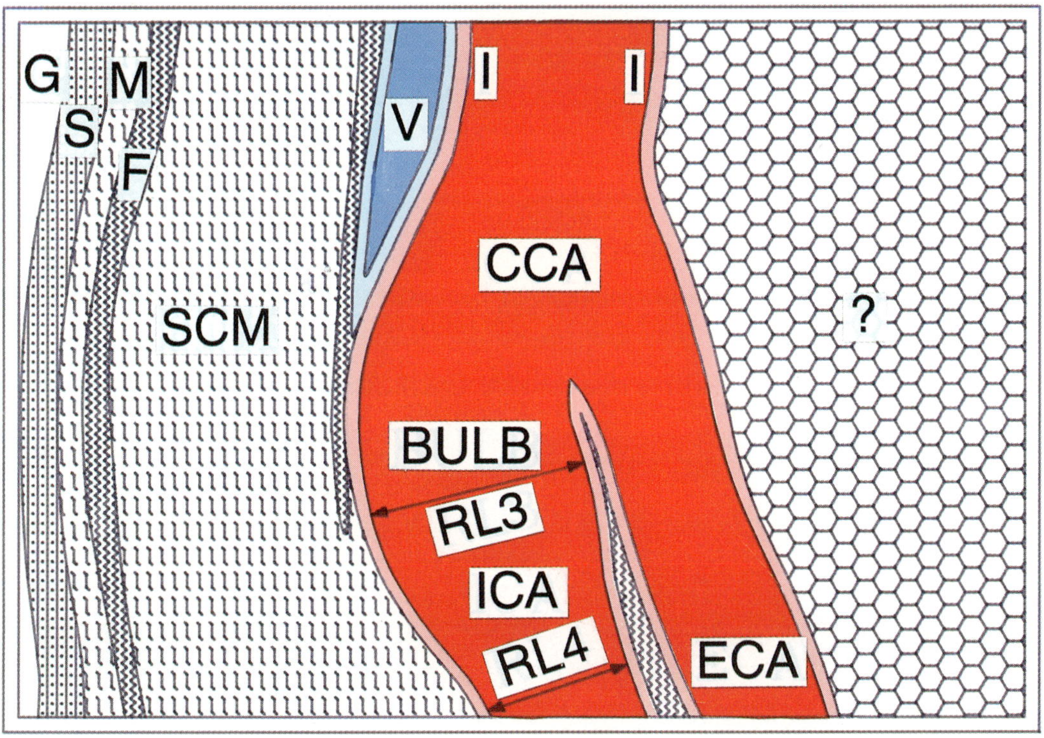

Figure 5. NORMAL LEFT BIFURCATION

This photograph is taken still farther beyond the level of the bifurcation at as high a level as can be achieved in this patient. Note the tapering of the internal carotid artery (ICA) distally which, at the very bottom of the picture, begins to curve out of plane giving rise to some back wall (BW) echoes. The superficial wall of the internal carotid is extremely faint in that portion abutting the internal jugular vein (V). Nevertheless, the residual lumen considered to be most representative of the distal ICA is drawn as RL4. Note the thinner appearance of the "intimal stripe" (I) in the ICA to the right of the cursor in comparison with the larger common carotid artery in Figure 3. The deep wall of the external carotid artery (ECA) appears to have a thicker "intimal stripe," but again this is partly due to the curvature of the vessel out of plane, as it travels distally. S = skin, M = platysma muscle, F = fascia, SCM = sternocleidomastoid muscle, CCA = common carotid artery, ? = tissue of uncertain composition.

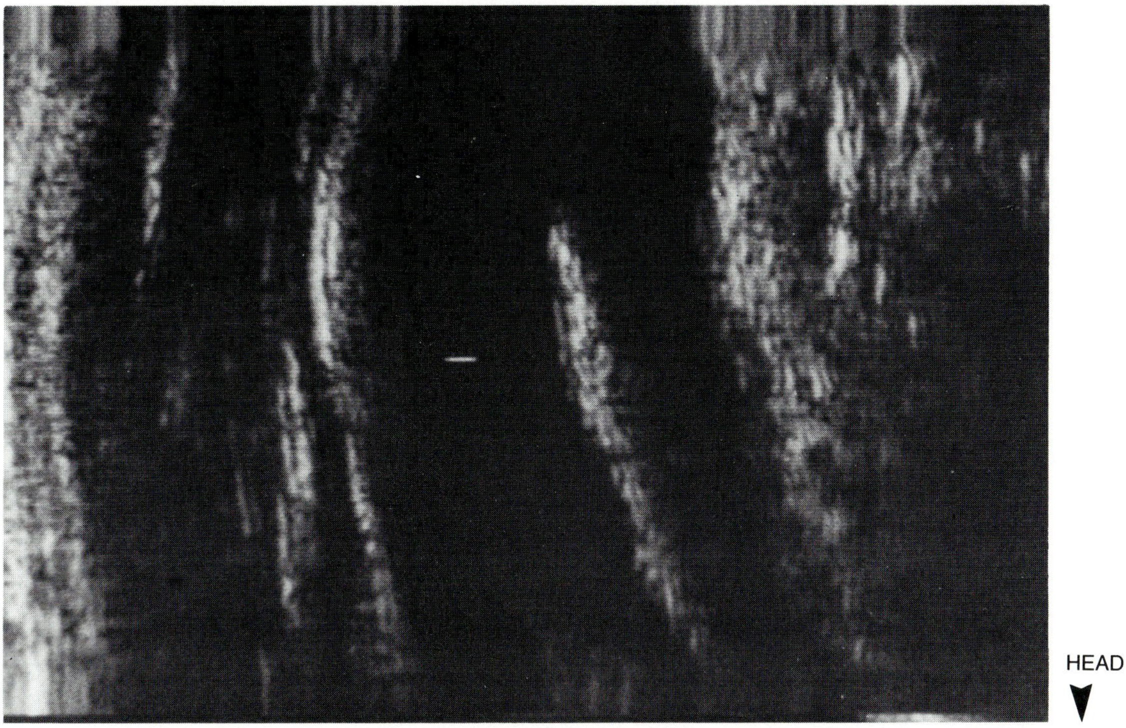
HEAD

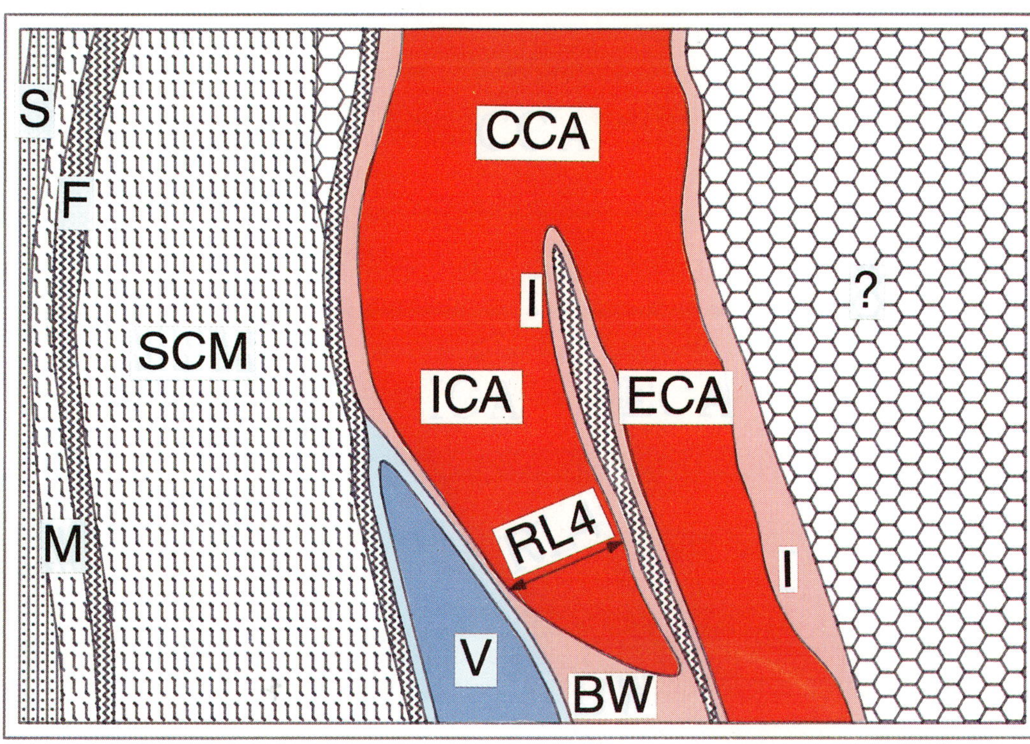
S
F
M
SCM
CCA
I
ICA
ECA
?
RL4
I
V
BW

Figure 6. NORMAL LEFT BIFURCATION

The same left internal and external carotid arteries (ICA and ECA) are seen just above the bifurcation at a level corresponding to the center of the photograph in Figure 5. Line 1 represents the plane of the ultrasound beam used to obtain the longitudinal view seen in Figure 5. Note the typical appearance of the ICA, which is slightly larger and located above (lateral) and superficial to the ECA. Compare this 10-o'clock orientation to the other left carotid bifurcations seen in Figures 9, 10, and 11. The deep portion of this photograph is all black because of the gain settings used to bring out the composition of the more superficial tissues. Because of the overall low gain settings, parts of the artery walls appear to be missing. Nevertheless, note the short sections of "intimal stripe" seen at the 3-o'clock position along the deep wall of both arteries. This is the typical appearance of an "intimal stripe" visualized in transverse view that is not usually visualized along the top and bottom "back walls." S = skin, M = platysma muscle, F = fascia, SCM = sternocleidomastoid muscle, SQ = subcutaneous tissue, IJV = internal jugular vein.

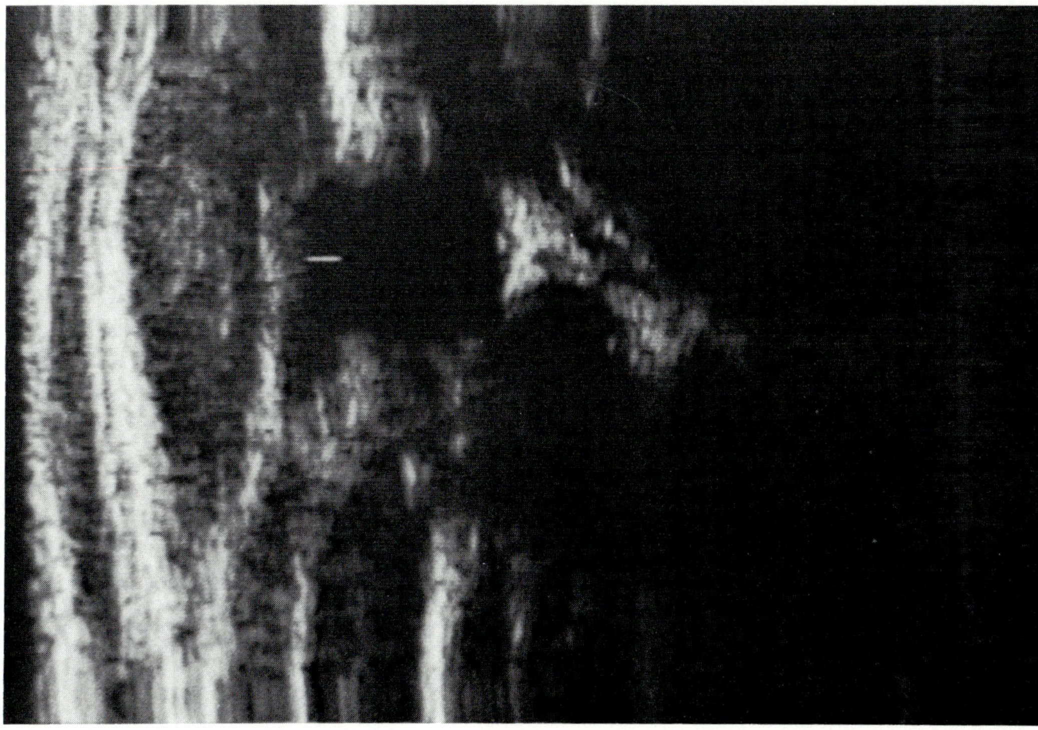

MEDIAL

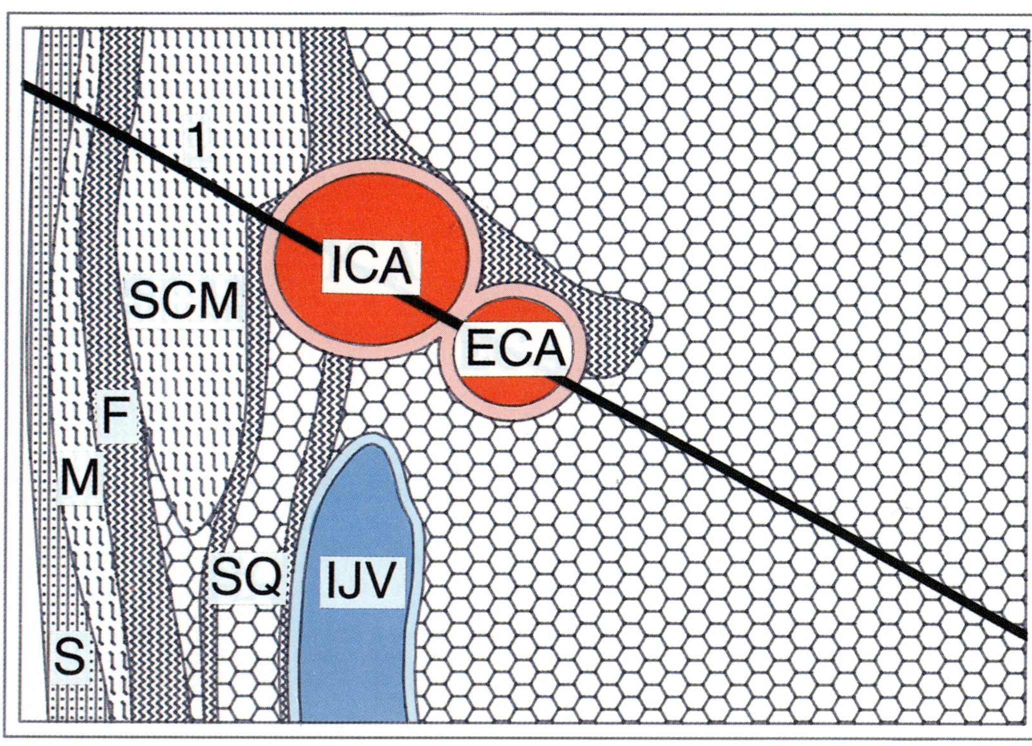

Figure 7. NORMAL RIGHT CAROTID BIFURCATION

This is a longitudinal view of the right carotid bifurcation of the same patient in which the left carotid arteries are shown in Figures 3 to 6. Note the typical orientation of the internal carotid artery (ICA) deep to the external carotid (ECA). Note also the substantial dilatation of the internal carotid bulb and its overall contour relative to the smaller common carotid artery (CCA) seen at the bottom of the photograph, which widens in the center of the photograph to reach a maximum diameter of 10.5 mm at the crotch of the bifurcation. By definition, the CCA ends and the internal and external arteries begin at this crotch. Plaque is measured separately in terms of stenosis in regard to each vessel. S = skin, SQ = subcutaneous tissue, M = muscle (sternocleidomastoid), V = internal jugular vein, F = fascia, ? = tissue of uncertain composition.

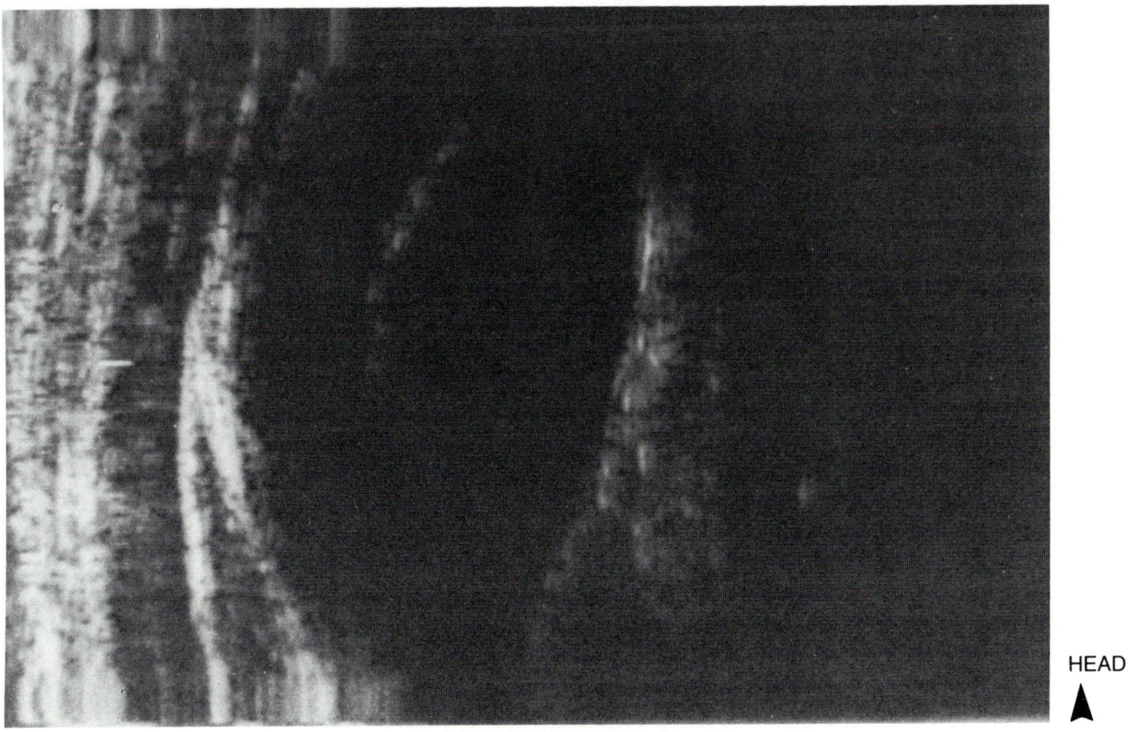
HEAD

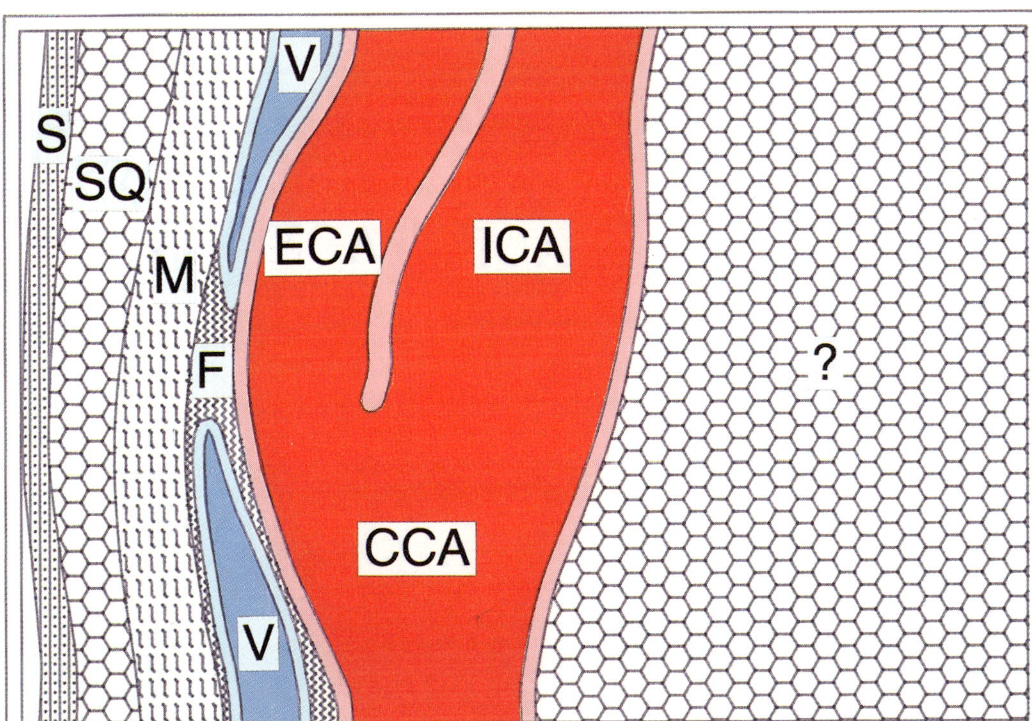
V
S
SQ
ECA
ICA
M
F
?
CCA
V

Figure 8. NORMAL RIGHT CAROTID BIFURCATION

This is a transverse view just above the crotch of the bifurcation seen in Figure 7. The Doppler cursor (C) resides within the internal carotid bulb (ICA). The end points of this cursor do not quite reach the "intimal stripes" of the normal vessel, which are not visualized in this particular view. Note the typical orientation of the external carotid artery above (medial) and to the left of (superficial to) the internal carotid. The internal jugular vein (V) has been partially compressed by the probe and is of small size. S = skin, M = platysma muscle, SQ = subcutaneous tissue, SCM = sternocleidomastoid muscle, F = fascia.

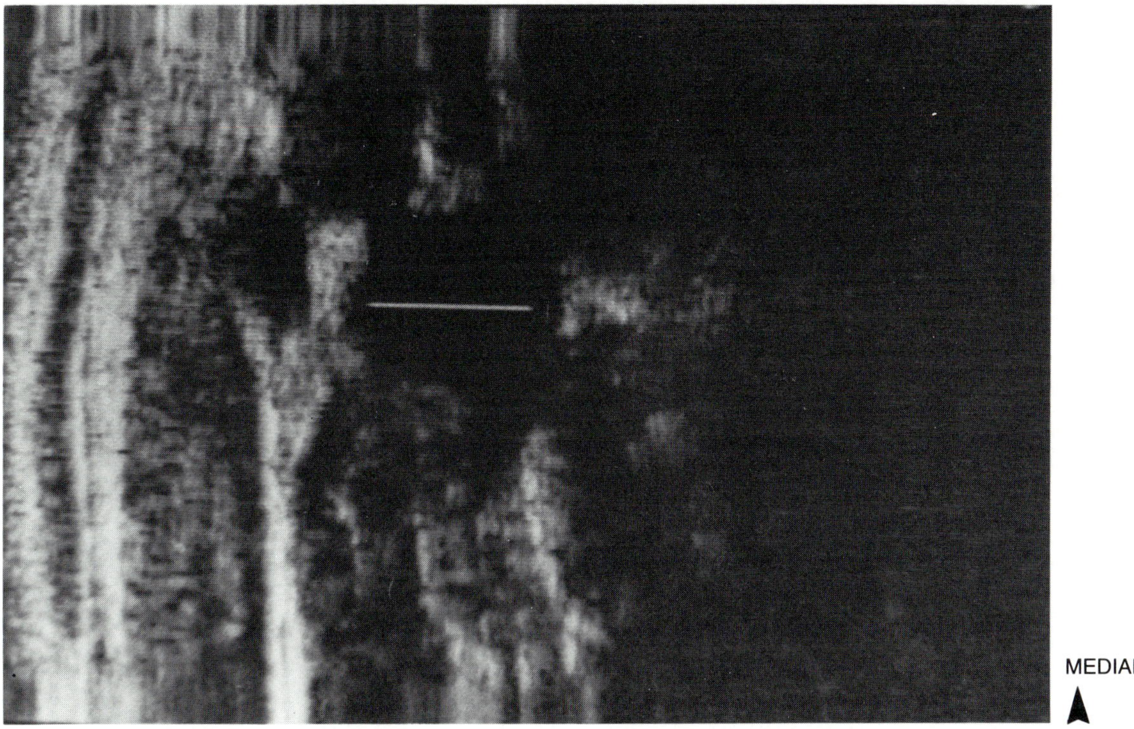
MEDIAL

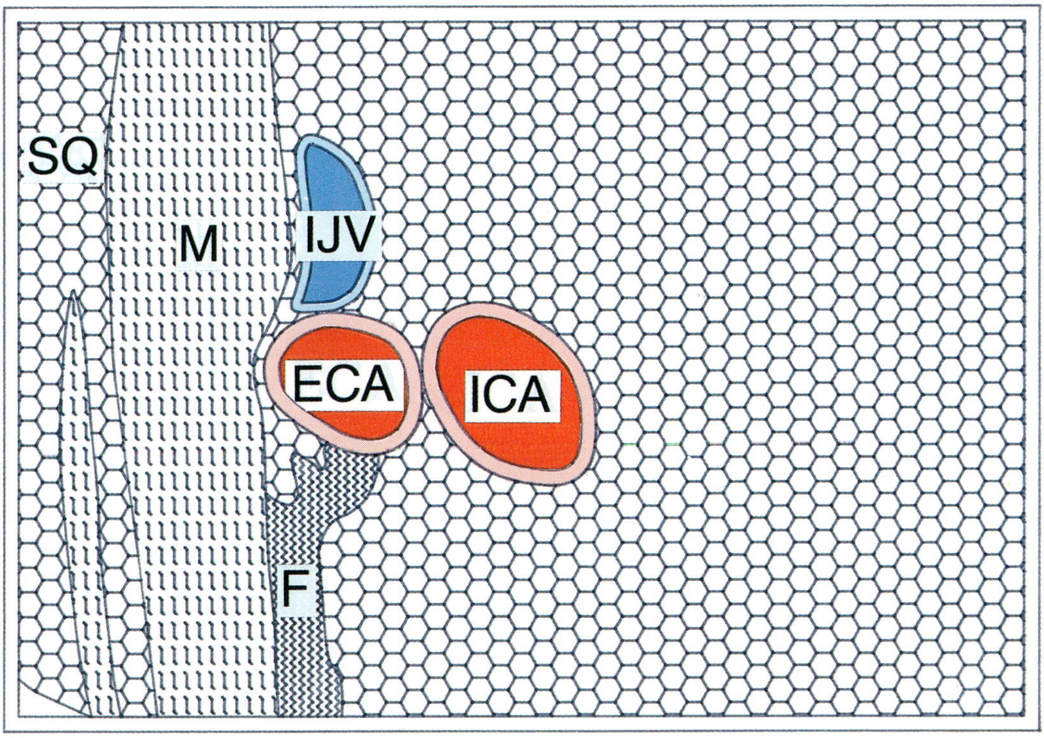
SQ
M
IJV
ECA
ICA
F

Figure 9. NORMAL LEFT TRANSVERSE ORIENTATION

This is an example of a normally oriented internal carotid artery (ICA) and an external carotid artery (ECA). The platysma (M) and the medial edge of the sternocleidomastoid (SCM) muscles are seen quite well in this view with the internal jugular vein (IJV) tucked behind the SCM at the top of the image. Note the larger diameter of the internal carotid bulb seen at this level. The arteries are normal, and the grayish material in them is an image processing artifact; there is no plaque. The ICA has a normal orientation above the ECA in which lies the Doppler cursor (not drawn). In this particular view the ICA lies at one o'clock relative to the external carotid. S = skin, SQ = subcutaneous tissue.

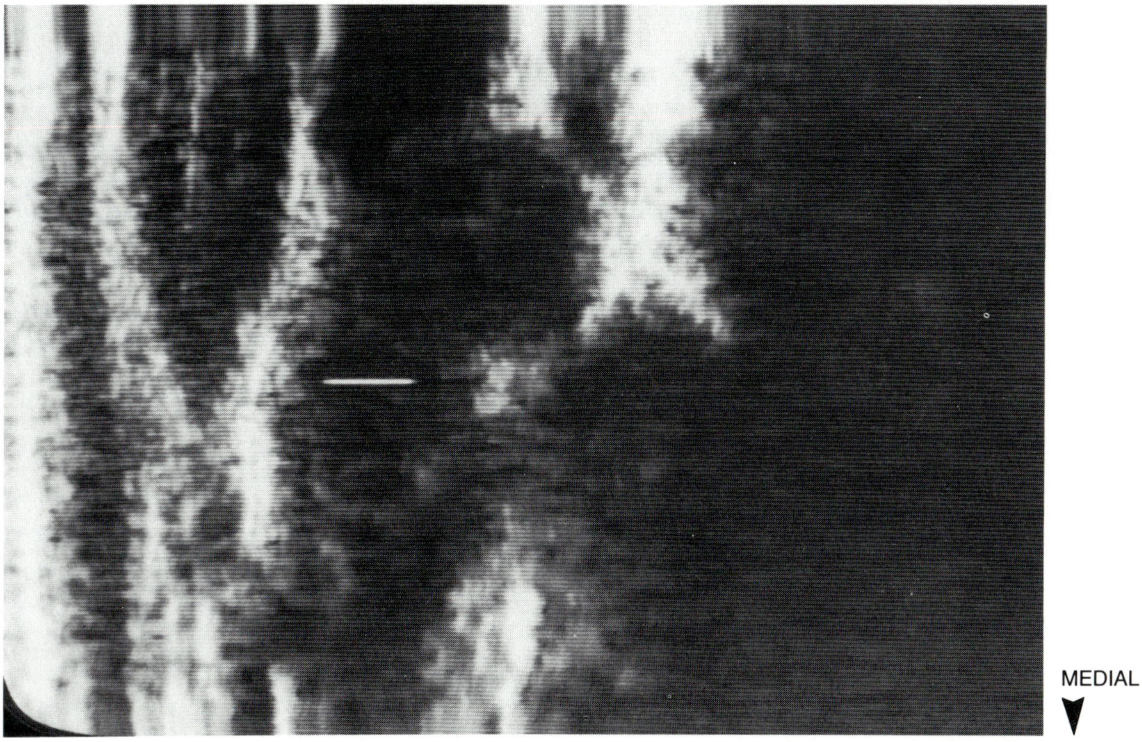
MEDIAL

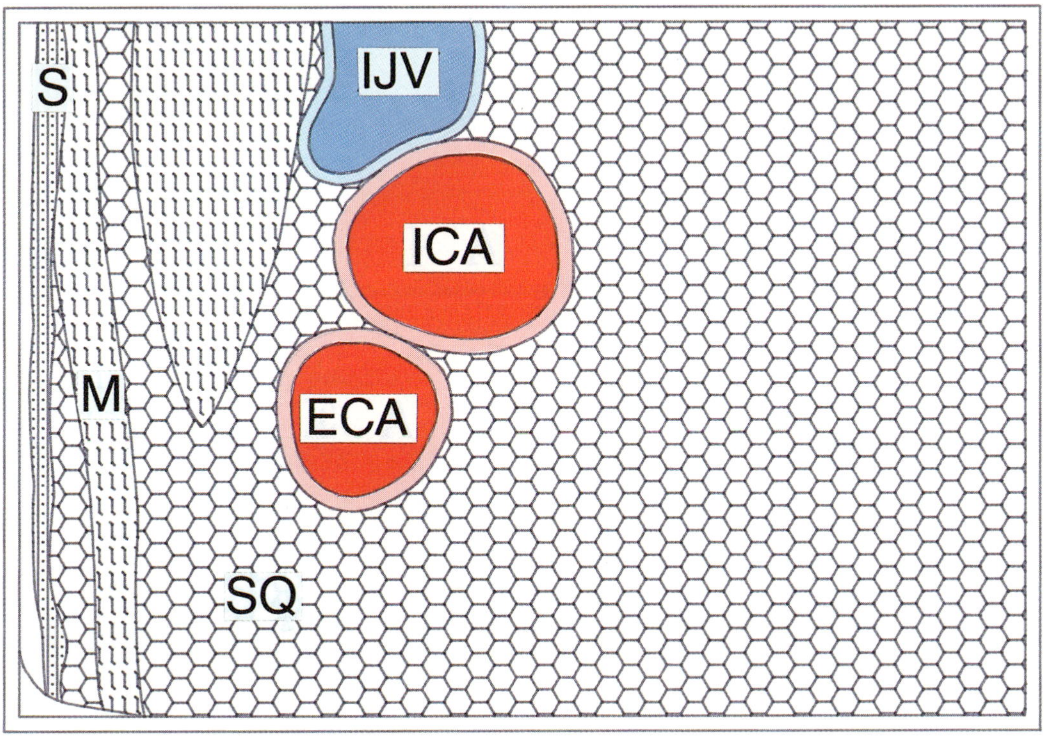
S
IJV
ICA
M
ECA
SQ

Figure 10. LEFT TRANSVERSE VIEW-ROTATED BIFURCATION

In another patient the left internal carotid artery (ICA) and external carotid artery (ECA) are seen in transverse view but are rotated out of the usual orientation as seen in the first photo. The ICA is oriented at 3 o'clock relative to the external carotid where the Doppler cursor (not drawn) is located. The two vessels are also of more equal size. Proper identification was made in this case by Doppler signal characteristics and distal position above the level of this view. The internal jugular view (IJV) is seen above the ECA and is compressed and therefore small. The arteries are somewhat elliptical in this view because they are beginning to dive into the deeper tissues and are not quite at right angles to the orientation of the probe. SQ = subcutaneous tissue, M = muscle (platysma and sternocleidomastoid), F = fascia.

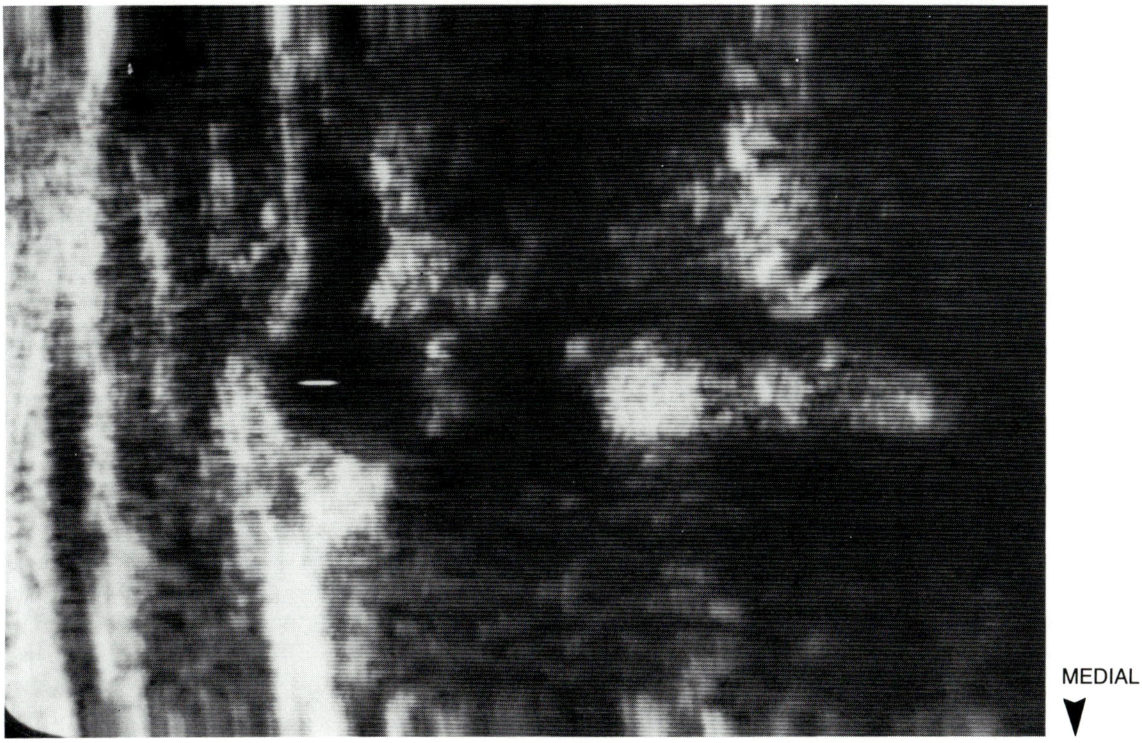
MEDIAL

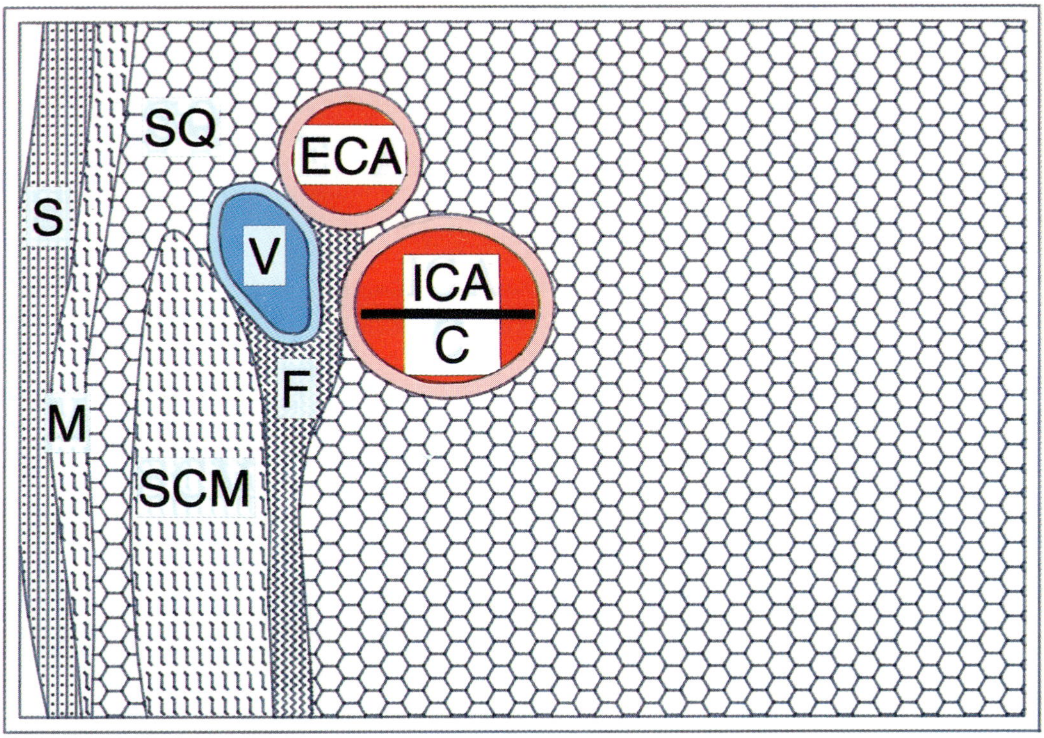
SQ
ECA
S
V
ICA
C
F
M
SCM

Figure 11. LEFT TRANSVERSE-REVERSED BIFURCATION

In yet another patient, the left internal carotid artery (ICA) and external carotid artery (ECA) are seen to be rotated even farther relative to each other in what is termed "reversed bifurcation," with the ICA below (medial to) the ECA. This is not a particularly good photograph in terms of quality of imaging of the vessels because of overlying acoustic shadowing (AS) across the bottom of the ECA. Nevertheless, the ICA can be seen at the 4-o'clock position relative to the ECA. The proper vessel identification in this case was dependent upon other factors, including relative size, distal direction, and Doppler signal characteristics. This example reinforces the principle of vessel identification by multiple criteria. There are five basic criteria by which one can identify the two arteries. The most frequent criterion is a relative orientation in transverse view. This holds true in perhaps 90% of cases. We use the mnemonic *RIB* to remember *R*ight *I*nternal *B*ottom and *LIT* to remember *L*eft *I*nternal *T*op. The second criterion is relative size just above the bifurcation. The ECA generally does not have a bulb as does the ICA. The third criterion is Doppler signal characteristic; a more monophasic signal is obtained in the ICA because of a low outflow resistance into the brain. The fourth criterion is distal direction. Although the arteries appear to be reversed at the level of the bifurcation, by following them distally they are sometimes seen to cross back over, and one can appreciate the ICA lying more laterally than the ECA at a higher level. The final criterion is the presence of branches of the ECA. The ICA has no branches in the neck. SQ = subcutaneous tissue (including platysma muscle), M = sternocleidomastoid muscle.

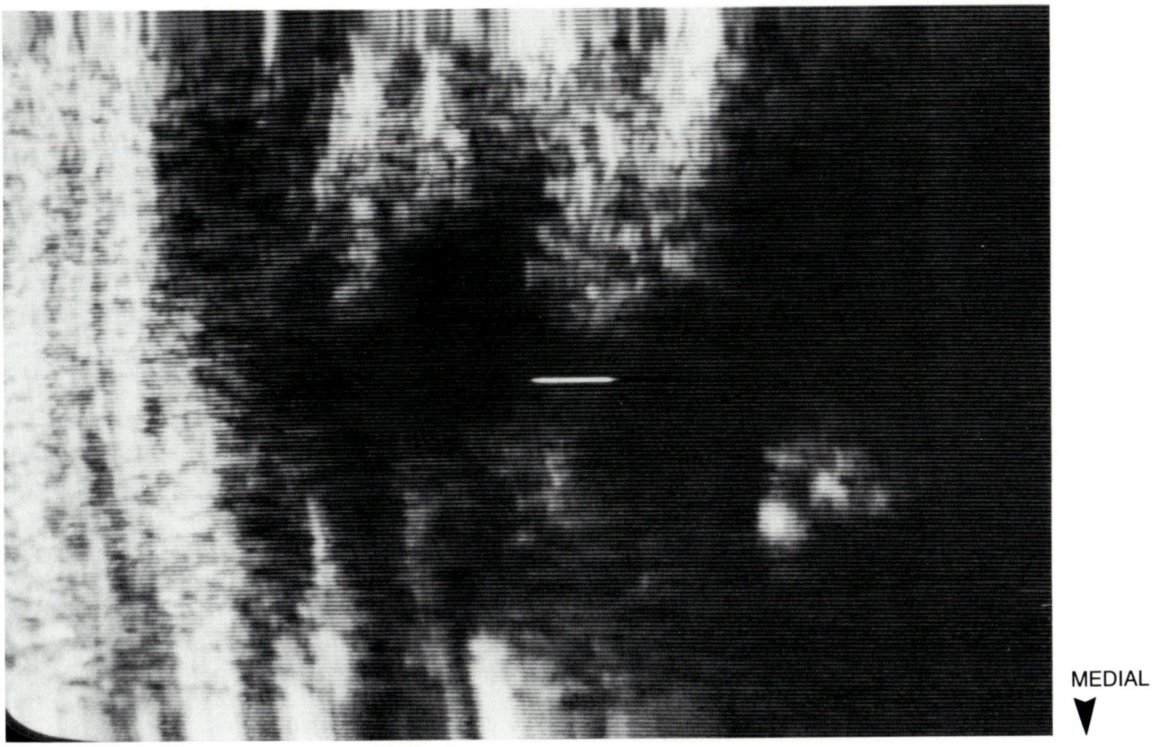
MEDIAL

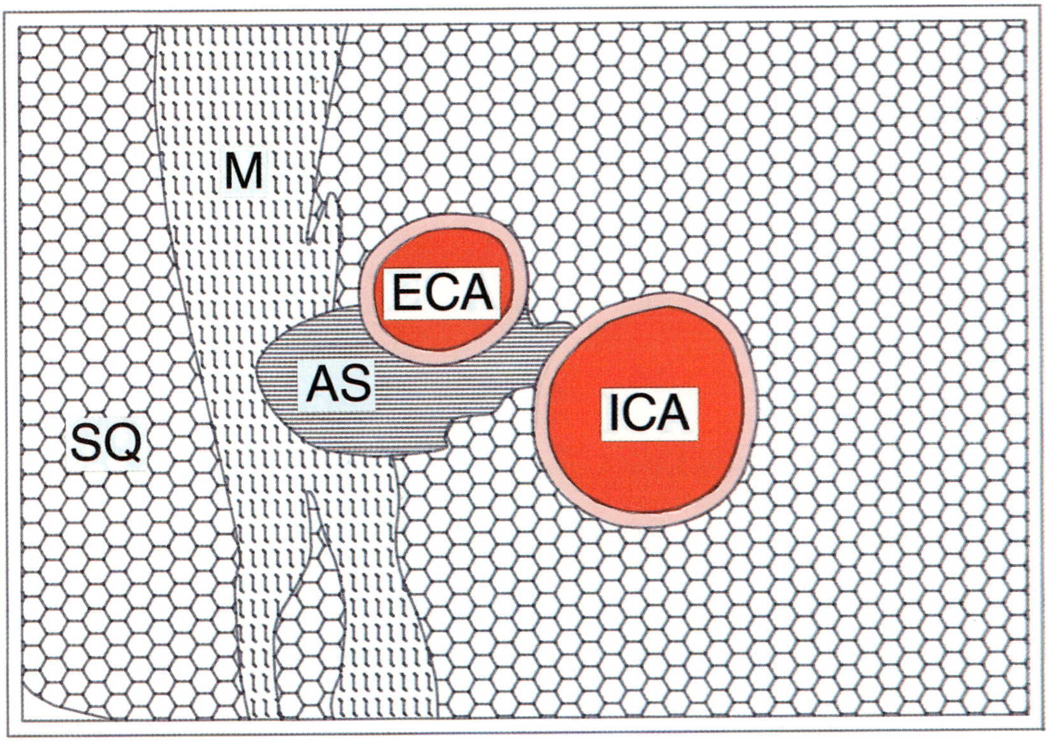
M
ECA
AS
ICA
SQ

Figure 12. EXTERNAL CAROTID BRANCHES

This is a longitudinal view of a right carotid bifurcation in which one can properly identify the external carotid artery (ECA) by means of its branches. The superior thyroid (ST), ascending pharyngeal (AP), and lingual (L) arteries are visualized at their origins. It is uncommon to have all these arteries in the same plane as shown here. Some artifact (AF) is seen due to reverberation tailing from the superficial wall of the common carotid artery (CCA). The internal carotid artery (ICA) is somewhat out of plane, with much of the artifact at its origin due to back wall contact by the ultrasound beam. S = skin, SQ = subcutaneous tissue, SCM = sternocleidomastoid muscle, F = fascia, V = internal jugular vein (filled with artifact), C = Doppler cursor, ? = tissue of uncertain composition.

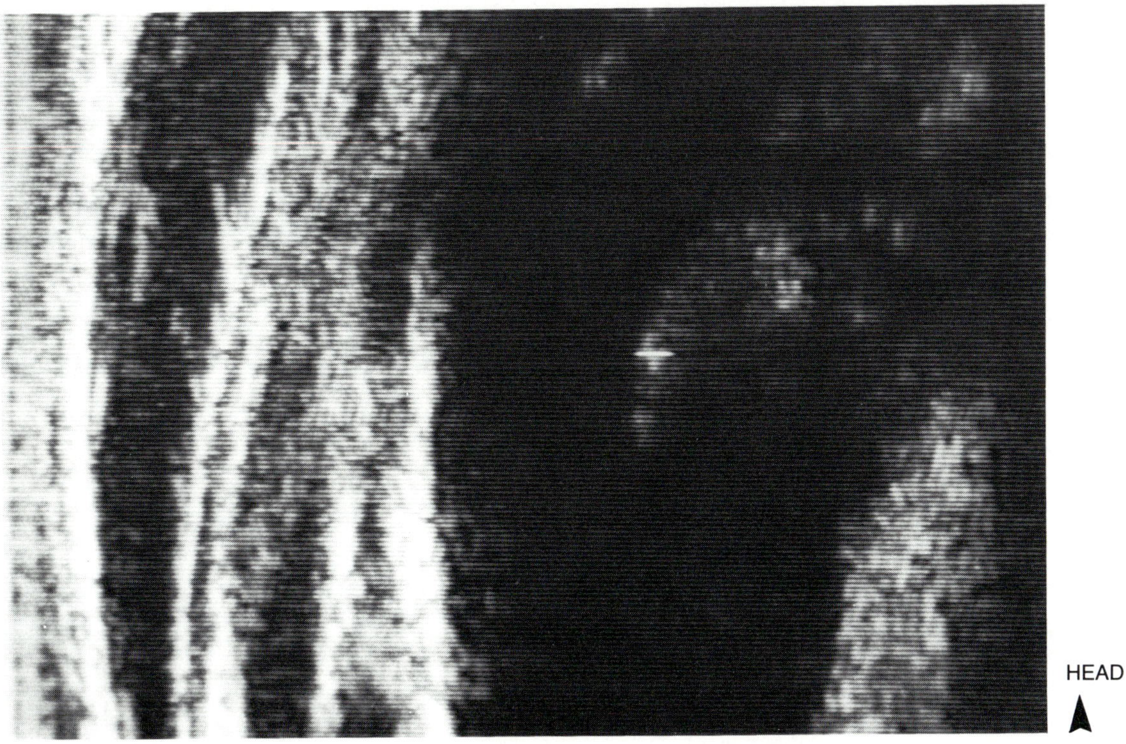
HEAD

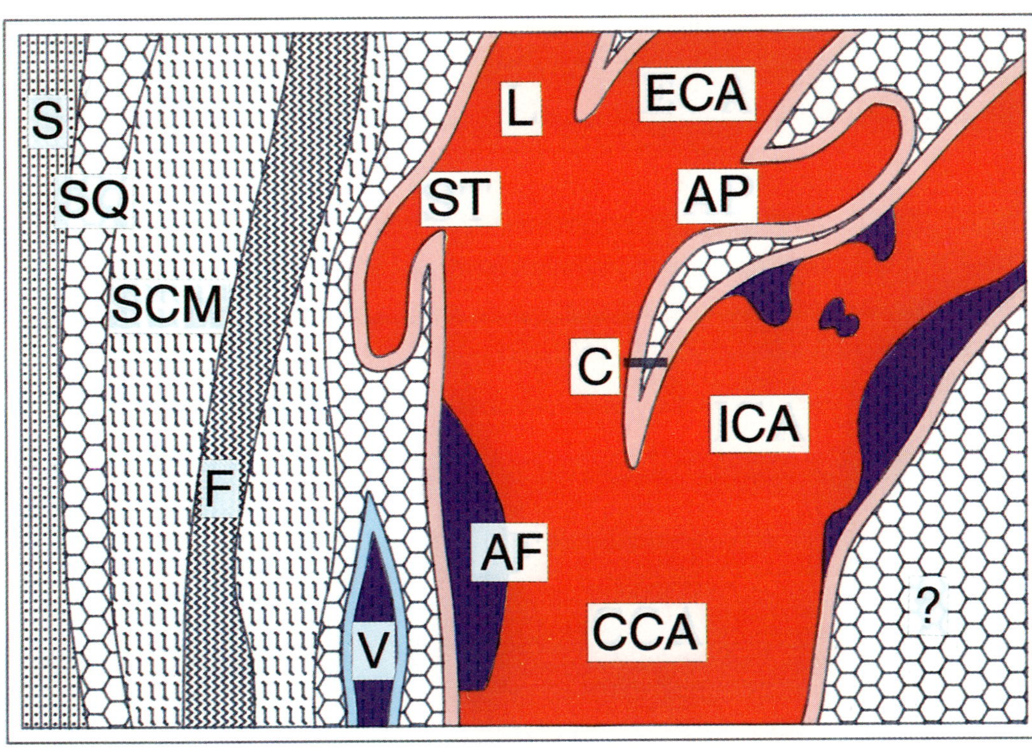
S
SQ
SCM
F
V
L
ST
ECA
AP
C
ICA
AF
CCA
?

Figure 13. EXTERNAL CAROTID BRANCHES

In this second example of a branching external carotid artery (ECA), only the origins of the arterial branches are seen. Although the lingual artery (L) has a definite tubular appearance, the superior thyroid (ST) and ascending pharyngeal (AP) arteries are seen only as round craters beyond the surface of the external carotid. This "wall defect" in the parent artery is the more common way to spot an arterial branch since most of the time the branches travel quickly out of plane. When trying to identify arterial branches, one should not expect to see long segments. Again, some artifact (AF) appears at the origin of the internal carotid artery (ICA), owing to back wall contact. S = skin, SQ = subcutaneous tissue, SCM = sternocleidomastoid muscle, V = internal jugular vein (containing some artifact at bottom), F = fascia, CCA = common carotid artery.

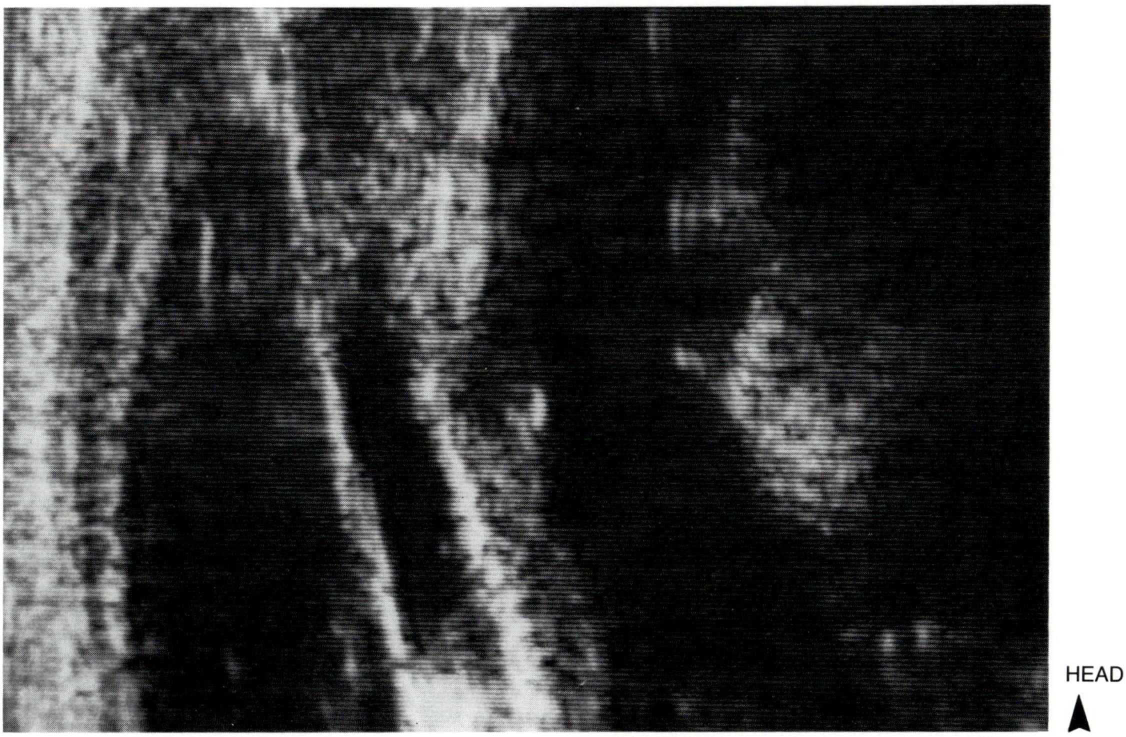
HEAD

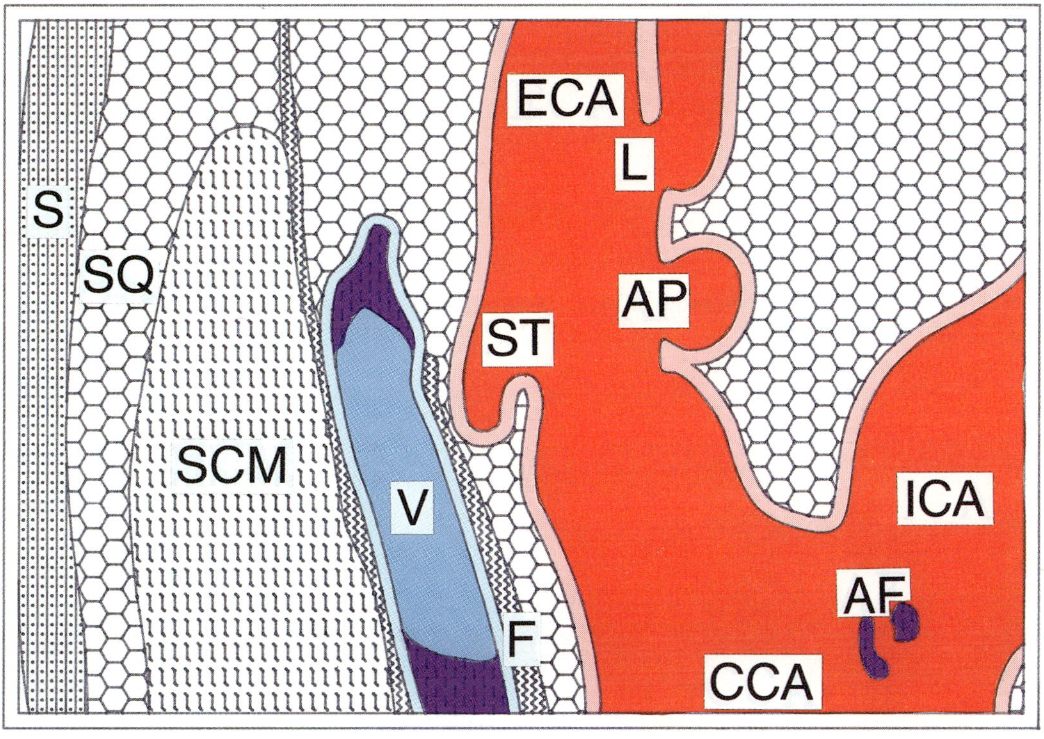
ECA
L
S
SQ
AP
ST
SCM
V
ICA
AF
F
CCA

Figure 14. CAROTID BIFURCATION—TRANSVERSE

The following four photographs, in Figures 14, 15, 16, and 17, are shown to illustrate the appearance of a typical carotid bifurcation as seen in the longitudinal view, as the probe is rocked from lateral to medial. The term "rocking the probe" is defined as pivoting the probe around its central point of contact with the skin. It does not involve moving the probe to a new location on the skin. Longitudinal carotid views are routinely performed from three different locations on the neck, anterior, lateral, and posterior to the belly of the sternocleidomastoid muscle. The following photographs were taken from a lateral position on the neck, but with rocking the probe so that a more medial or lateral view of the bifurcation was obtained. This example uses the left carotid bifurcation with the internal carotid artery (ICA) seen above and to the left of the external carotid artery (ECA), and the internal jugular vein (IJV) is seen below. There is some plaque (P) on the deep wall of the internal carotid bulb. Lines 1, 2, and 3 indicate the planes through which the following three views are taken. S = skin, M = muscle (platysma and sternocleidomastoid), F = fascia.

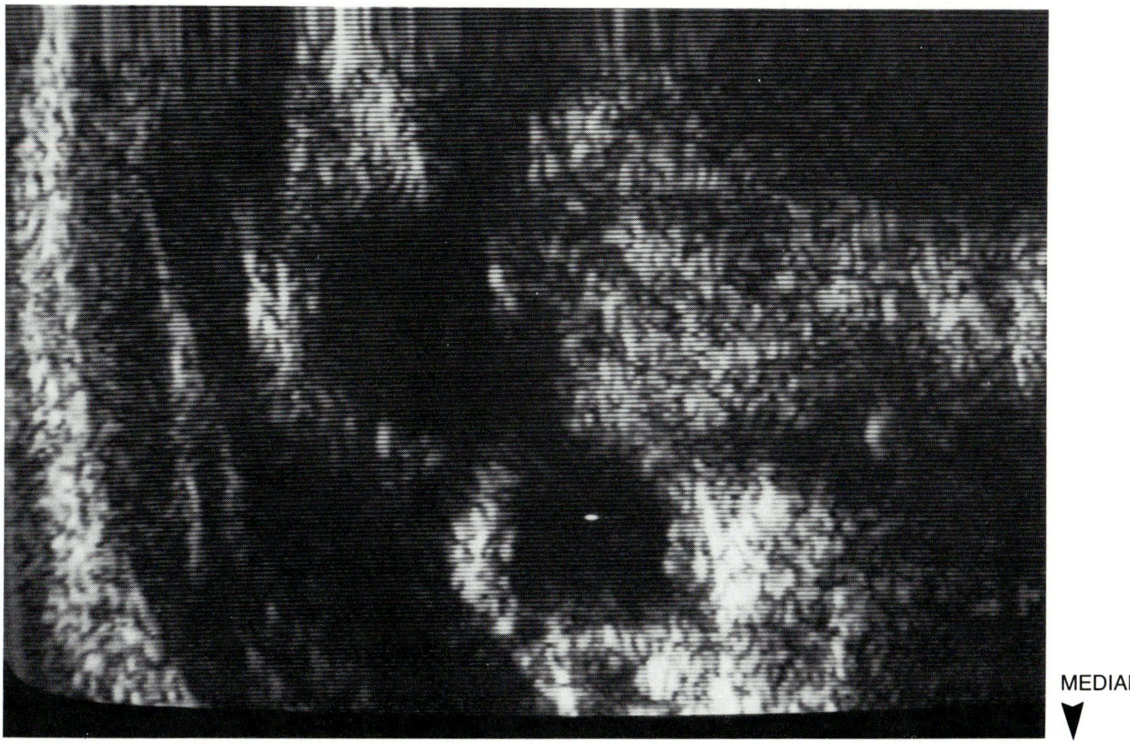
MEDIAL

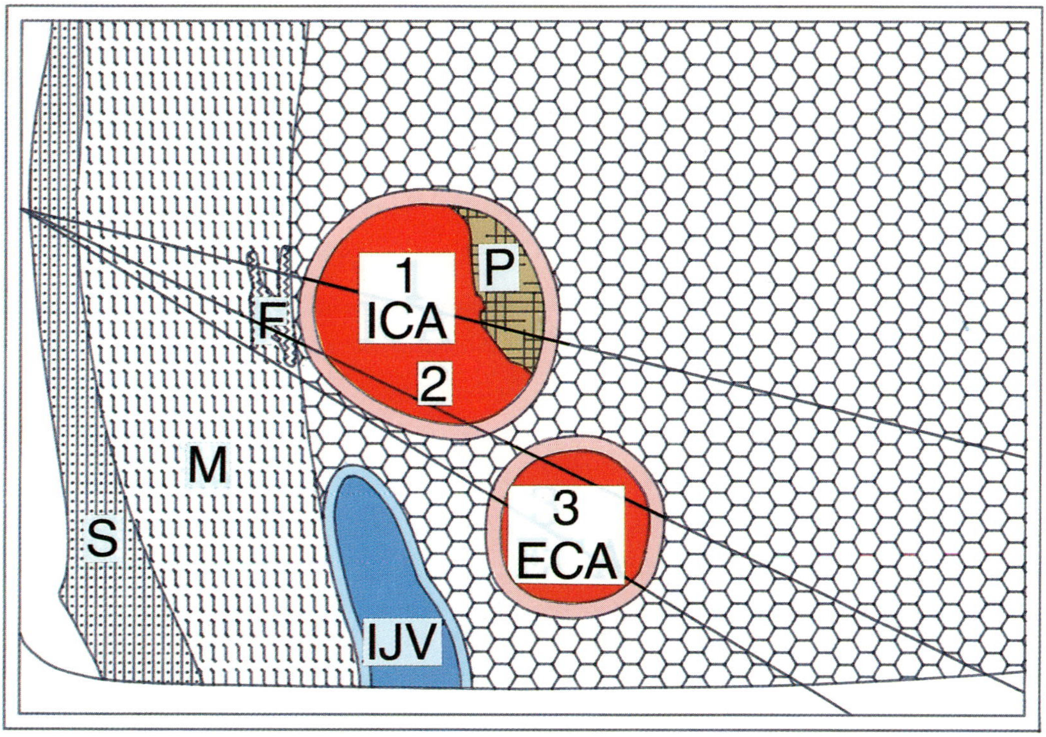
P
1
ICA
F
2
M
3
ECA
S
IJV

Figure 15. BIFURCATION—POSTEROLATERAL

This is a longitudinal view of the same bifurcation seen in Figure 14. The effect of rocking the probe from lateral to medial will be demonstrated. As one begins with a more posterolateral tilt to the probe (line 1 in the transverse view), the internal carotid artery (ICA), as it originates from the common carotid artery (CCA), is clearly seen. There is some plaque (P) on the deep wall of the internal carotid bulb, as is also seen in the transverse view. The constriction of the artery at its origin is caused not by plaque, however, but by the appearance of the back wall (BW) of the artery as it indents at the bifurcation. G = gel, S = skin, M = muscle (platysma and sternocleidomastoid), F = fascia, TV = border of the television screen, ? = deep tissues (uncertain composition).

HISTORY *This 82-year-old male presented with syncope. The ultrasound scan was obtained to rule out significant carotid disease. The patient had a history of atrial fibrillation and congestive heart failure with a mitral regurgitation and an ejection fraction of 14% by subsequent workup. He remained asymptomatic over the following 5 months.*

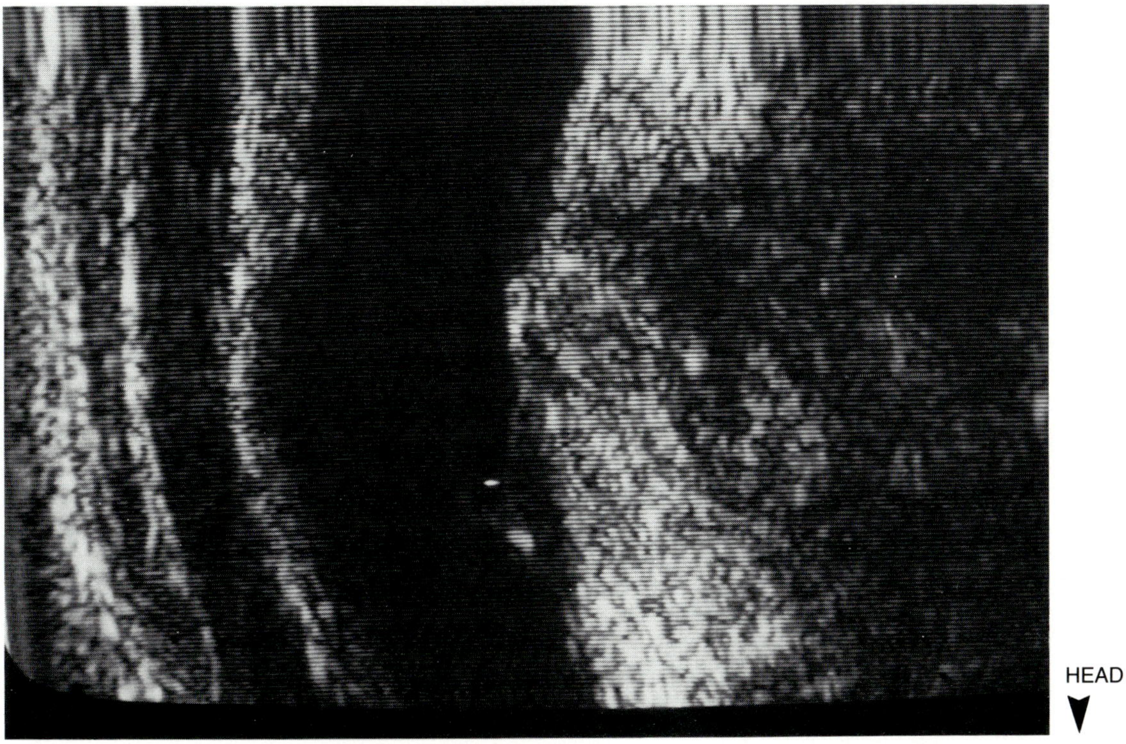
HEAD

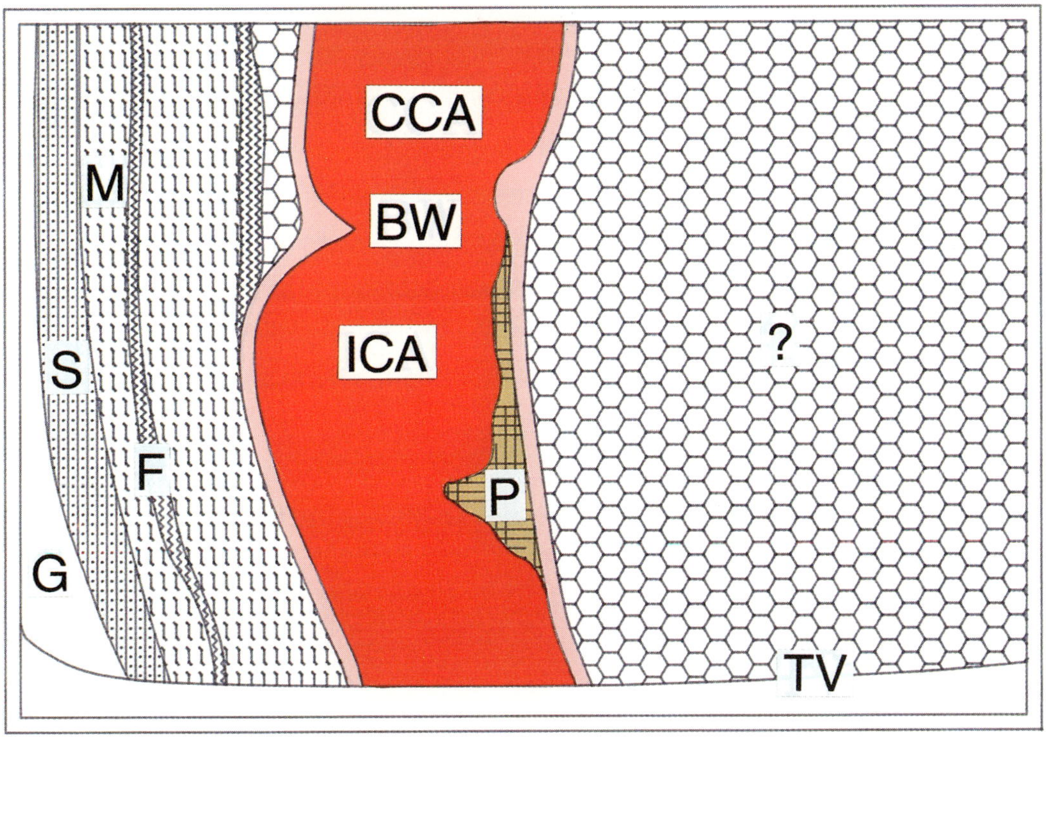
CCA
M
BW
ICA
?
S
F
P
G
TV

Figure 16. BIFURCATION—MIDDLE POSITION

Midway through the rocking motion (cut #2 in the transverse view) the external carotid artery (ECA) begins to come into view as the side or back wall (BW) of the internal carotid artery (ICA) begins to fade from view. In a still photograph such as this, the BW is difficult to distinguish from plaque, but in real time one is able to appreciate this as a gradual disappearance of the artery. In this cut, which is not centered through either artery, neither the internal nor the external carotid arteries reach their maximal diameters. The common carotid artery (CCA), however, is quite well seen with some plaque (P) on the deep wall and a smaller amount on the superficial wall of the bifurcation. S = skin, M = muscle (platysma and sternocleidomastoid), F = fascia.

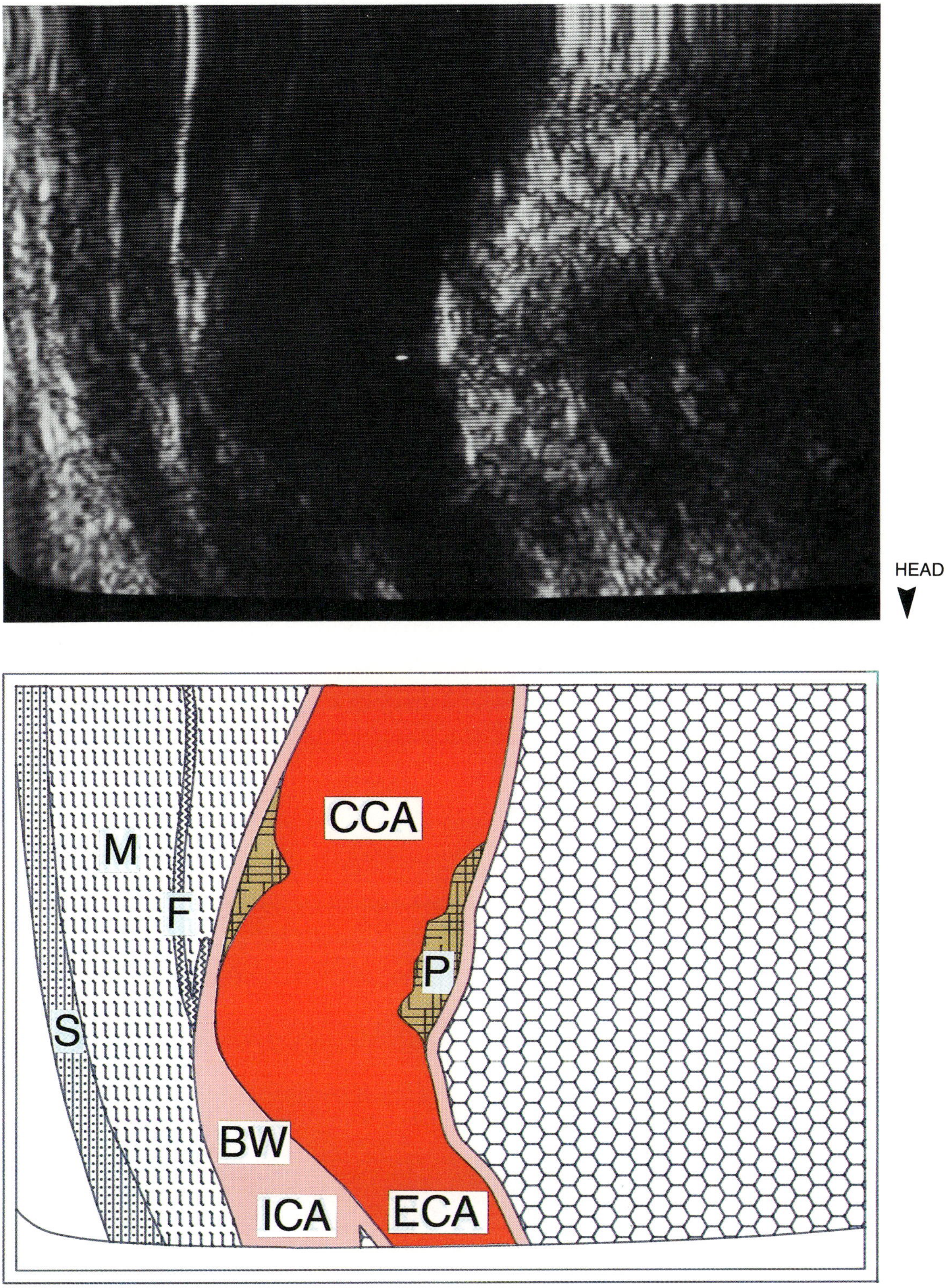
HEAD
CCA
M
F
P
S
BW
ICA
ECA

Figure 17. BIFURCATION—MEDIAL POSITION

If the probe is rocked further medially, the external carotid artery (ECA) comes fully into view with just a trace of the back wall (BW) of the artery extending from the deep wall of the artery. This view is due to the crotch of the arterial bifurcation and not to plaque. A quick comparison of this view and the view into the internal carotid artery (ICA) as seen in Figure 15 does not reveal a striking difference in appearance between the arteries. When the ICA and ECA are at equal distances from the skin, the interpreting physician may be unable to determine which vessel the technician is examining unless the technician specifies a medial or lateral rock of the probe. It is also important to perform this rock slowly and smoothly so that the transition between the two arteries is clearly seen. Otherwise, the two vessels can be misidentified. G = gel, S = skin, M = muscle (platysma and sternocleidomastoid), SQ = subcutaneous tissue.

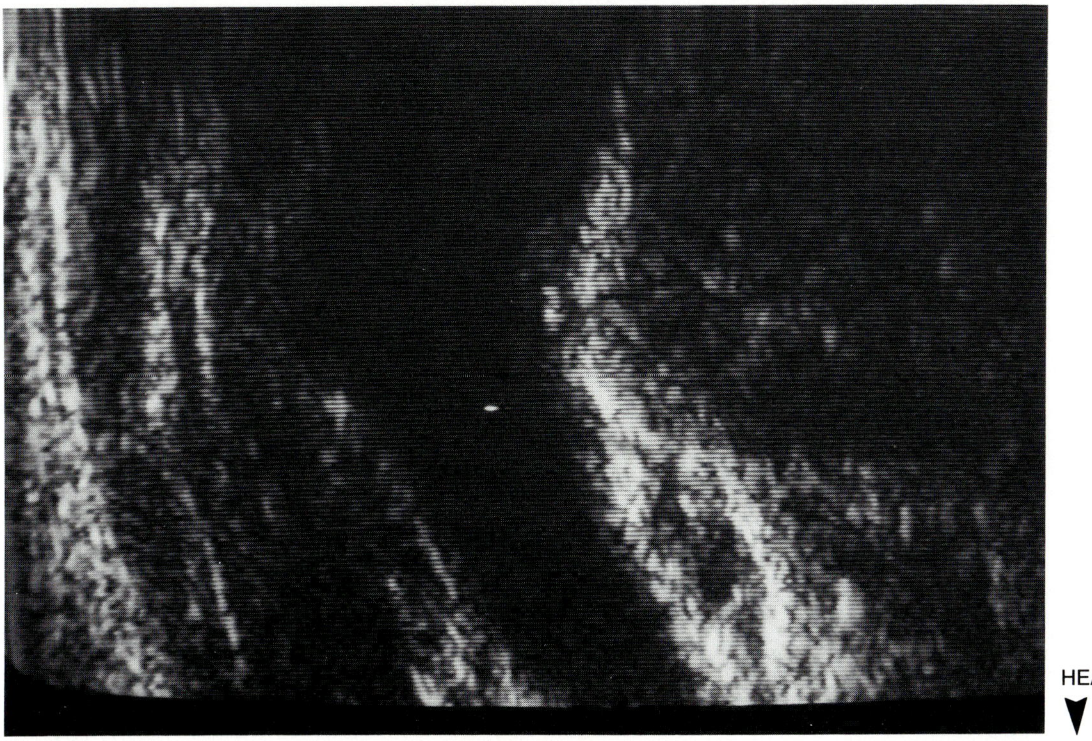
HEAD

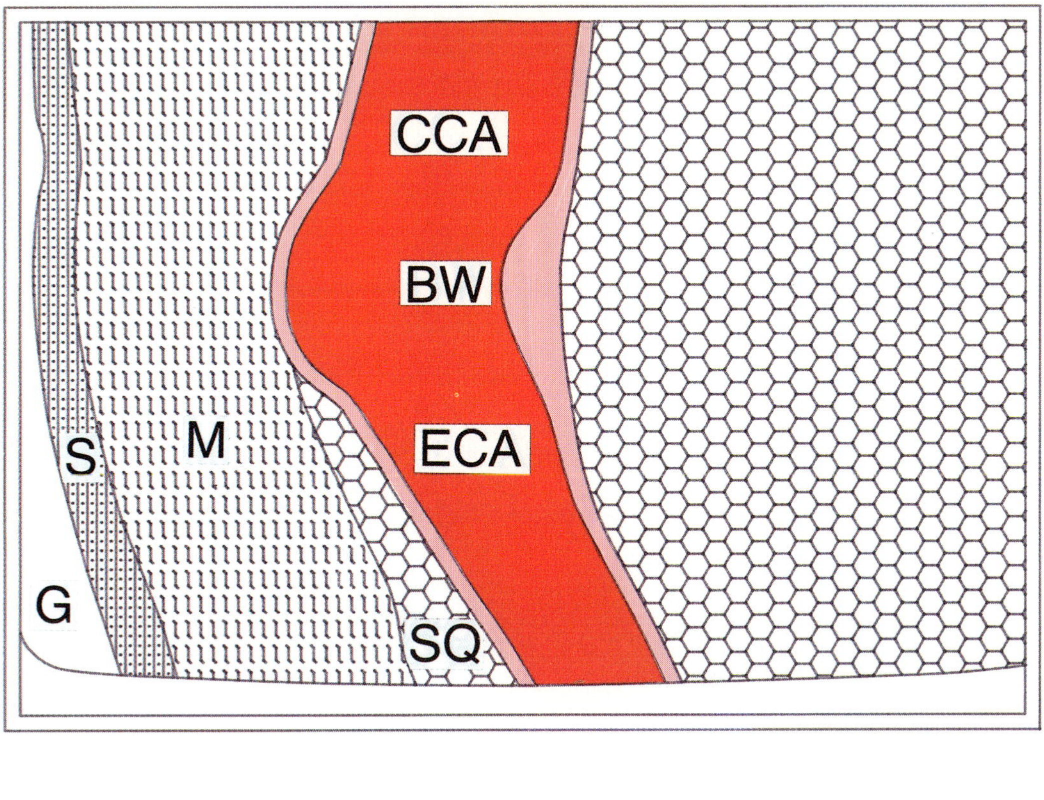
CCA
BW
ECA
S
M
G
SQ

Figure 18. 4 MHz VIEW OF BIFURCATION

This is a longitudinal view of a right carotid bifurcation using the 4 MHz probe. The Doppler cursor (C) lies within the lumen of the external carotid artery (ECA). There is a small amount of plaque (P) on the deep wall of the internal carotid artery (ICA) extending down to the bifurcation. The common carotid artery (CCA) appears to end abruptly toward the lower part of the photograph, as the CCA curves out of plane. The superficial wall of the internal carotid bulb appears to cause a septum across the orifice of the ECA. This appearance is caused by the somewhat thicker slice of tissue imaged with the 4 MHz probe. The beam with this slice thickness is encompassing both a portion of intact superficial wall as well as the open origin of the ECA, which is slightly out of plane. Details regarding plaque morphology and accurate measurement of small residual lumens are more difficult to resolve using this probe. It does, however, have advantages not only in imaging deep lying arteries but also in obtaining an idea of the overall contour and location of plaque. The view is sometimes actually superior to an 8 MHz probe when there is an excessive amount of tissue artifact or when there is shadowing due to calcification encountered with the higher frequency probe. We, therefore, currently follow a routine protocol of obtaining at least one single longitudinal view of the carotid arteries using the 4 MHz probe even though in many cases this view can be omitted. G = gel, SQ = subcutaneous tissue, SCM = sternocleidomastoid muscle.

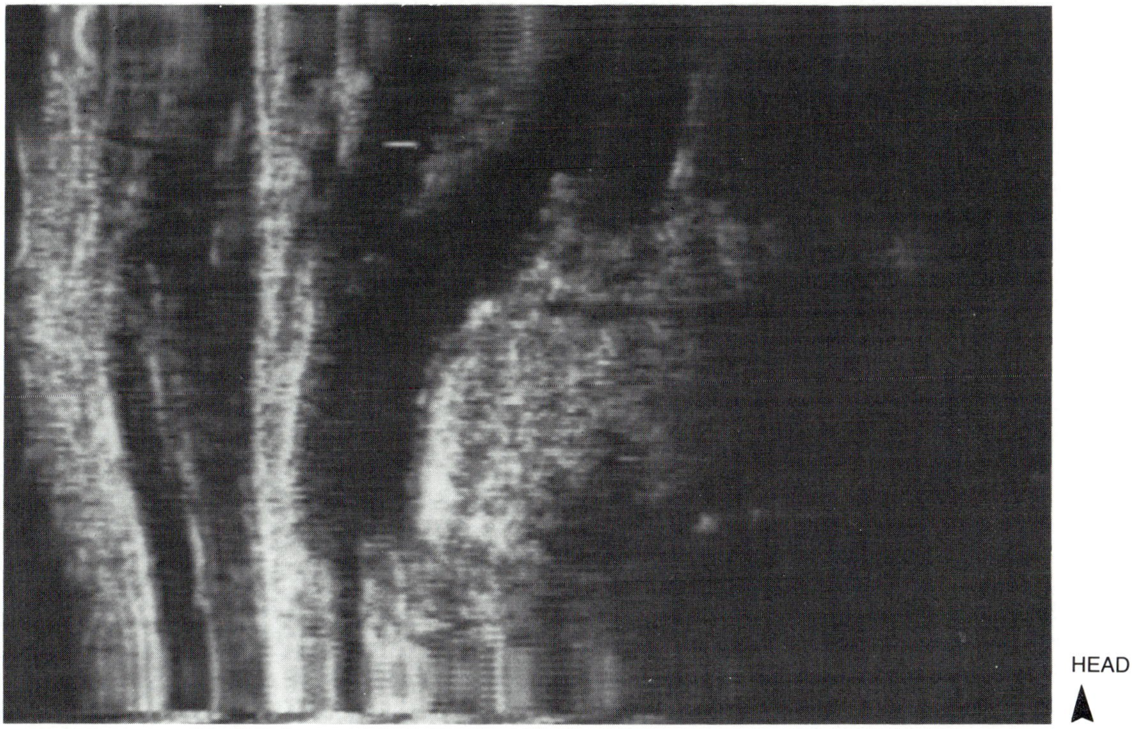
HEAD

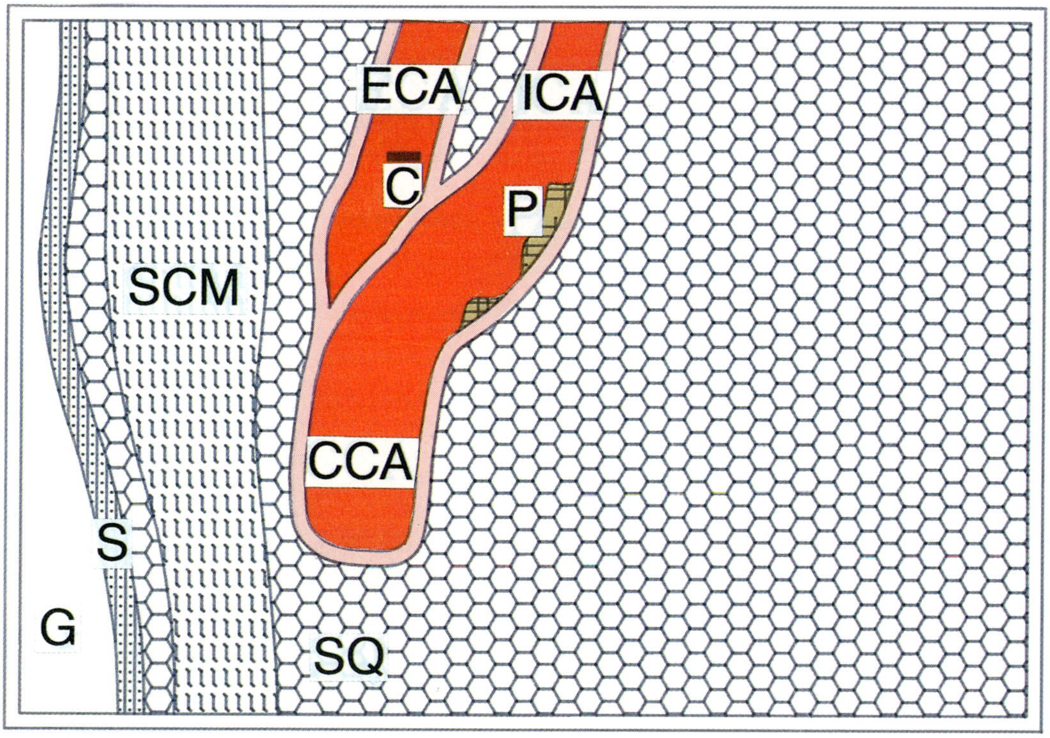
ECA
ICA
C
P
SCM
CCA
S
G
SQ

Figure 19. HYPOPLASTIC CAROTID ARTERY

This 31-year-old female (height, 5′2″, and weight, 160 lb) was found to have a hypoplastic carotid arterial system on the right and a somewhat small carotid arterial system on the left, although not as striking as the system on the right. The majority of carotid diameters by ultrasound range from 6.0 to 8.0 mm for the common carotid artery (CCA), 3.5 to 4.5 mm for the distal internal carotid artery, and 3.0 to 4.0 mm for the external carotid artery in women. The carotid diameters are approximately 0.5 to 1.0 mm larger in men. This is a magnified and cropped photograph of her right CCA, which is free of plaque but quite small in diameter, measuring 3.5 mm. This same artery tapered down to a smallest diameter of 2.5 mm. The CCA on the opposite side of the neck measured 4.5 mm in diameter at the same level. The distal internal carotid artery measured only 2.0 mm in diameter on this side and 4.0 mm in diameter on the opposite side. The internal jugular vein (IJV) is immediately below in the picture. The vagus nerve (VN) is located deep to the artery. The thyroid gland is seen to the upper right but is not drawn except for a portion of its capsule indicated by fascia. S = skin, M = muscle (platysma and sternocleidomastoid), F = fascia.

HISTORY *This patient presented with right arm paresis and intermittent dizziness suggestive of a subclavian steal syndrome. Six weeks later the scan was repeated, confirming the small diameters of these vessels. There was still an open lumen but very poor Doppler signals. An arteriogram at the time of the follow-up scan showed no visualization of the internal or external carotid arteries with an innominate artery occlusion. Two weeks later the patient underwent an endarterectomy of the occluded innominate artery and an operative arteriogram, revealing essentially no plaque at the bifurcation but very tiny vessels. This artery did not become larger following endarterectomy and thrombectomy of the innominate artery. The patient became asymptomatic and has remained so over the past 2 years. This example illustrates the usefulness of ultrasound in confirming the patency of arteries distal to an occlusion, which therefore cannot be visualized in an arteriogram.*

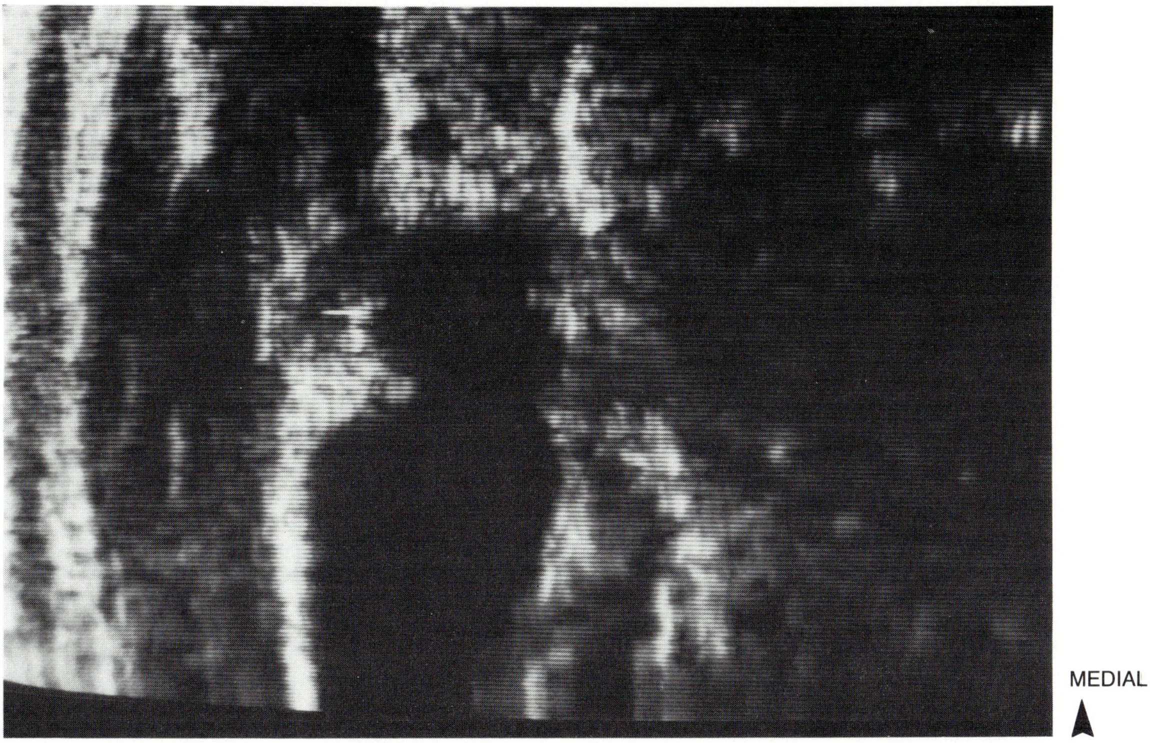
MEDIAL

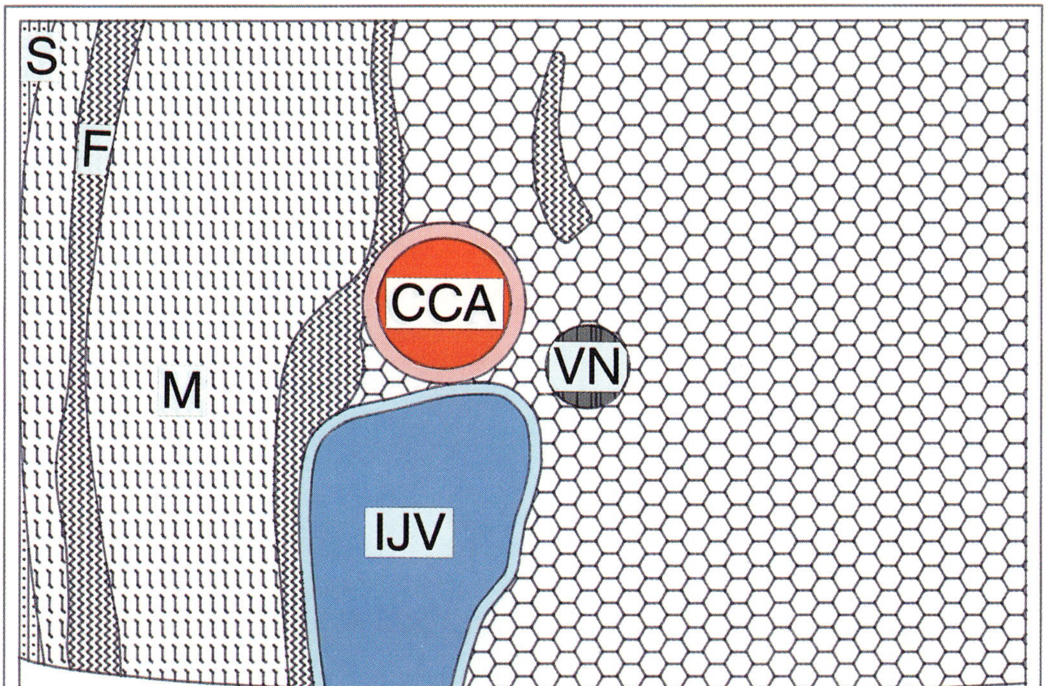
S
F
M
CCA
VN
IJV

CHAPTER 2

MEASUREMENT OF STENOSIS

Figure 20. WHAT % STENOSIS?

One should adopt a consistent scheme in quantifying the degree of stenosis of an artery. In this figure, three different arteries, A, B, and C, are illustrated with the arterial wall in pink, flowing blood in red, and plaque in a brown hound's-tooth check pattern. The arteries are shown in transverse view above and longitudinal view below, with the dashed line through the middle of the longitudinal section representing the plane from which the transverse views were taken. The first decision is whether the degree of stenosis ought to be quantified in terms of diameter or area. Most experts have chosen to use measurement of stenosis based upon diameter since noninvasive tests are compared with arteriograms as the "gold standard." Transverse views of stenoses are virtually never obtained with x-ray studies, and direct measurements of areas are not possible on longitudinal views. In a recent survey of vascular surgeons, most reported that the hourglass-shaped stenosis caused by the plaque in artery A is equal to a 50% diameter stenosis and have, therefore, based their calculations on the percentage of diameter reduction rather than area reduction. There was less agreement, however, in regard to arteries B and C. In the case of artery C, the residual lumen is 2 mm regardless of the vantage point used to show the longitudinal view. If one uses diameter stenosis, artery C is 50%. Many clinicians, without hesitation, call artery C a 75% stenosis. This three-quarters, pie-type lesion is, in fact, a 75% stenosis on the basis of residual area. Thus, in this case, many respondents instinctively used residual area rather than diameter. Indeed both artery A and artery C have exactly the same degree of stenosis whichever system one wishes to use since they are both a 50% diameter stenosis and a 75% area stenosis.

Artery B presents another problem. It is clearly a 50% area stenosis on the basis of the transverse view, but this view is not available with arteriograms. If biplanar longitudinal views at right angles to each other were obtained, one would see either a 50% stenosis or a 0% stenosis depending upon the vantage point. Thus, one is forced to make a choice. On the one hand, artery B could be considered to be a 50% stenosis because the minimum residual diameter measures 2 mm in a 4-mm vessel. On the other hand, one would then have to conclude that there is no difference in the degree of stenosis among arteries A, B, and C.

One can base the degree of stenosis upon minimum residual diameter and decide to report arteries A, B, and C as having equal degrees of stenosis. We have chosen, however, to use the average residual diameter. By this method of calculation, the residual diameter is equal to 3 mm since it is equal to 2 mm in one transverse direction and 4 mm in the other transverse direction. The method of utilizing average residual diameter seems to give a reasonable indication of stenosis in arteries A, B, and C while maintaining the concept of taking measurements by diameter. This method can be applied to both arteriograms and ultrasound images and is preferable to area measurements that have to be calculated rather than measured and require transverse views. If one does not adopt either an area stenosis or an average residual diameter stenosis, then the degree of stenosis is not closely related to the degree of blood flow reduction one might expect as a result of the plaque.

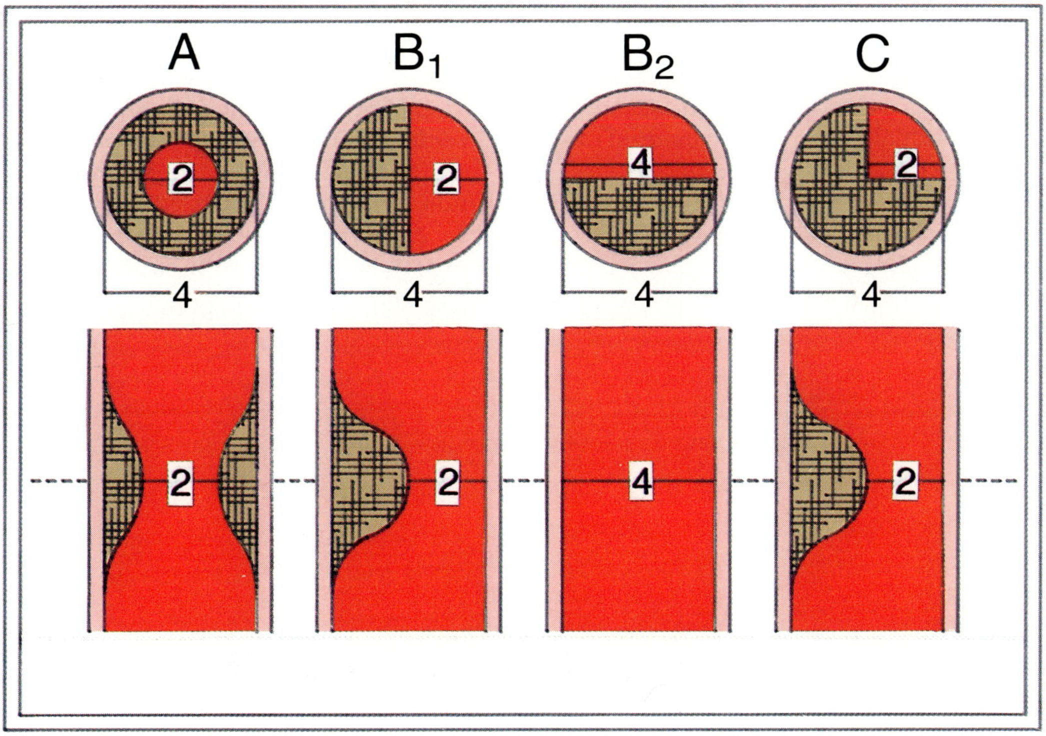
A
B1
B2
C
2
2
4
2
4
4
4
4
2
2
4
2

Figure 21. WHAT % STENOSIS?

In this figure, artery A is assessed as having a 50% diameter stenosis, and artery C has a normal lumen or 0% stenosis. Artery B contains plaque with an elliptical residual lumen. By the method of average residual diameter, this plaque produces an average residual lumen of 3 mm, and the degree of stenosis is, therefore, equal to (1 − 3 / 4) × 100% = 25%. The formula for the area of an ellipse is A = pi × r − 1 × r − 2, where r − 1 and r − 2 are the major and minor radii of the ellipse. If one, therefore, wishes to report stenosis in terms of area, then artery B has a 50% stenosis.

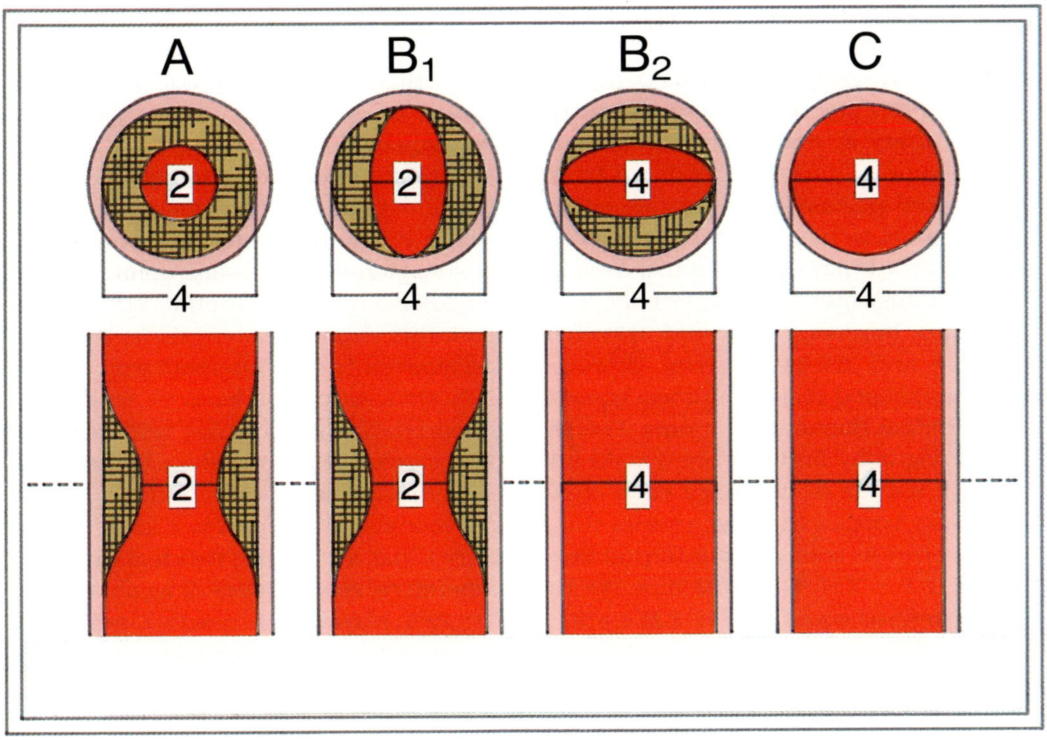
A
B1
B2
C
2
2
4
4
4
4
4
4
2
2
4
4

Figure 22. WHAT % STENOSIS?

Actually, plaques are not perfectly smooth. Although artery A contains a 50% diameter stenosis, how does one quantitate arteries B and C? In an arteriogram of artery B, one might see an hourglass-shaped stenosis with a bright inner column of contrast, bordered by a more grayish zone, and represented by the dotted portion of the plaque where the contrast fills the crevices. As one uses calipers to measure the degree of stenosis in this artery, one could consider it either a 1-mm residual lumen or a 3-mm residual lumen, depending upon whether one measures from inner edge to inner edge or outer edge to outer edge of the fuzzy borders. One could, therefore, assess this degree of stenosis as between 25% and 75% by diameter. However, in an attempt to be consistent, we call this star-shaped residual lumen equal to a 50% stenosis on the basis of an average residual diameter of 2 mm. Therefore, in correlating noninvasive tests with arteriography findings one would need to be careful in placing the calipers from the middle of the fuzzy edge of contrast across to the middle of the opposite fuzzy border. In small arteries this factor becomes critical and is a large source of error in comparing interpretations. Artery C has an average residual diameter of $(2.2 + 3.5) / 2 = 2.85$ mm. We would, therefore, report artery C as containing a stenosis equal to $(1 - 2.85 / 4 \times 100\% = 29\%$. However, in practical terms, we would round this and report artery C as containing a 30% diameter stenosis.

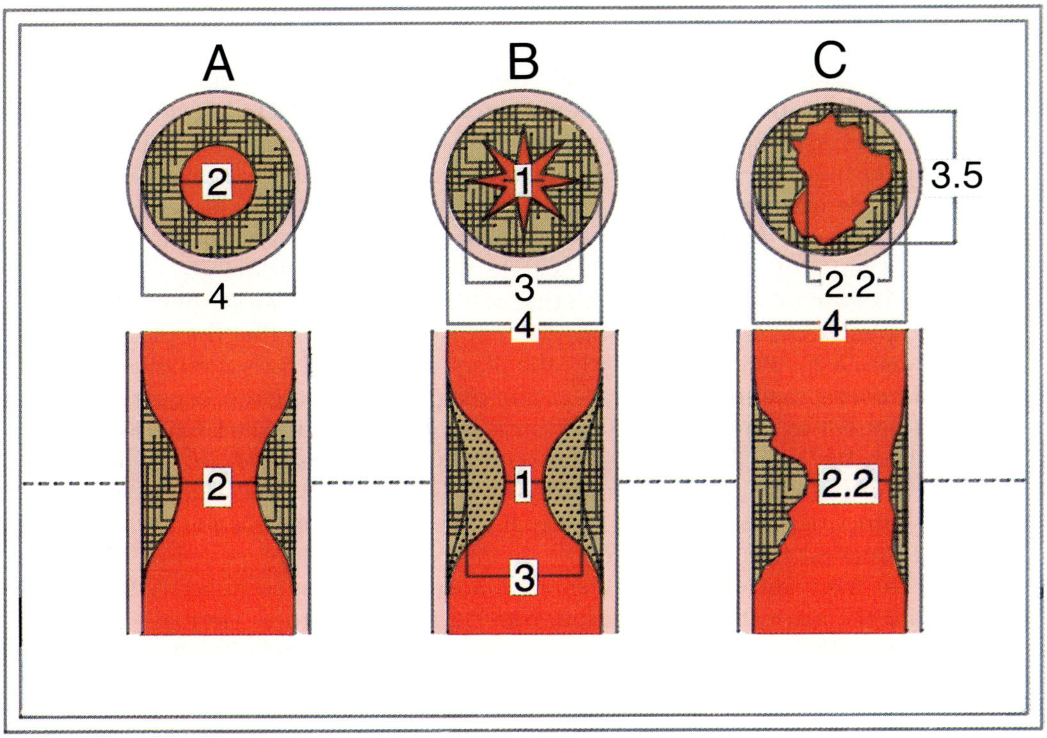
A
B
C
2
4
2
1
3
4
1
3
3.5
2.2
4
2.2

Figure 23. WHAT % STENOSIS?

In this diagram, artery A is an artery that tapers from a diameter of 4 mm at the bottom of the image to a diameter of 2 mm at the top of the image. This finding often occurs at the carotid bifurcation where the internal carotid bulb is quite a bit larger than the diameter of the artery distally. How, then, should one quantify the degree of stenosis of the plaques at level A_1 and A_2? In fact, the plaque at level A_2 is seen to narrow the column of blood to no greater degree than the normal taper of the artery immediately above. Therefore, the plaque at level A_2 should cause no significant reduction of blood flow to whatever tissue this artery is supplying. On the basis of this rule, we would suggest that the plaque at level A_2 causes a 0% stenosis. Similarly, the plaque at level A_1 causes no greater degree of narrowing than the plaque at A_2. The plaque at A_1, therefore, causes no greater impediment to flow than the plaque at A_2 and should likewise be called a 0% stenosis. We therefore propose a second rule that has been recommended by others as follows: the degree of stenosis caused by a plaque should be assessed as a comparison between the residual lumen within that plaque and the artery at its smallest normal diameter.

For the same reasons, the aneurysm that is illustrated in artery B also contains a 0% stenosis. By definition, one cannot measure a "normal" arterial diameter within an aneurysm because the artery is not "normal" at this point.

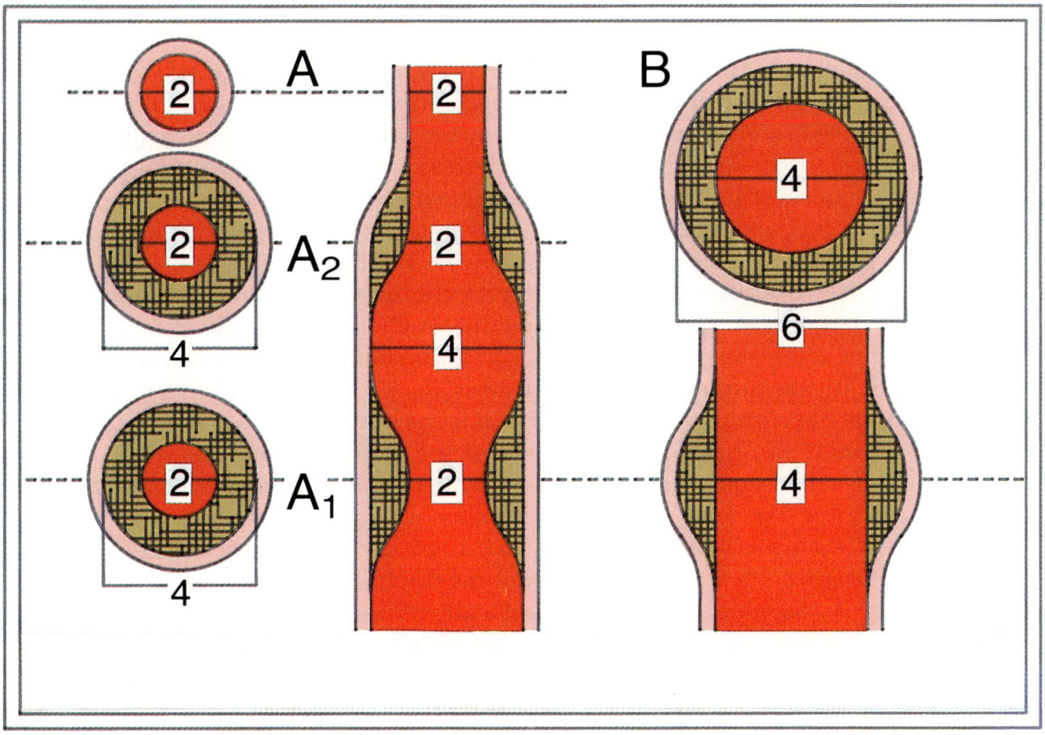
A
2
2
A2
2
2
4
4
A1
2
2
4
B
4
6
4

Figure 24. WHAT % STENOSIS?

If one concludes that artery A has a stenosis of 0%, what can be said of artery B? This artery bifurcates into two smaller branches. Should one then compare the 2-mm residual diameter to the diameter of one of the branches at 2.8 mm? This comparison would lead to the decision that all plaque within an artery demonstrates a 0% stenosis because somewhere in the distal tree there will be an arterial diameter equal to the stenosis in question. Obviously, this decision is unacceptable and leads to a third following rule: one should pick the value of the smallest normal arterial diameter as the denominator in the equation for stenosis only when the artery remains unbranched. By this rule, therefore, artery A contains a 0% stenosis because it is unbranched, but artery B contains a 50% stenosis. In the human body, it is almost always true that at major arterial bifurcations the sum of the cross-sectional areas of the arterial branches at a distal level exceeds the cross-sectional area of the parent artery. Therefore, there is little increase in total resistance to blood flow at any degree of branching until the arterioles. The flow reduction, therefore, caused by the plaque in the parent artery in example B is substantial and much greater than that caused by the plaque in artery A, which remains unbranched with a distal taper. The plaque in artery A causes a relatively insignificant reduction in flow based mostly on local turbulence, which is difficult if not impossible to quantitate and which is therefore ignored.

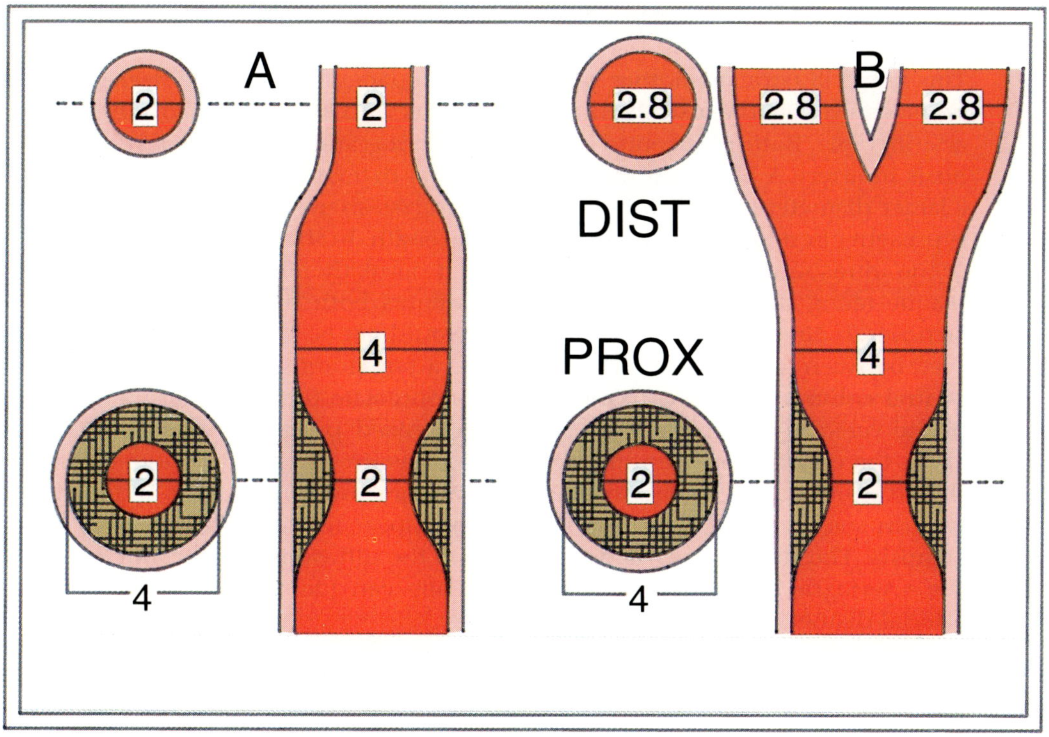
A
2
2
4
2
2
4
B
2.8
2.8
2.8
DIST
PROX
4
2
2
4

Figure 25. WHAT % STENOSIS?

This figure illustrates another source of discrepancy between the degree of stenosis shown by the use of ultrasound scans and that shown by the use of arteriograms. Both ultrasound scans and arteriograms would suggest a 0% stenosis in artery A based upon average residual diameter. Artery B, however, has a larger diameter but in addition to the hourglass-shaped stenosis below, plaque is present circumferentially along its entire length. In this example, the accuracy of the ultrasound scan is superior in that it correctly identifies the presence of plaque along the entire vessel and quantitates both the proximal and distal stenoses as 50% diameter reduction. One would not be able to distinguish, however, between artery A and artery B on the arteriogram since all one sees is the central column of contrast. One may not appreciate the true internal diameter of the vessel by arteriography. The unrecognized presence of smooth plaque along the entire vessel would lead one to measure the "normal" lumen as less than it truly is and give rise to a falsely low degree of stenosis. This is the reason why, in some cases, ultrasound scans may appear to "over read" the degree of stenosis. The discrepancy is not an error of the ultrasonographer, but rather of the arteriographer in presupposing that one can identify a proper "normal" arterial diameter.

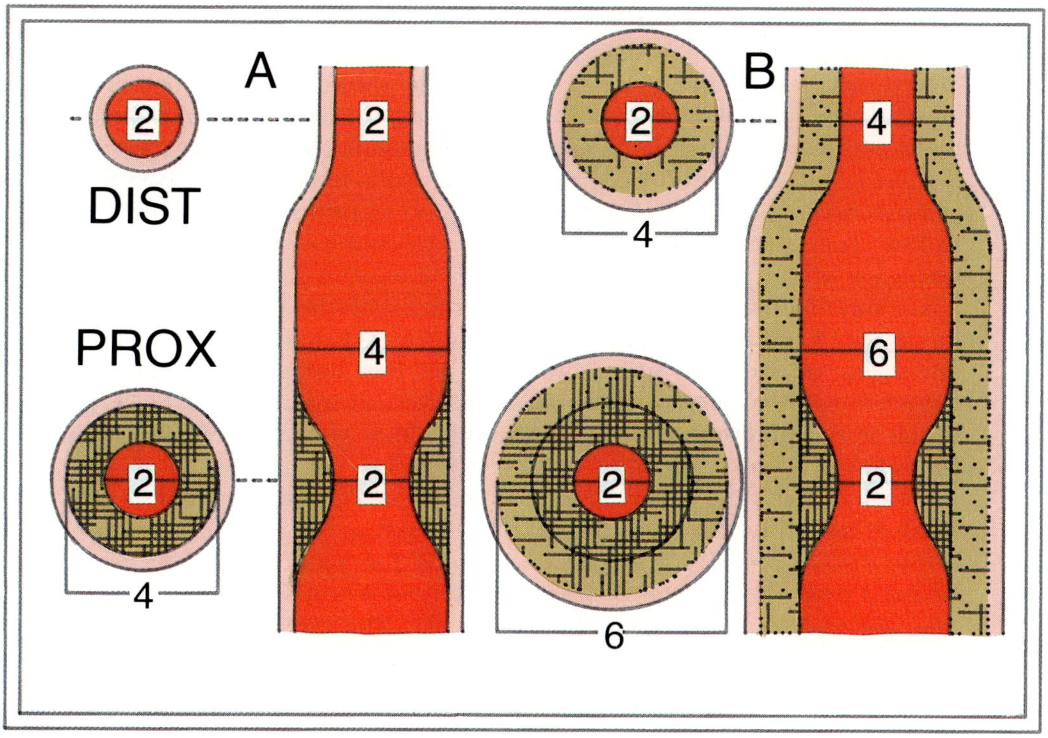
A
B
DIST
PROX
2
2
4
2
2
4
2
4
6
2
2
4
2
6

Figure 26. IDEALIZED CAROTID BIFURCATION

This diagram illustrates the variability of interpretation among observers. This particular diagram has been shown to a number of surgeons and radiologists in our community as well as to vascular surgeons nationwide and has produced reports of internal carotid stenosis ranging from 12% to 81%, external carotid stenosis ranging from 0% to 90% and common carotid stenosis ranging from 0% to 75%. The interpreting physician was instructed to assume that the residual diameters of the plaque at its narrowest points were given as illustrated in the boxes and that the plaque was circumferential, with the same residual diameters in all planes. By the method of average residual diameter, the internal carotid artery has an average residual lumen of 3.5 mm compared with a distal unbranched internal carotid diameter of 4.0 mm, giving rise to a 12.5% stenosis which is rounded to 15%. This is the value that would be reported from our laboratory.

In a neighboring hospital, the same diagram was interpreted as a 3.5-mm residual lumen within an 8-mm diameter vessel at the point of stenosis, giving rise to a 55% stenosis. In yet another hospital, this same plaque was assessed as having a residual diameter of 3.5 mm within an 8-mm artery; these values were then squared to give an area stenosis of 80%. The radiologists in reporting an 80% internal carotid stenosis did not inform the clinician that this value was based upon area, and they assumed that the clinician knew the radiologists' method of interpretation.

A referring physician who sends a patient for carotid evaluation, unaware of the method of calculating stenosis in the hospital that performs the testing, may receive a report of a 15%, a 55%, or an 80% internal carotid stenosis. The physician may come to the conclusion that the patient has "nothing to worry about" with a 15% stenosis; may recommend frequent repeat examinations upon receiving a report of a 55% stenosis; or may send the patient to a vascular surgeon upon receiving a report of an 80% stenosis, with concern that the patient is in imminent danger of carotid occlusion. It is distressing to note this variability in reporting. The best that can be recommended at this point is adherence to a consistent system of interpretation and to clearly define the method used. Diagrams of the plaque that include measurements are very important in communicating the extent of lesions with accuracy (see Appendix). Again, using the method of average residual diameter stenosis compared with the smallest normal diameter of the unbranched artery, the external carotid artery is best reported as containing plaque with a 2.5-mm residual lumen in a 3.5-mm vessel equal to a 30% stenosis. The distal external carotid diameter of 2.5 mm should not be used because this diameter is measured beyond the origin of the superior thyroid artery. The common carotid stenosis is calculated employing the 5.5-mm residual diameter in comparison with the 7.0-mm diameter of the artery at the base of the neck. This is a 20% common carotid stenosis since there are no intervening branches.

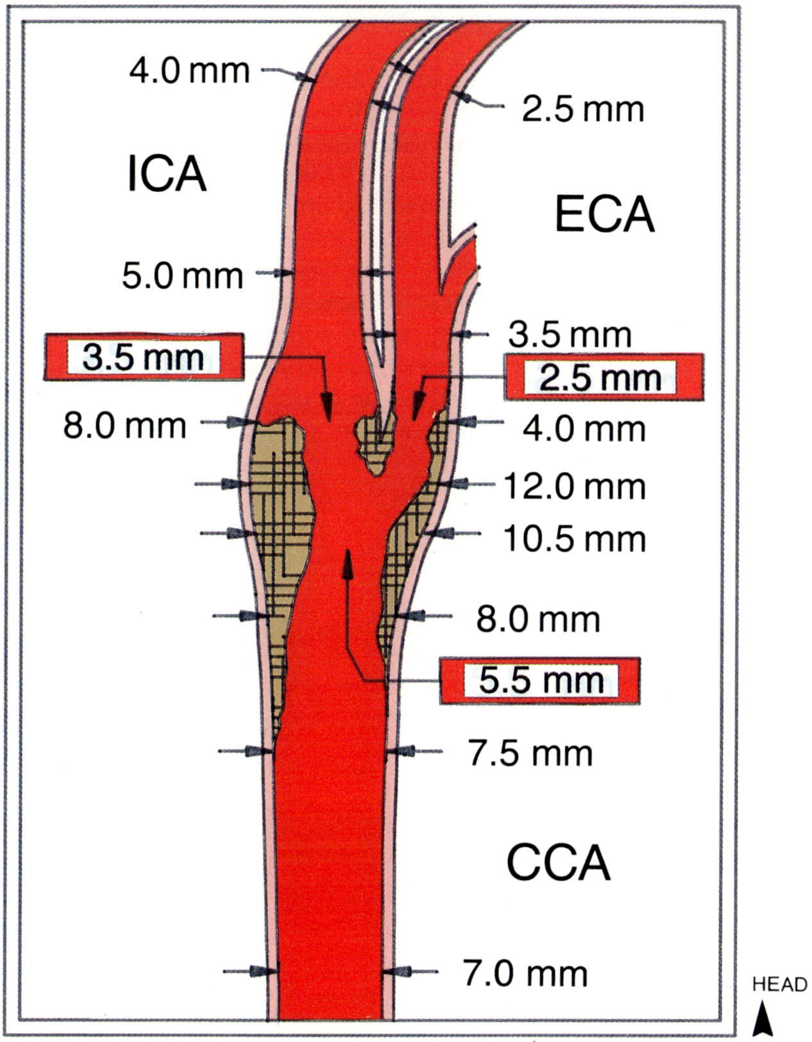

Table 1. RULES IN MEASURING ARTERIAL STENOSIS

1. Find the point of maximal narrowing caused by plaque in the artery in question.
2. Use diameter, not area.
3. Use average residual diameter, not minimum or maximum residual diameter.
4. Find the diameter of the normal artery at its smallest point.
5. Do not go beyond bifurcations in obtaining this normal diameter.
6. Calculate the percent stenosis as equal to (1 − average residual diameter / normal arterial diameter) * 100%.

Figure 27. COMMON CAROTID—LOWER NECK

The following two ultrasound scans demonstrate the effect of arterial tapering upon the calculation of the degree of stenosis. Figure 27 is a transverse view of a right common carotid artery (CCA) near the base of the neck shown for purposes of comparison with Figure 28. The Doppler cursor (C) measures 7.4 mm in length. However, the left end of the cursor extends midway into the "intimal stripe" of the superficial wall of the CCA. The right end of the cursor extends almost beyond the adventitial portion of the deep wall of the CCA. The actual diameter of the CCA at this level is 6.3 mm. The top and, particularly, the bottom walls of the CCA are obscured by artifact within the widely patent normal lumen. (This artifact is not drawn.) F = fascia, SCM = sternocleidomastoid muscle, IJV = internal jugular vein, THYROID = thyroid gland, ? = tissue of uncertain composition.

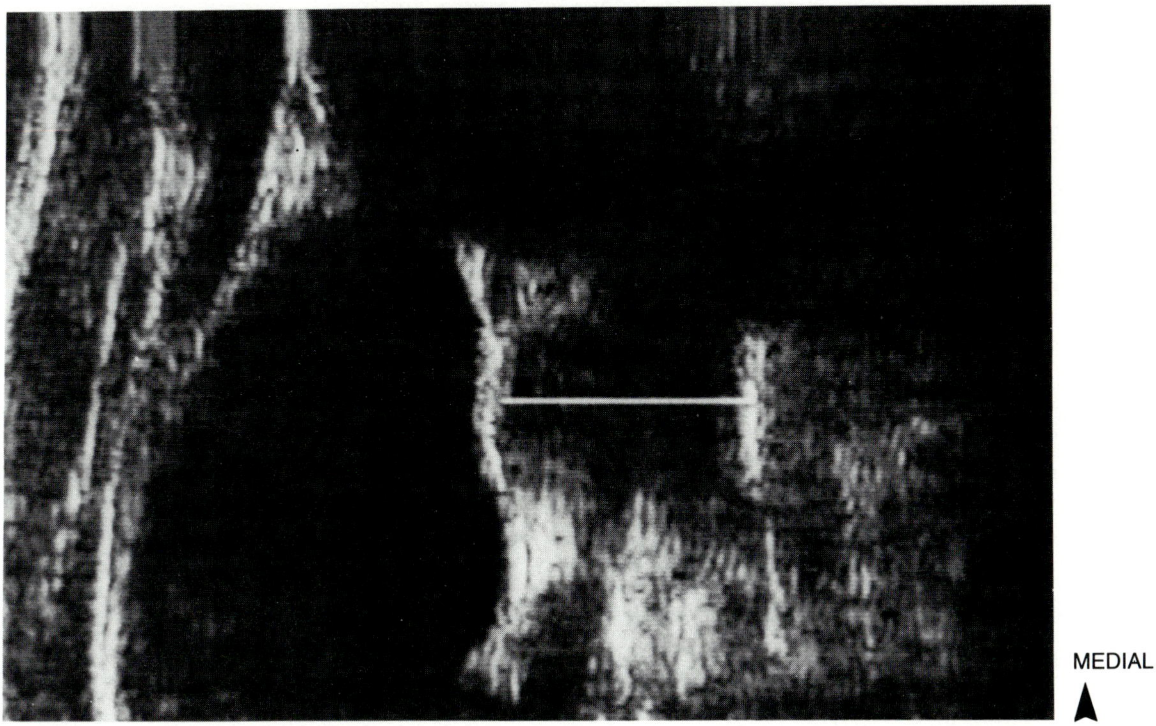
MEDIAL

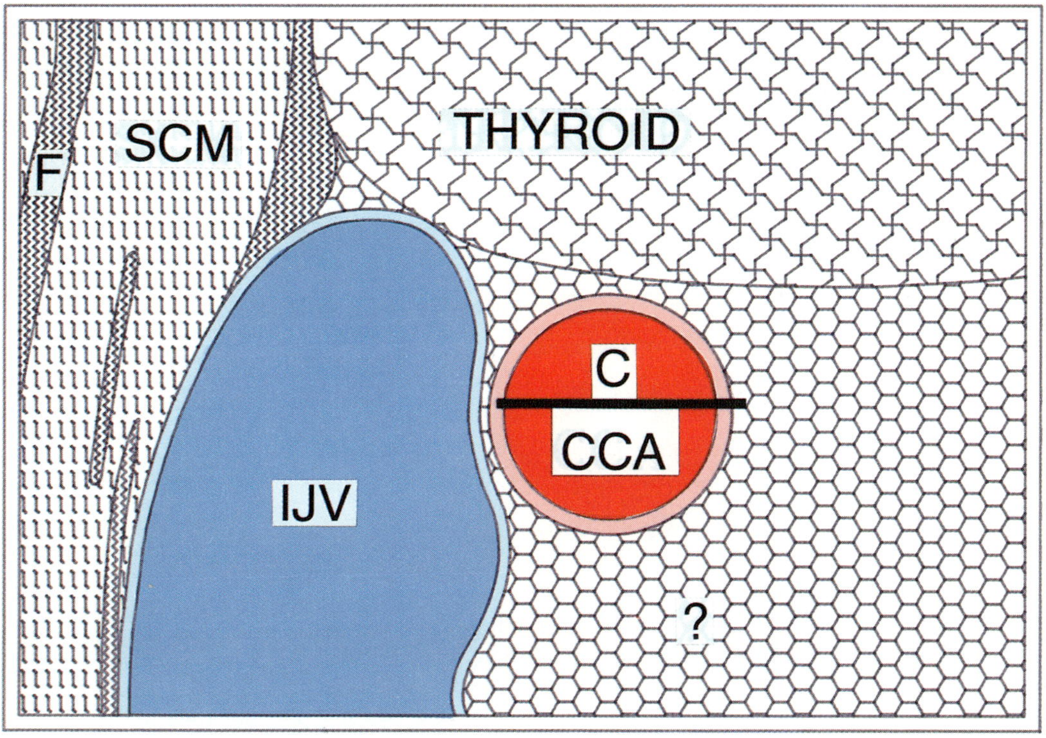
F
SCM
THYROID
C
CCA
IJV
?

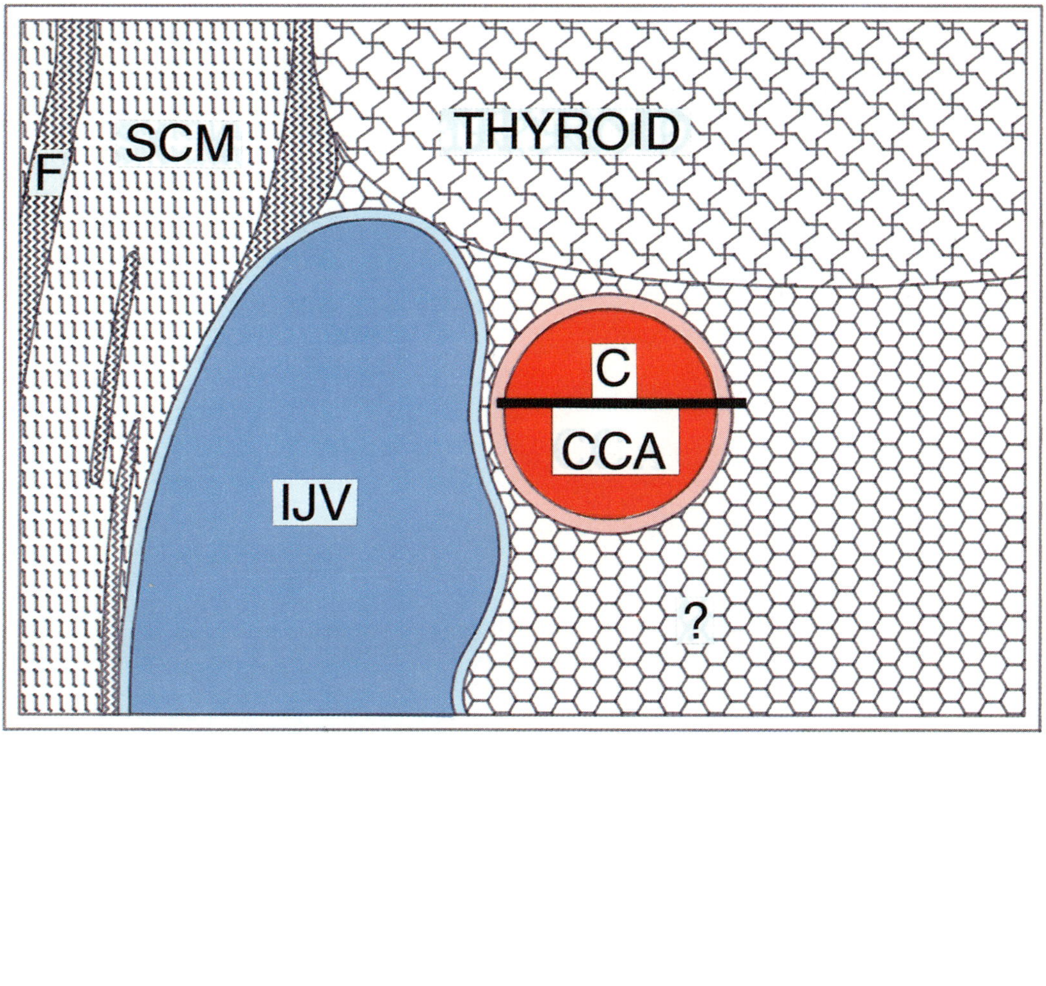

Figure 28. COMMON CAROTID—UPPER NECK

In the upper neck proximal to the bifurcation, the common carotid artery (CCA) has enlarged slightly to a diameter of 8.0 mm. There is moderately echogenic, moderately heterogeneous plaque (P) with a smooth surface occupying three quarters of the circumference of the artery, leaving a residual lumen that is 5.0 mm by 6.5 mm in horizontal and vertical diameters, respectively. (The Doppler cursor (C) measures 4.1 mm in length.) The average residual lumen of 5.8 mm in diameter causes only an 8% stenosis relative to the proximal artery, which we would round to 10% (see Figure 27). If one uses the arterial diameter of 8.0 mm at this level as the normal arterial diameter, there is a 27.5% stenosis which we would round to a 30% stenosis by diameter. One of the additional advantages to be gained by utilizing the proximal common and distal external and internal carotid arteries for normal arterial diameters is that usually at these levels, the arteries are relatively free of plaque, and an accurate diameter measurement of the artery can be obtained. In comparing this set with Figure 27, note the relative difficulty one would have in deciding where the plaque ended and the normal arterial wall began when obtaining a transverse diameter measurement of the artery at this level. Sometimes, with highly echogenic plaque, the deep wall of the artery cannot be visualized at all. It is better to measure an arterial diameter at a different level than to guess. SCM = sternocleidomastoid muscle, F = fascia, IJV = internal jugular vein.

HISTORY *This 76-year-old female presented with multiple transient ischemic attacks with expressive aphasia and was found, by ultrasound scan, to have an ulcerated plaque on the left that was confirmed by subsequent carotid endarterectomy. However, she has remained asymptomatic over the 6 months following this ultrasound scan on the right side.*

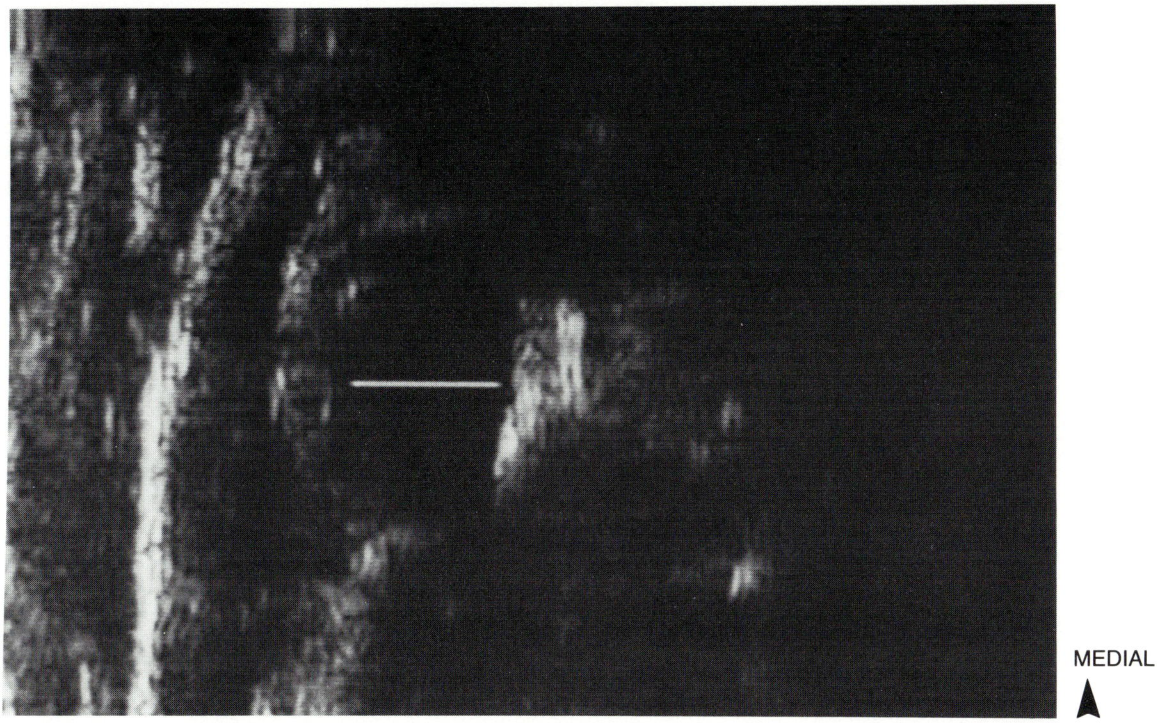
MEDIAL

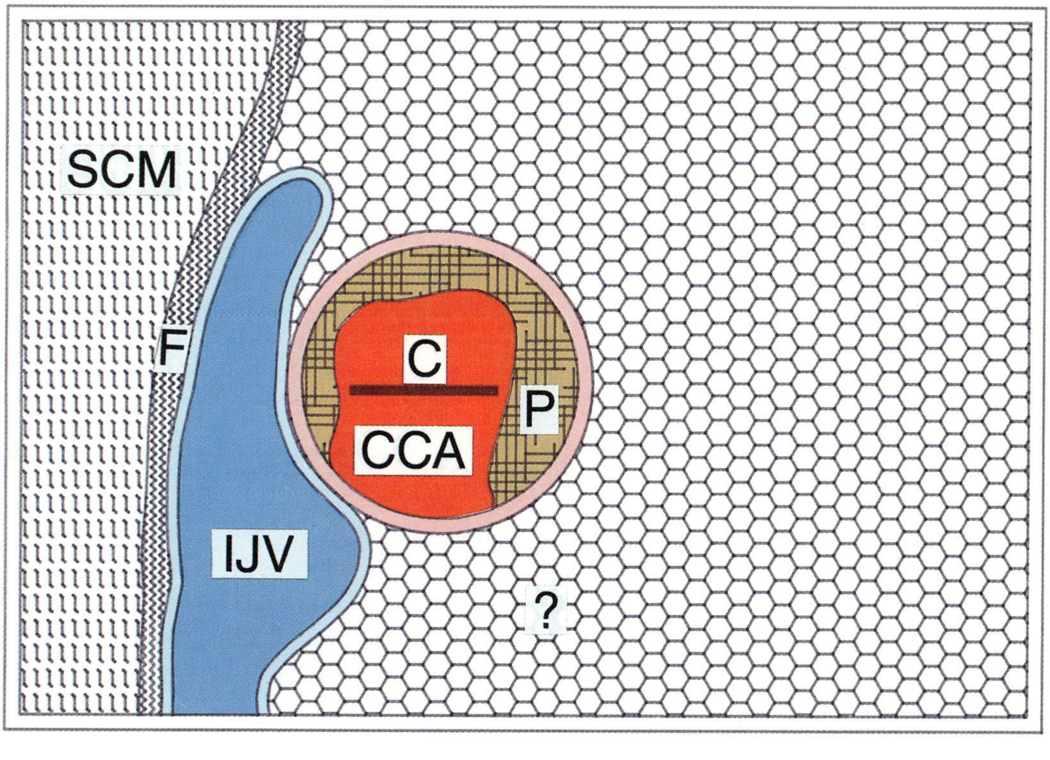
SCM
F
C
P
CCA
IJV
?

Figure 29. PROXIMAL COMMON CAROTID

A second example of the effect of arterial tapering on the calculation of stenosis is shown in the following. This view is provided for comparison with the ultrasound scan that follows, showing the right common carotid artery (CCA) low in the neck at its smallest diameter. The Doppler cursor (C) has been placed so that the left-hand edge is properly against the "intimal stripe" on the superficial wall, but the right-hand edge does not reach the "intimal stripe" of the deep wall. The cursor measures 6.0 mm in length, and the arterial diameter is actually 6.5 mm. In real time, it is very difficult for the technician to place the cursor perfectly within the residual lumen of the artery because of arterial pulsation and other movement. The arterial diameter in real time varies between systole and diastole. SQ = subcutaneous tissue, SCM = sternocleidomastoid muscle, IJV = internal jugular vein, THYROID = thyroid gland, VN = vagus nerve, HL = "hard-line" artifact.

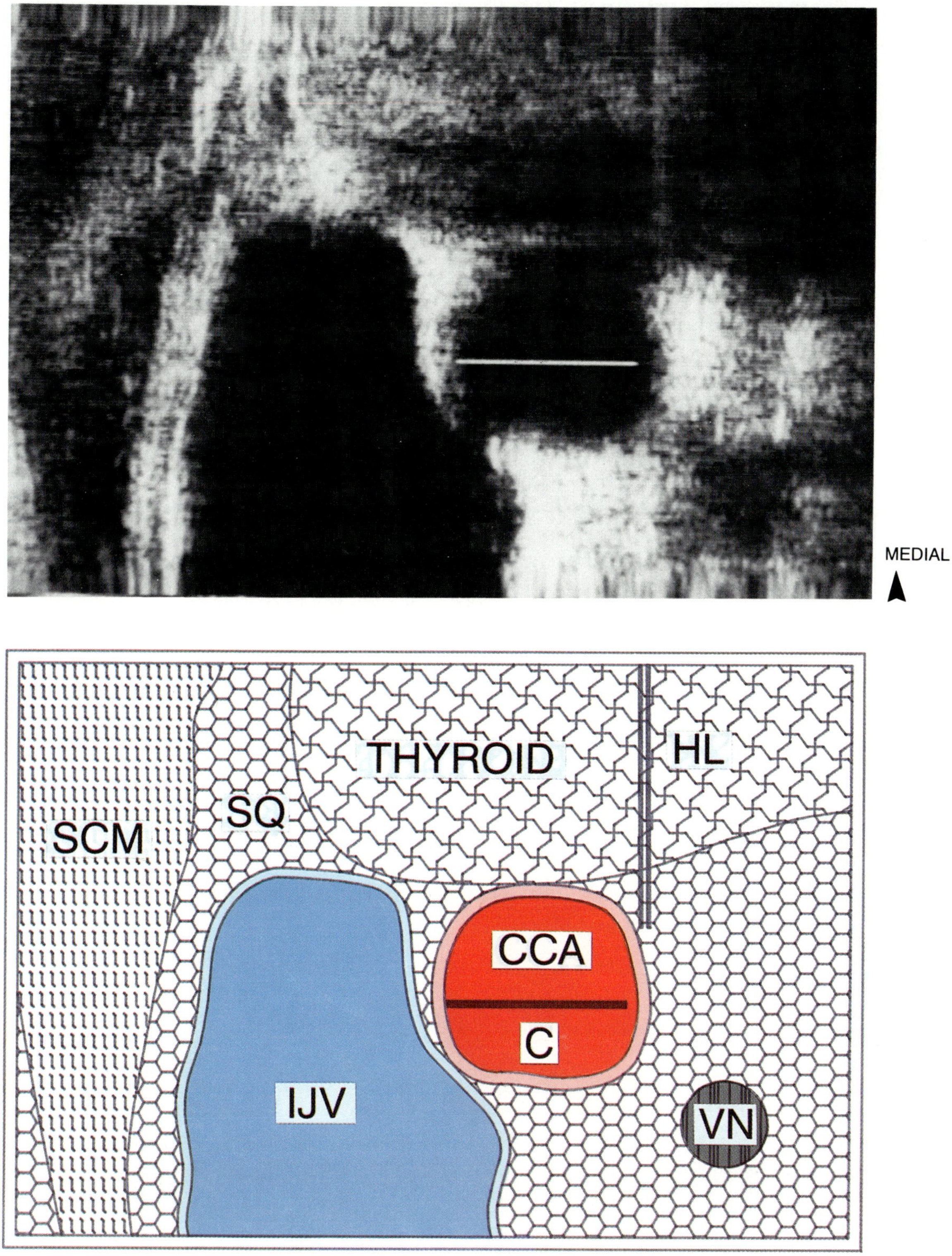
MEDIAL
THYROID
HL
SQ
SCM
CCA
C
IJV
VN

Figure 30. RESIDUAL LUMEN AT BIFURCATION

This same right common carotid artery (CCA) as in Figure 29 is followed up to the bifurcation where the origins of the external carotid artery (ECA) and internal carotid artery (ICA) are beginning to form. There has not yet been a separation of the internal and external carotid arteries. The level of this ultrasound scan, therefore, still corresponds to the CCA. Note the difficulty, however, in assigning a uniform diameter to the residual lumen created by the faintly echogenic plaque (P). Measuring from upper left to lower right, the long axis of the residual lumen is 11 mm in diameter. As measured from lower left to upper right, however, the residual lumen has minimum and maximum widths of 2.5 and 6.0 mm. Certainly, one would be able to fit a diameter of 6.0 mm within the lower right portion of the residual lumen. By adding the portion beginning to split off toward the ECA, one might say this residual lumen is equivalent to a 6.5-mm or 7.0-mm diameter residual lumen overall. Therefore, the plaque in this common carotid bifurcation is equivalent to a 0% stenosis by diameter in comparison with the smaller more proximal common carotid, according to the principles outlined previously. SQ = subcutaneous tissue, SCM = sternocleidomastoid muscle, IJV = internal jugular vein, THYROID = thyroid gland, C = Doppler cursor, HL = "hard-line" artifact, AS = acoustic shadowing. (See Figure 68. The acoustic shadowing is quite prominent in this scan, but from the top and bottom side walls of the artery, i.e., the "pigtail effect," and is not due to plaque.)

HISTORY *This 88-year-old male was admitted following an episode of syncope with a residual neurologic deficit of aphasia that disappeared over the next 2 days. A subsequent computed tomography scan showed cortical atrophy. A cardiac workup revealed a complex arrhythmia, which the internist felt was responsible for this patient's symptoms.*

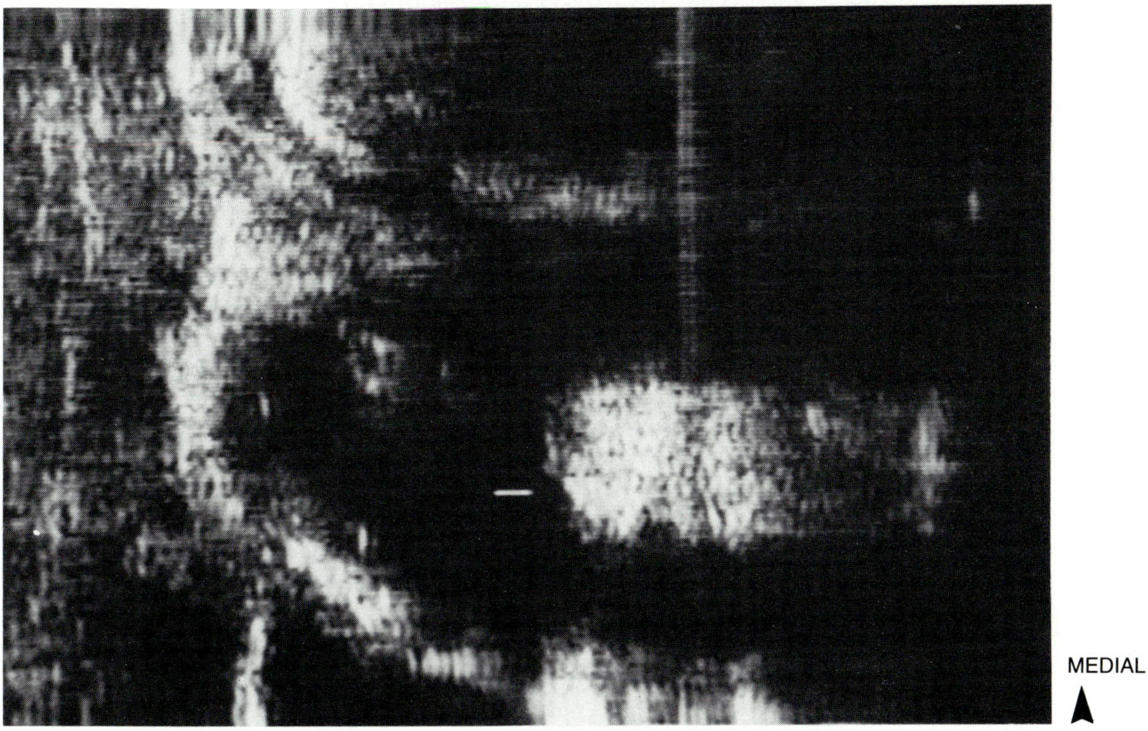
MEDIAL

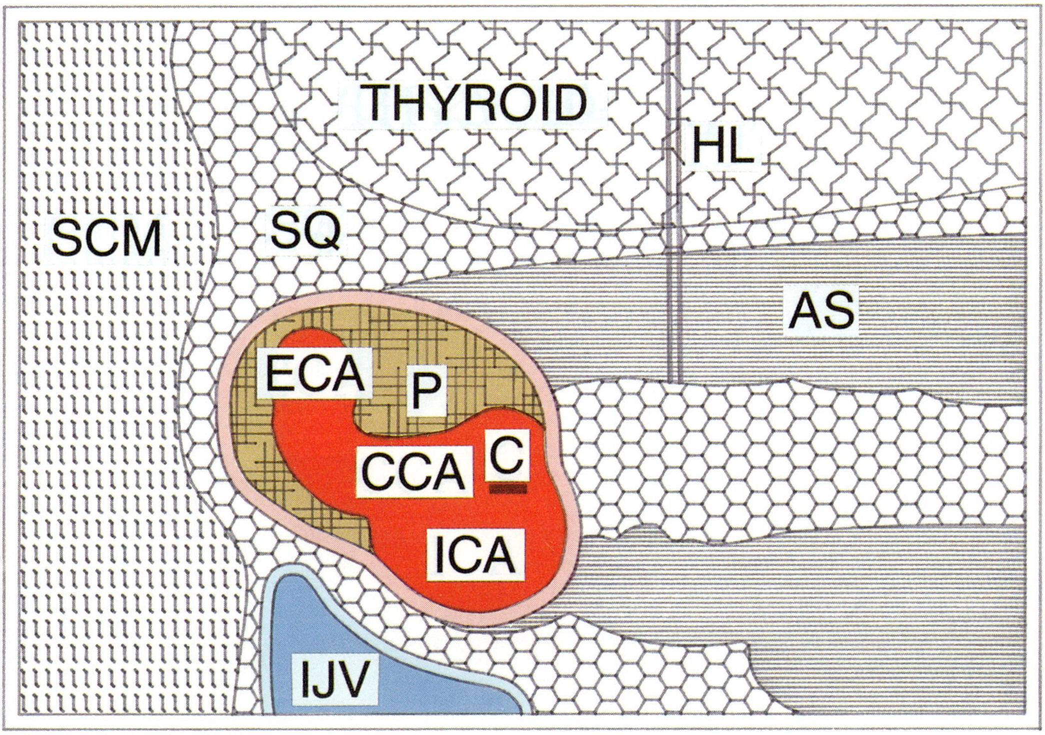
THYROID
HL
SCM
SQ
AS
ECA
P
C
CCA
ICA
IJV

Figure 31. 55% INTERNAL CAROTID STENOSIS

This is an example of the calculation of percent stenosis as seen in a transverse view of the distal left internal and external carotid arteries. The internal carotid artery (ICA) has a diameter of 5.5 mm with a smooth, circular residual lumen (RL) of 2.5 mm in diameter giving rise to a 55% stenosis based upon average residual diameter. This view was taken above the level of the internal carotid bulb where the ICA had already tapered to its smallest normal diameter. The shape of the arterial wall at this point is ovoid because the ICA is somewhat oblique rather than perfectly transverse to the beam. The plaque (P) surrounding the residual lumen is homogeneous and faintly echogenic. The external carotid artery contains a 3.3-mm diameter lumen within a 3.8-mm diameter artery corresponding to a 15% stenosis. S = skin, SQ = subcutaneous tissue (including platysma muscle), M = muscle (sternocleidomastoid), F = fascia, V = internal jugular vein.

HISTORY *This 55-year-old male with diabetes and bilateral carotid bruits presented with repeated episodes of vertigo and one episode of syncope 3 days prior to this ultrasound scan. Over the following 17 months the lesion progressed to greater than a 95% diameter stenosis with no visible residual lumen and a faint distal Doppler signal. Two weeks following the repeat ultrasound scan he underwent a carotid endarterectomy. The patient also had progression of stenosis on the opposite side from a 90% stenosis to a total occlusion in the intervening period between ultrasound scans.*

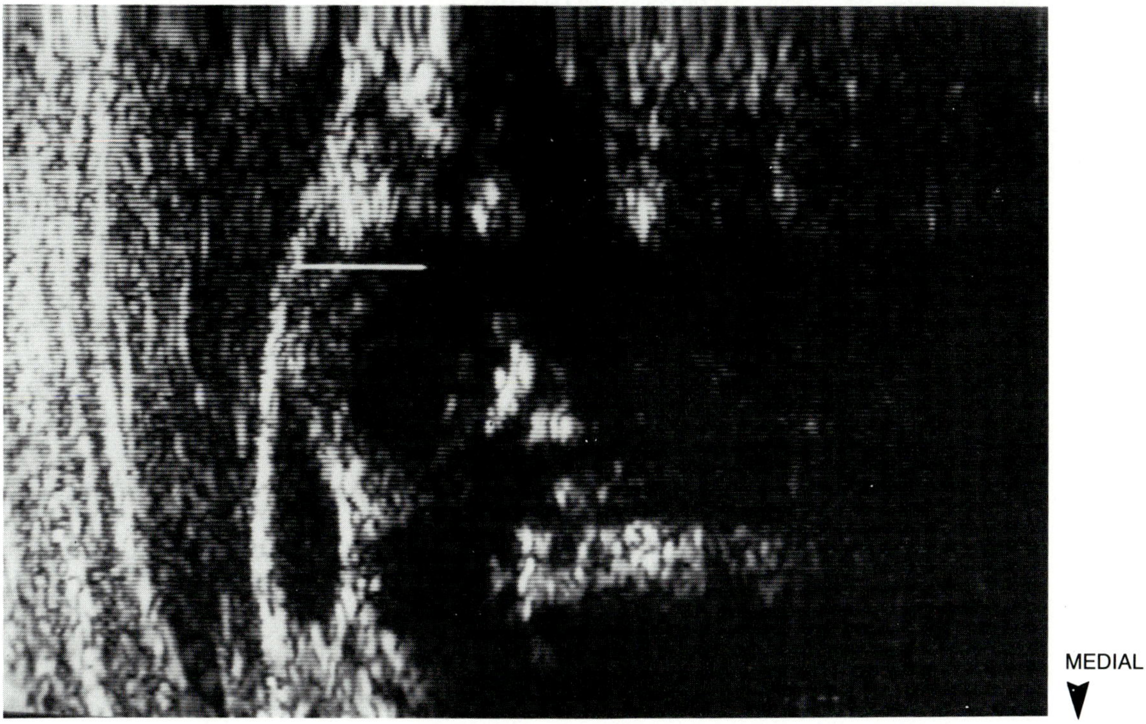
MEDIAL

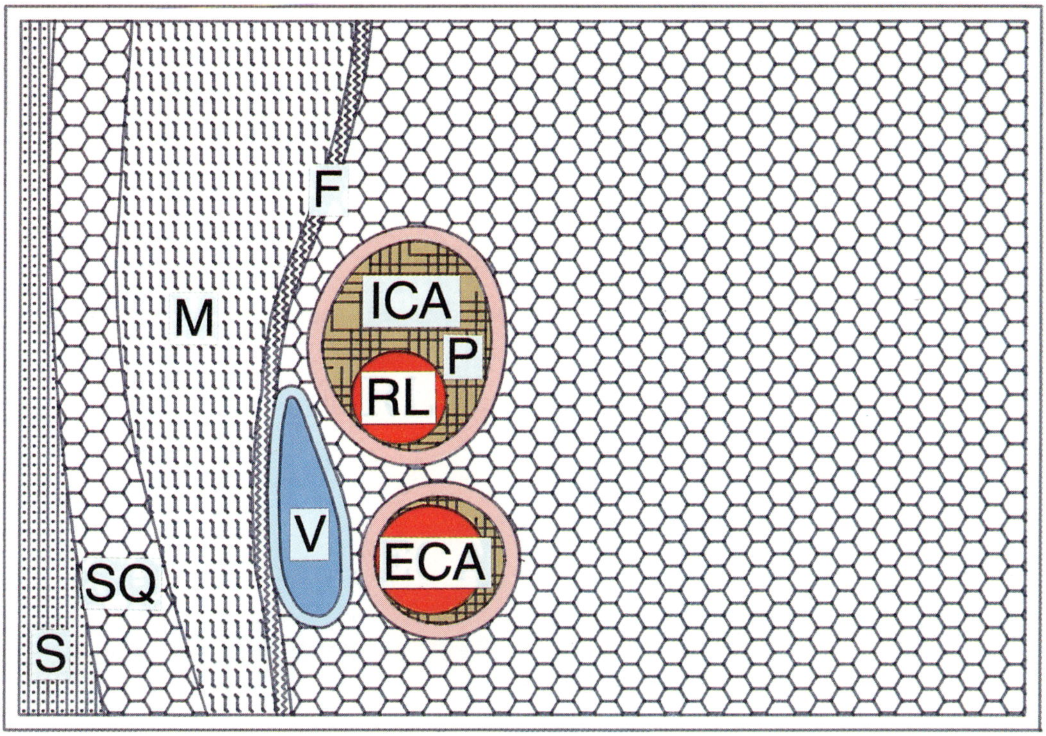
F
ICA
P
RL
M
V
ECA
SQ
S

Figure 32. 90% CAROTID STENOSIS

In this longitudinal view of the right carotid bifurcation a very tight stenosis of the internal carotid bulb caused by a very faintly echogenic and homogeneous plaque (P) is seen. The residual lumen measures only 0.5 mm across and, by comparison with the distal internal carotid diameter of 4.0 mm, causes an 87.5% stenosis which is rounded to 90% of the internal carotid artery (ICA). This is probably the most severe stenosis that can be measured. If smaller than this the residual lumen lies beyond the resolution of the instrument, and the only clue that this is not a total occlusion is the presence of a Doppler signal in the distal artery. In such severe degrees of stenosis, even a Doppler signal may be absent because of the tremendous slowing of blood flow, caused by viscosity effects, through a tiny residual lumen that overcomes the usual velocity increase associated with stenotic lesions. For these reasons we recently misdiagnosed one case, considering it to be a total occlusion of the artery when, in fact, it was proved to be patent both by arteriogram and subsequent endarterectomy. S = skin, SQ = subcutaneous tissue (including platysma muscle), M = sternocleidomastoid muscle, F = fascia, IJV = internal jugular vein, CCA = common carotid artery.

HISTORY *This is a 60-year-old male with a previous endarterectomy on the opposite side who presented with a transient ischemic attack, consisting of left hemiparesis shortly before this ultrasound scan was taken. Nine days later, the patient underwent a carotid endarterectomy at which time a near total occlusion was found. The plaque was characterized as atherosclerotic with both acute and chronic thrombi.*

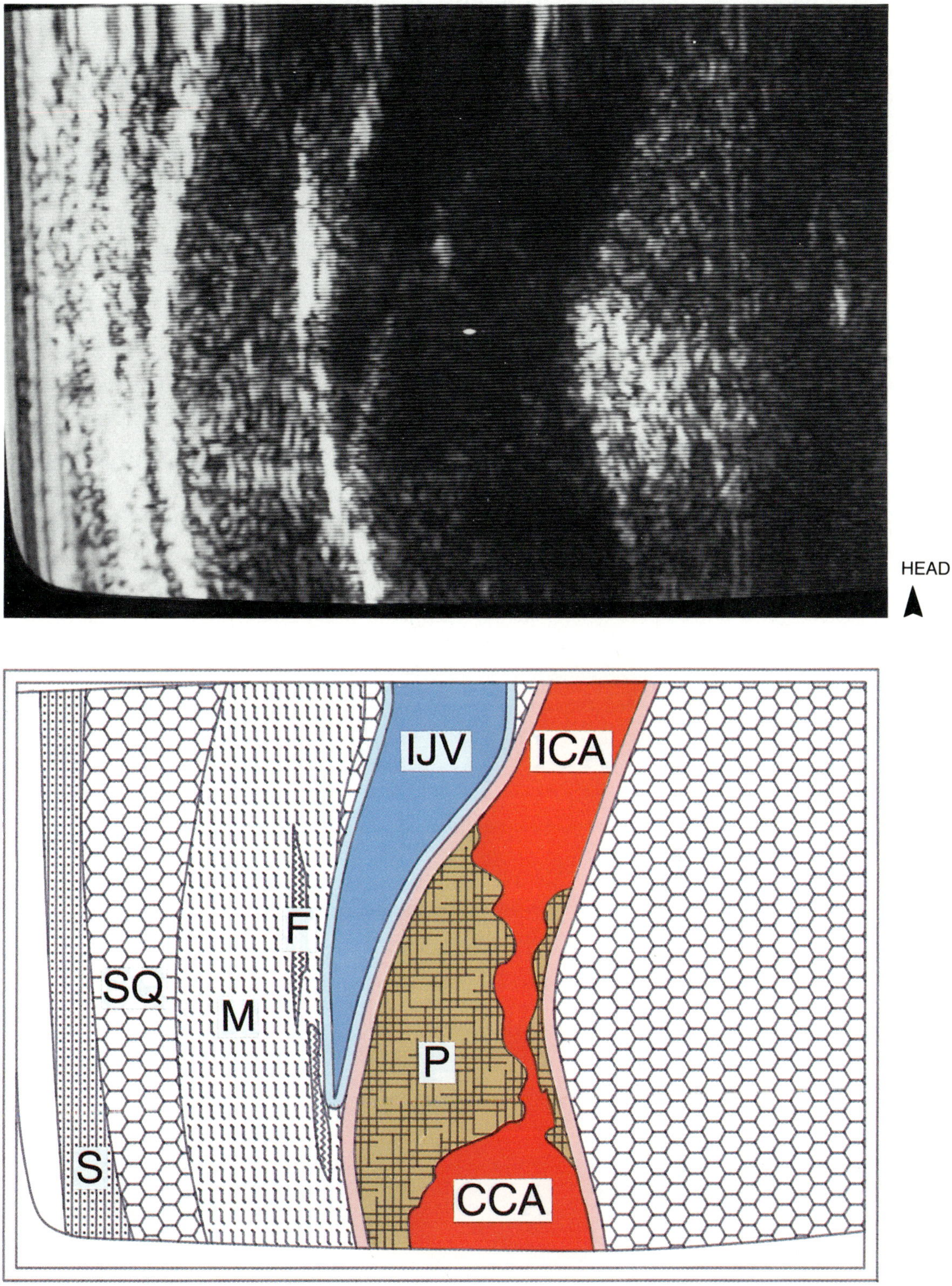
HEAD
IJV
ICA
F
SQ
M
P
S
CCA

Figure 33. CRITICAL STENOSIS—INTERNAL CAROTID

In this longitudinal view of the left internal carotid artery (ICA) there is faintly echogenic plaque (P) with a residual lumen (RL) of 1.0 mm in diameter. The distal ICA measures 5.5 mm in diameter just before it disappears under the mandible. The mandible causes blackening of the lower right-hand corner of the ultrasound scan but is not drawn. The percent stenosis of this ICA in this longitudinal view, therefore, appears to be 82% by diameter, which is rounded to 80%. This stenosis is equivalent to a 96% area stenosis. In fact, at the same level on transverse view, the degree of stenosis by diameter was equal to 90%. SQ = subcutaneous tissue (including some muscle that is not well defined).

HISTORY *This 44-year-old male originally presented with a perioperative stroke following an appendectomy. Shortly thereafter, he underwent a left carotid endarterectomy and had been followed at intervals by means of duplex scanning, with evidence of progressive stenosis until the time of this ultrasound scan 4 years following the endarterectomy. This plaque was confirmed by pathological examination to be atherosclerotic, following a repeat endarterectomy. At the time of operation 1 week following the ultrasound scan, the degree of stenosis was measured to be 85% by diameter.*

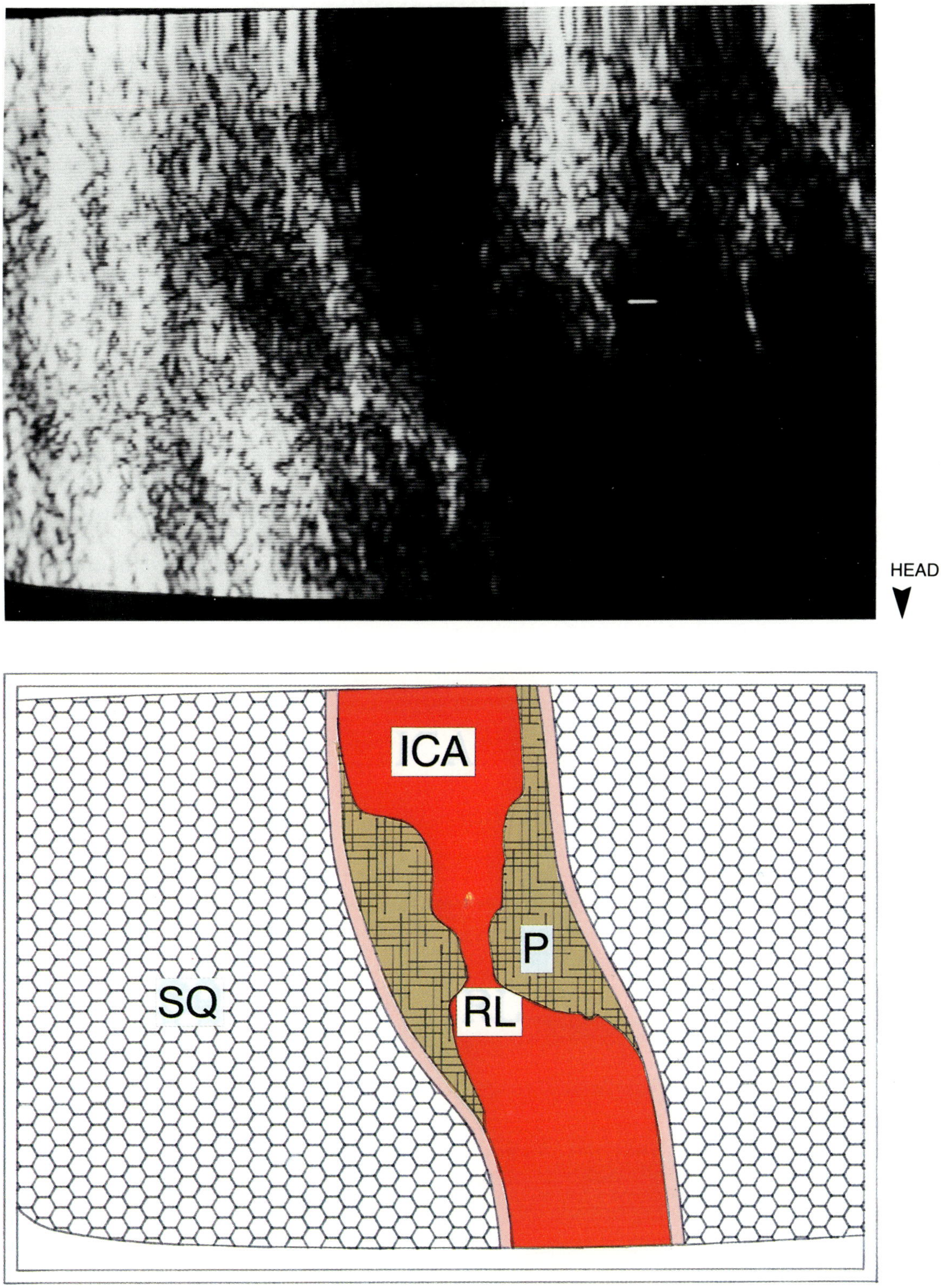
HEAD
ICA
P
SQ
RL

FIGURE 34. CRITICAL STENOSIS—VISIBLE FLOW

At a lower level within the common carotid artery (CCA) of the same bifurcation, in transverse view, visible flow (VF) is seen within the CCA as a faintly speckled snow-like pattern within the open lumen. In real time, this blood can be seen to swirl. The most important factor in determining whether or not blood flow is visible is its velocity. Visible blood flow, while quite frequently seen in veins, is very rarely seen in arteries. It is observed fairly frequently within aneurysms, owing to the pooling of blood within the very large residual lumen. This endarterectomized artery is somewhat large, being 12 mm in diameter. However, if the artery is of normal size, such visible blood flow carries an ominous implication. We have seen this phenomenon within the carotid arteries approximately a dozen times within the past 3 years. In all but two of these cases, the patient either had a total occlusion of the internal carotid artery or progressed from a very high grade stenosis to a total occlusion within a week of the ultrasound scan. Based on this experience, when visible blood flow is encountered within the carotid arteries and is not already associated with a total occlusion, the finding needs to be urgently communicated to the referring physician as an impending occlusion. SQ = subcutaneous tissue, M = muscle, P = plaque, LN = lymph node. To the right of the lymph node is another dark structure, possibly the vagus nerve, but identification is uncertain, and it is not drawn. Note the "pigtail" effect of acoustic shadowing from the top and bottom side walls of the common carotid (see Figure 68). The acoustic shadowing is not drawn in the diagram.

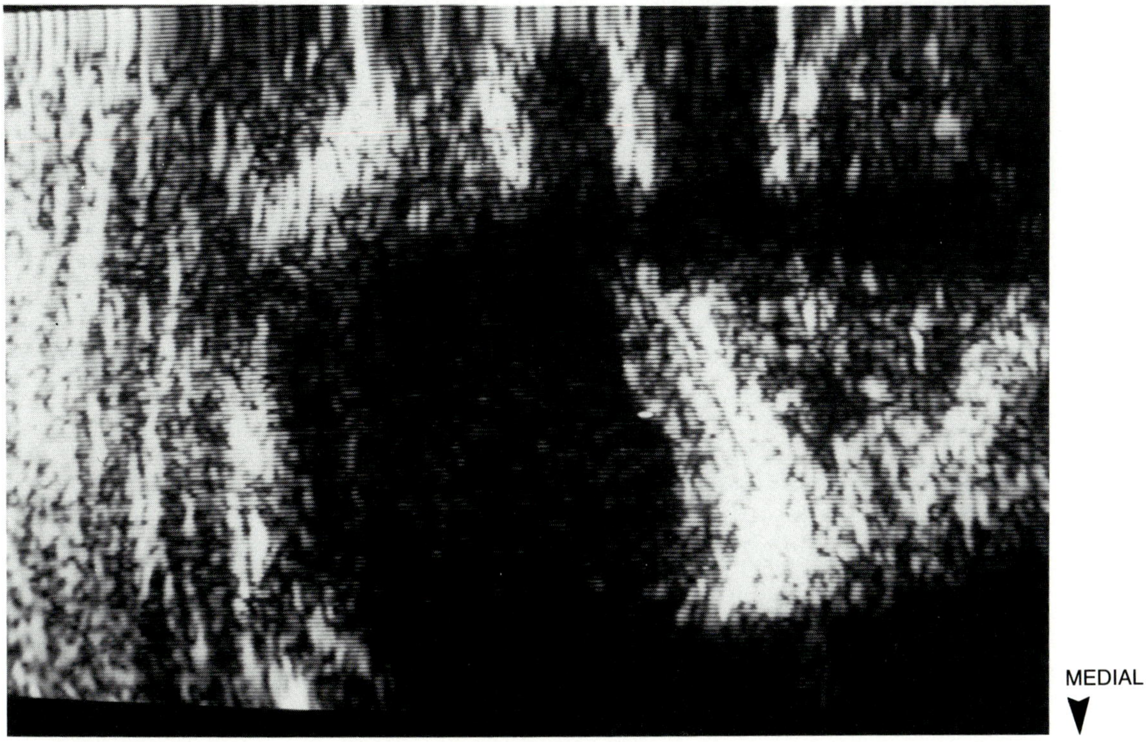
MEDIAL

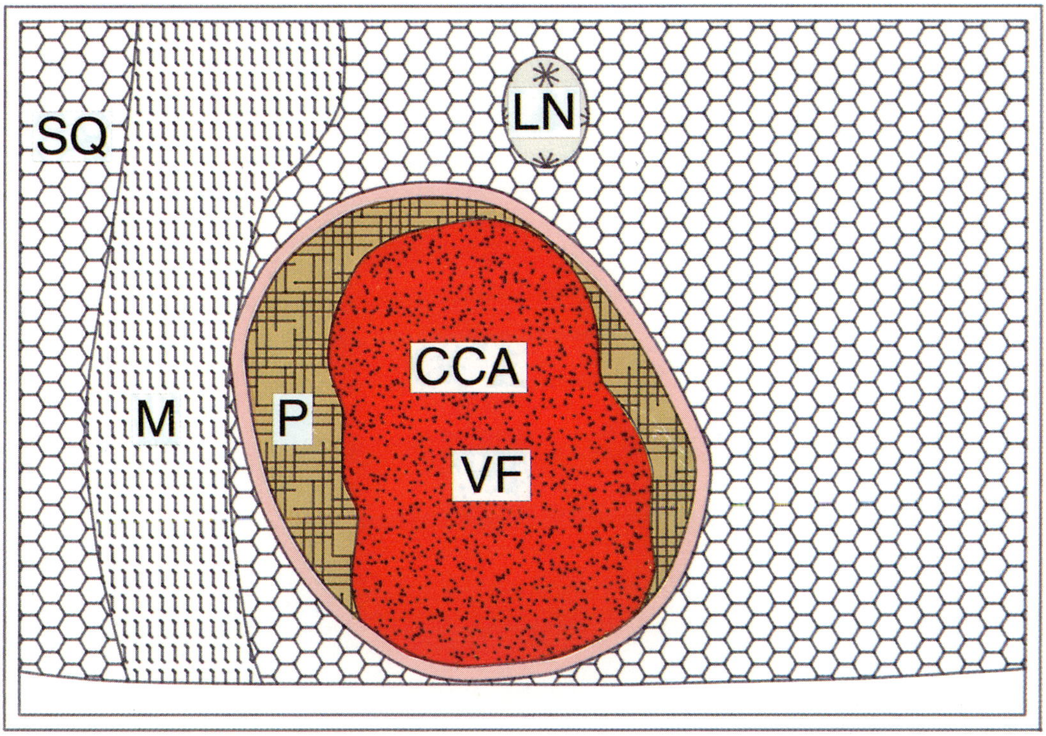
SQ
LN
M
P
CCA
VF

Figure 35. SEVERE INTERNAL CAROTID STENOSIS

This is a transverse view just above the left carotid bifurcation showing a severe stenosis. The Doppler cursor (C) is located near the bottom of the internal carotid artery (ICA). This vessel is nearly entirely filled in with plaque (P) of moderate echogenicity and moderate heterogeneity. The plaque causes the ICA to blend in quite well with the surrounding tissue and almost disappears from view. The tiny residual lumen is seen directly above the Doppler cursor and measures 0.7 mm in diameter in comparison with the cursor's width of 0.9 mm. The external carotid artery (ECA) is seen below and to the left with only a thin rim of plaque. This view is taken from the same artery seen in Figure 70. The 0.7-mm residual lumen in comparison with the 6.0-mm distal ICA qualifies as a 90% stenosis of this vessel. In a case such as this one, where the residual lumen is very small and difficult to see, it is helpful to first scan the artery longitudinally so as to be able to locate it. Then, while keeping the area of tightest stenosis in center field, rotate the probe into a transverse view as shown while maintaining eye contact so as not to lose the residual lumen. M = sternocleidomastoid muscle, F = fascia, IJV = internal jugular vein, V = facial vein, SQ = subcutaneous tissue, VN = vagus nerve.

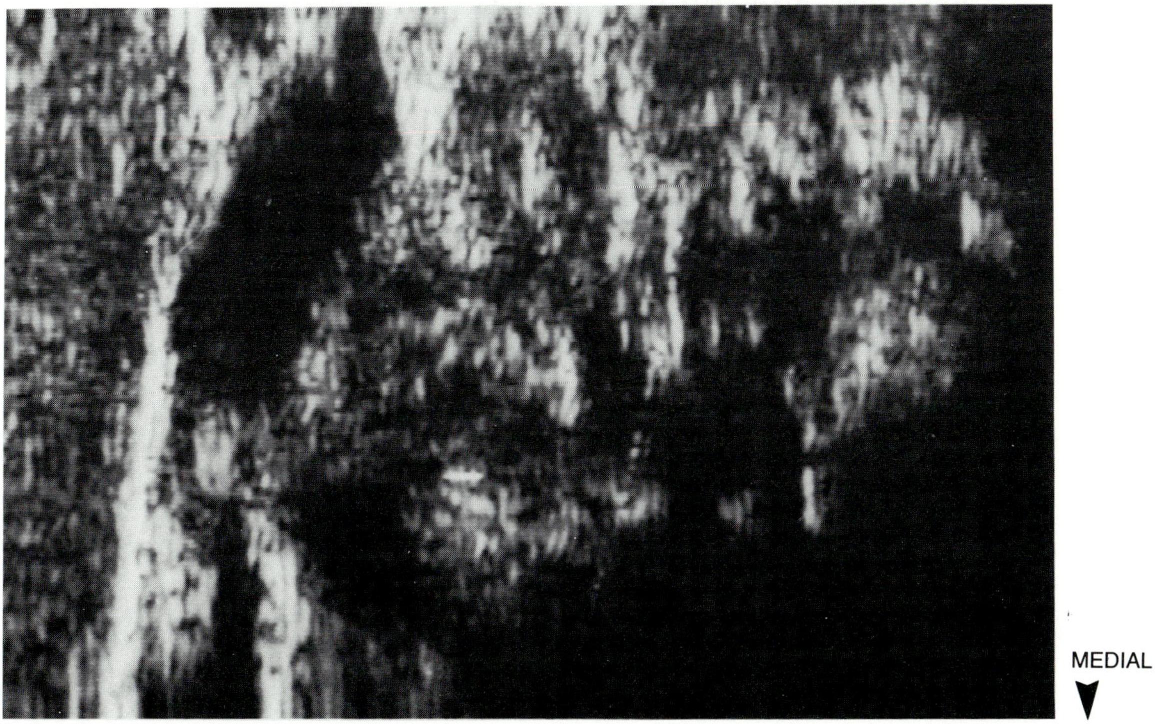
MEDIAL

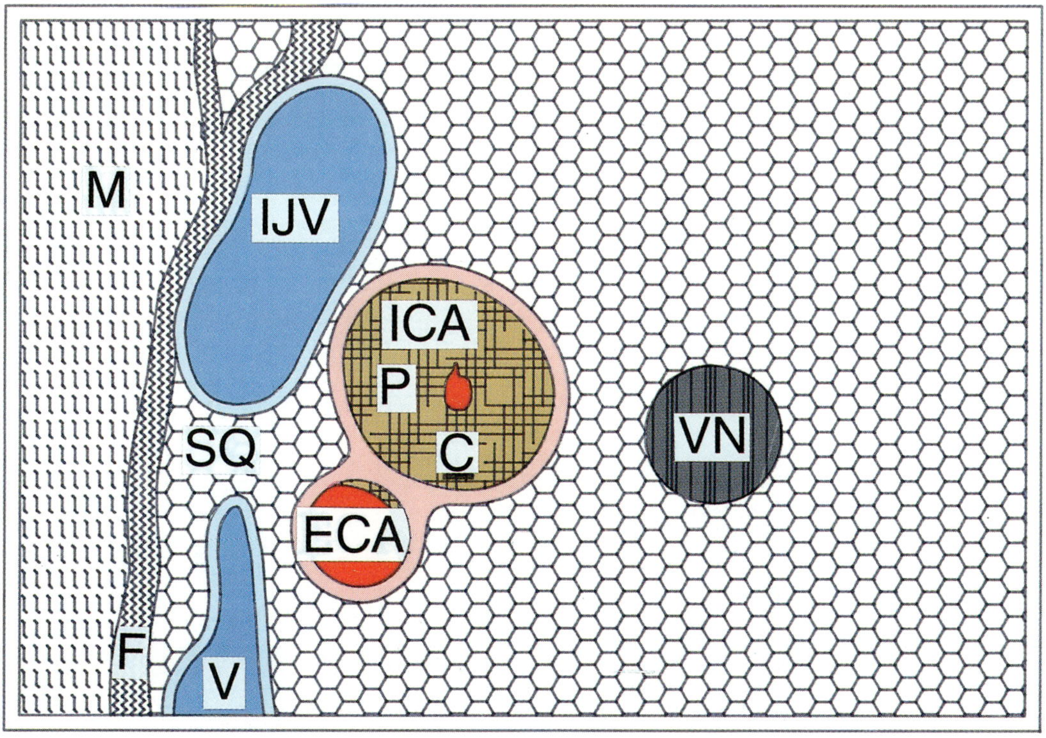
M
IJV
ICA
P
C
SQ
VN
ECA
F
V

Figure 36. CAROTID STENOSIS—TRANSVERSE VIEW

A transverse view of the left common carotid artery (CCA) is shown in order to make a point regarding the effect of rocking the probe as seen in the next two longitudinal views. There is plaque (P) within the artery at this level with an irregular lumen that has a depression near the bottom of the artery. The plaque immediately to the right of this groove is calcified with acoustic shadowing (AS) extending beyond the plaque to the right. The bone (B) to the right is part of one of the transverse cervical processes. Note the faintly visible vertical grid of lines superimposed on the ultrasound scan, which are spaced exactly 2.0 mm apart. The arterial diameter at this point measures 8.0 mm, and the residual lumen at its widest point from left to right measures approximately 6.0 mm. Along the vertical axis the residual lumen and normal arterial diameter are the same. Thus, with an average residual diameter of 7.0 mm in an 8.0-mm diameter vessel, the percent stenosis is only about 15% by diameter. M = muscle (platysma and sternocleidomastoid), F = fascia, SQ = subcutaneous tissue, V = internal jugular vein.

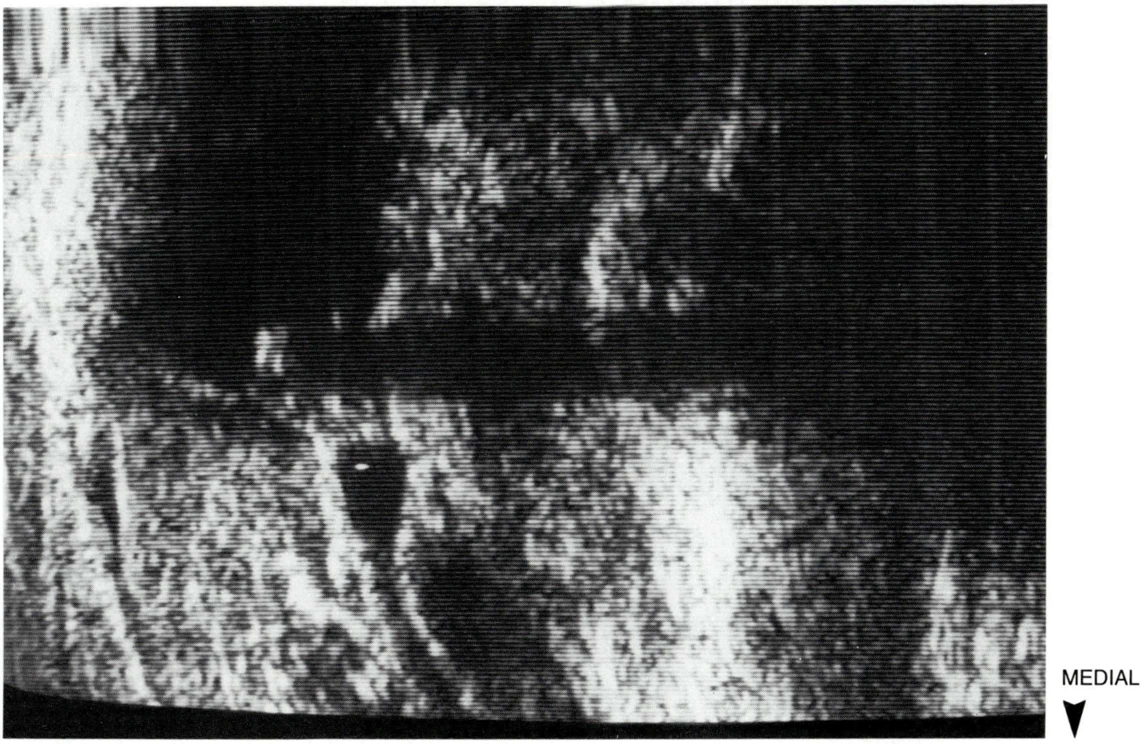
MEDIAL

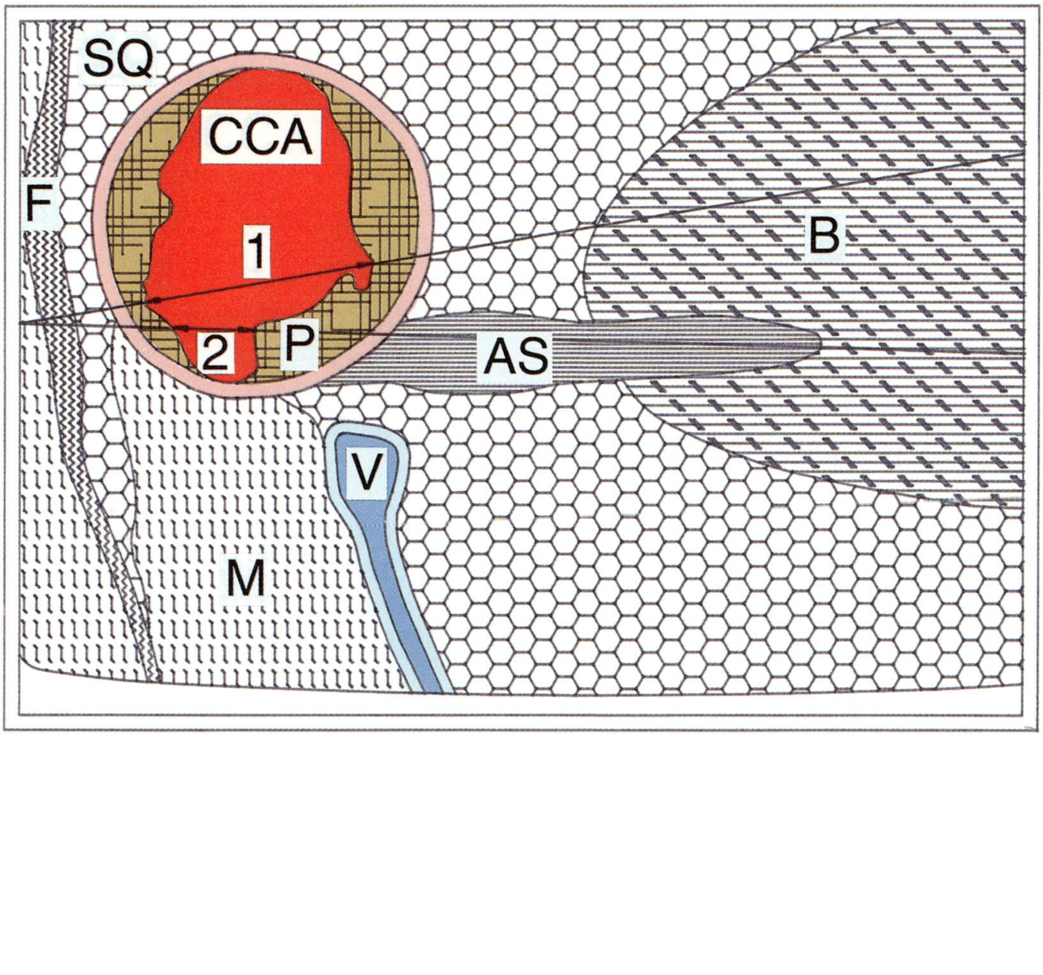
SQ
CCA
F
1
B
2
P
AS
V
M

Figure 37. STENOSIS WITH OFF-CENTER CUT

The same artery is seen in longitudinal view along a direction indicated in the transverse view by line #2. Notice the apparent severity of stenosis in this artery with a residual lumen (RL), measuring about 1.3 mm in diameter. This gives an apparent stenosis of about 80% relative to the 6-mm diameter artery. However, this apparent residual lumen is actually only a groove-like channel in the surface of the plaque (P), which is located along the bottom ("back") wall of the artery. SQ = subcutaneous tissue, M = muscle (sternocleidomastoid), CCA = common carotid artery, AS = acoustic shadowing.

HISTORY *This 89-year-old female complained of generalized weakness but no specific cerebrovascular symptoms.*

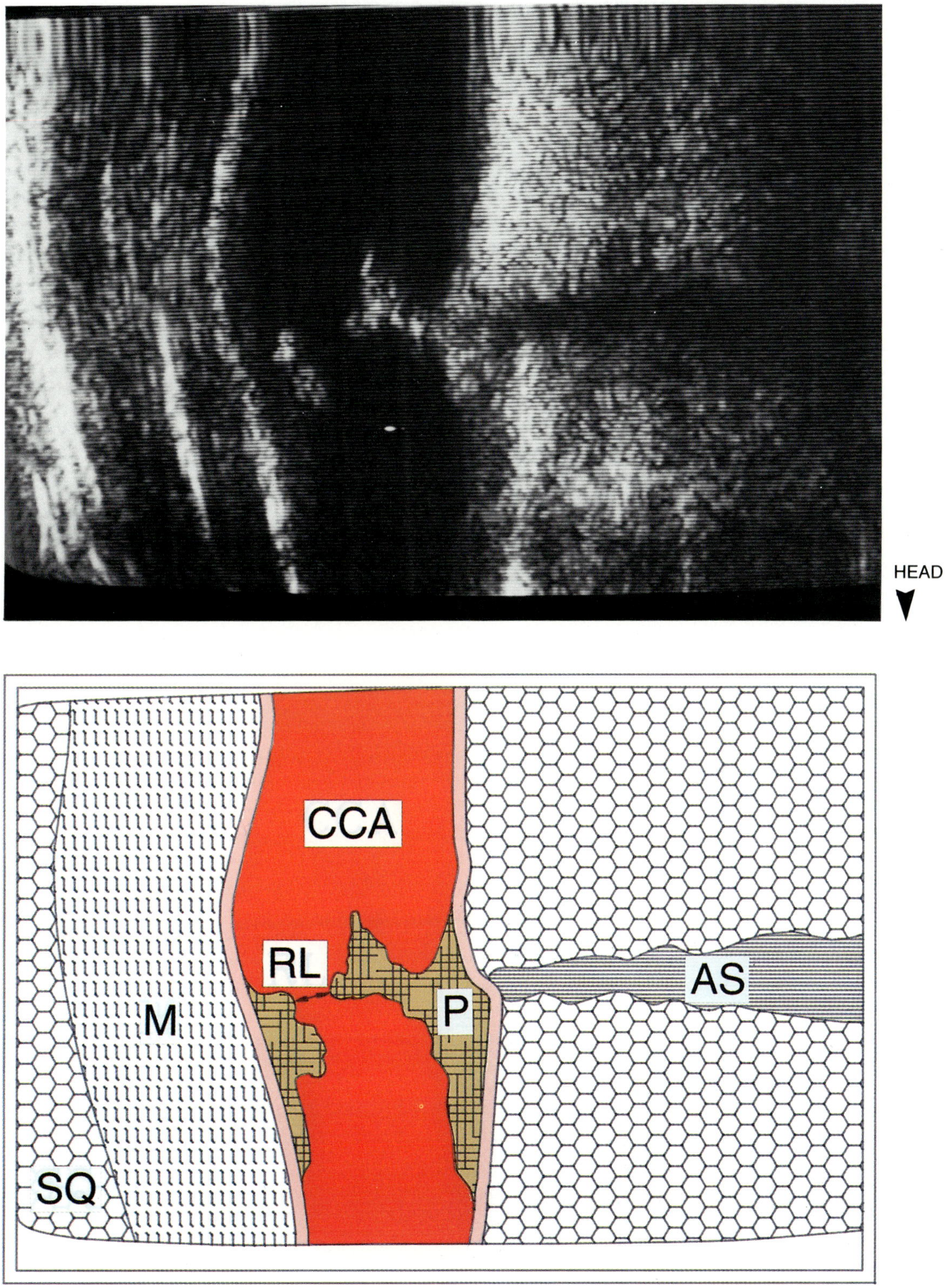
HEAD
CCA
RL
P
AS
M
SQ

Figure 38. CAROTID STENOSIS—CENTERED CUT

As the probe is rocked more toward the center of the vessel (direction #1 in the transverse view), this same plaque (P) appears to cause a much less severe—in fact, rather minimal—stenosis. The residual lumen (RL) in this view is slightly more than 4.0 mm. This finding emphasizes the importance of rocking the probe sideways across the vessel while in longitudinal view so as to maximize the residual lumen. Even in this longitudinal view the residual lumen is not as large as it is in the transverse view, and the true center of the vessel has not been reached. Thus, any single longitudinal scan of a stenosis can be very misleading when indicating the severity of disease. A transverse view, if of acceptable quality, is almost always better than a longitudinal view for measuring the percentage of stenosis. SQ = subcutaneous tissue, CCA = common carotid artery, M = muscle (sternocleidomastoid), AS = acoustic shadowing.

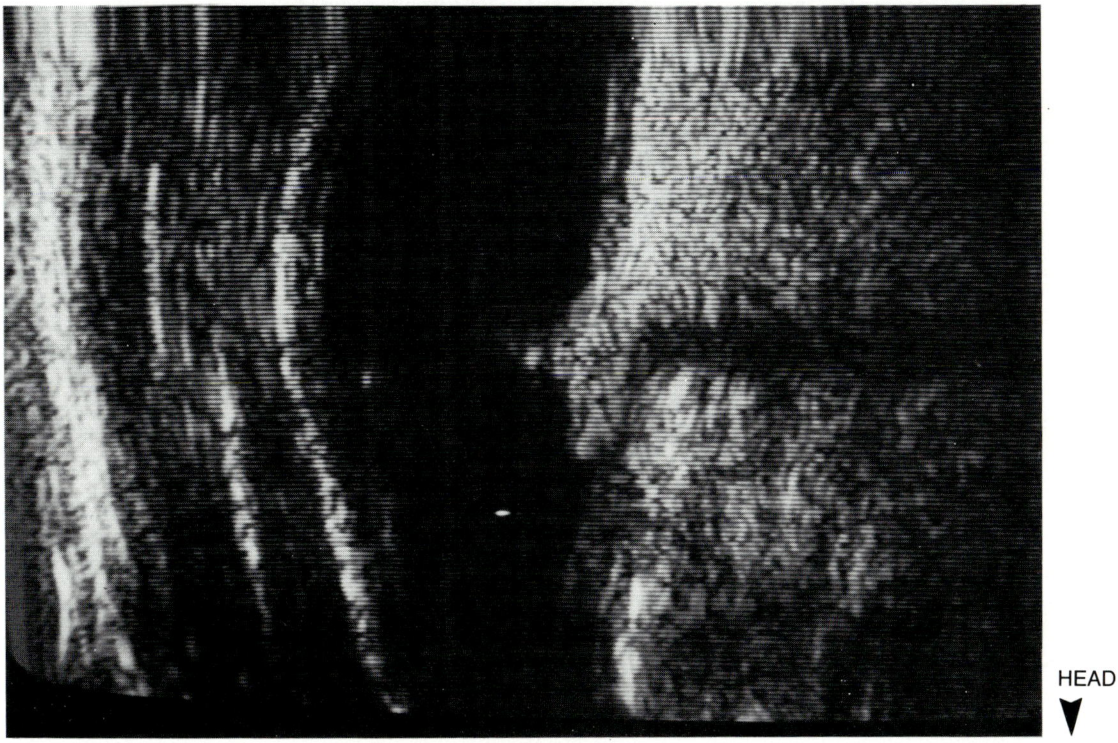
HEAD

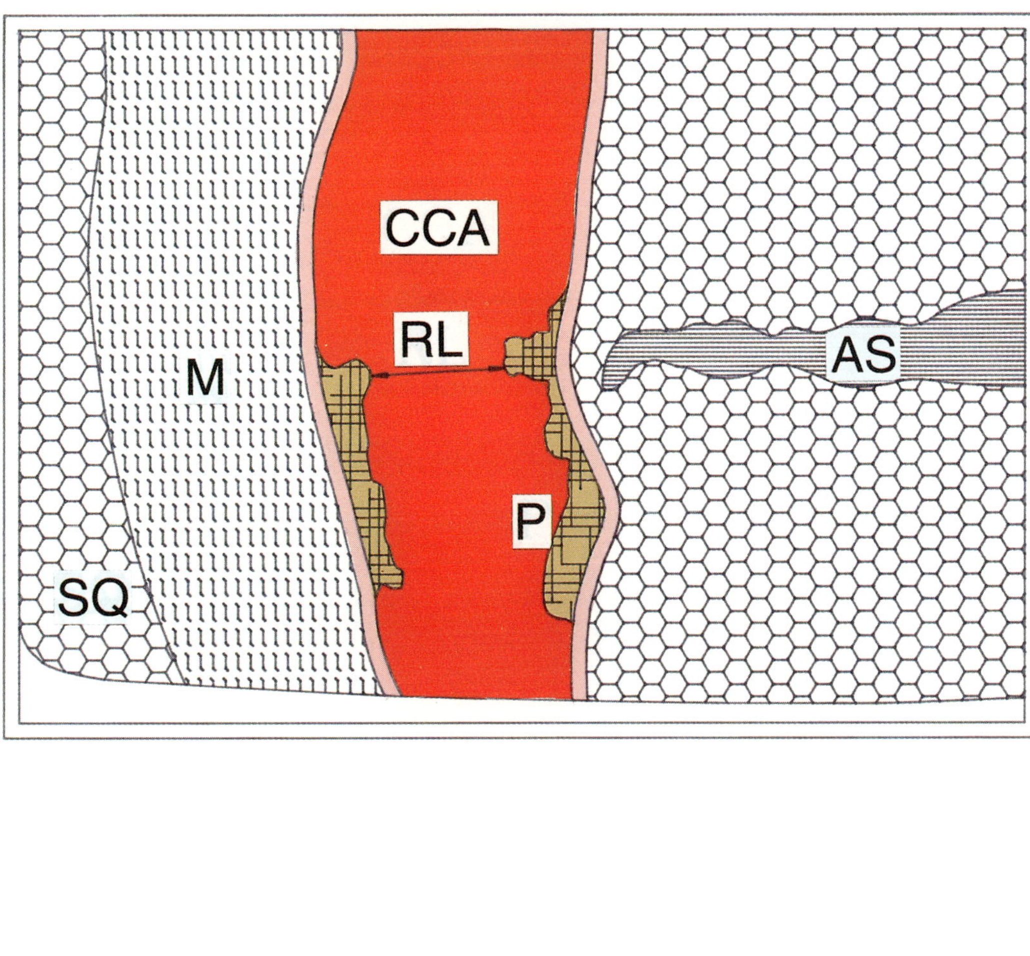
CCA
RL
M
AS
P
SQ

Figure 39. MILD STENOSIS—TRANSVERSE VIEW

In this view of a right internal carotid artery (ICA) above the bifurcation, there is a relatively small amount of plaque (P) at the Doppler cursor (not drawn). In this view, the degree of stenosis is only 15% by diameter and 25% by area. The external carotid artery (ECA) is above and to the right and not well seen because of an artifact of vertical smearing at the top and bottom edges of the ultrasound image. Line #1 corresponds to the plane of the following view in Figure 40. S = skin, M = platysma muscle, SQ = subcutaneous tissue, F = fascia, SCM = sternocleidomastoid muscle, ? = tissue of uncertain composition.

HISTORY *This 84-year-old female was screened for an asymptomatic left carotid bruit.*

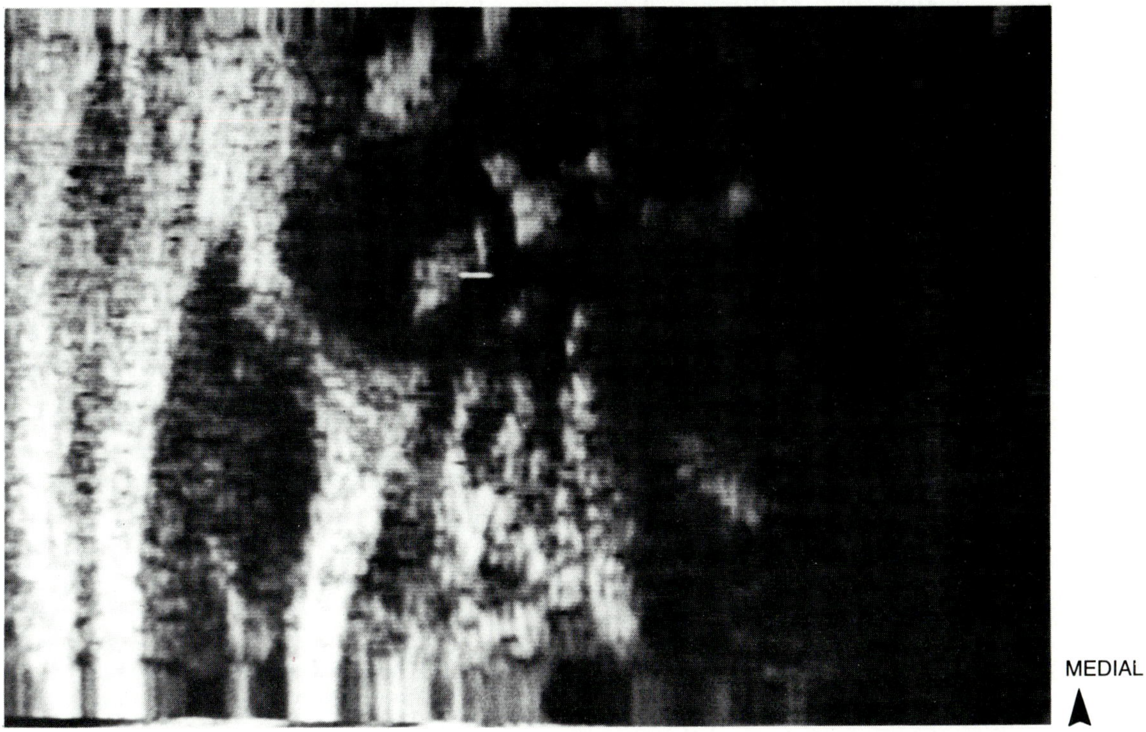
MEDIAL

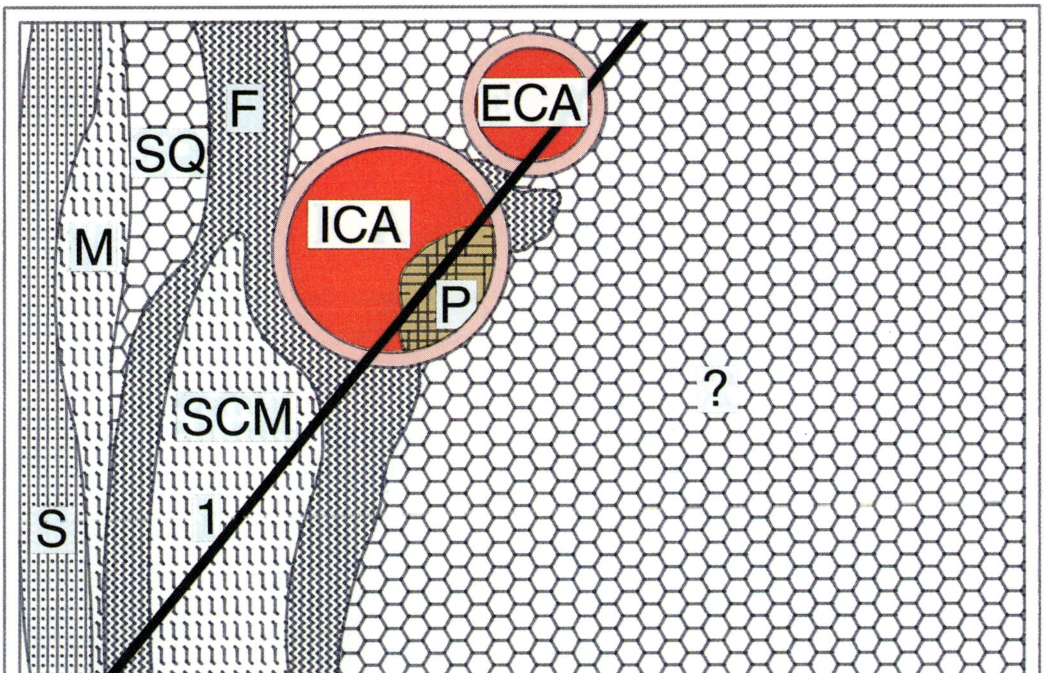
F
ECA
SQ
ICA
M
P
?
SCM
1
S

Figure 40. APPARENT "SEVERE" STENOSIS

In a corresponding longitudinal view, by directing the ultrasound beam along the direction of line #1 of the previous view, the technician is able to make this mild internal carotid stenosis appear to be a quite severe stenosis. An outline of plaque (P) is seen within the artery. To the left is a residual lumen (L) of only 0.7 mm in width with acoustic shadowing (AS) extending behind the plaque, in the midst of which is located the Doppler cursor (C). As can be seen on the more reliable transverse view, this longitudinal view obtained by rocking the probe somewhat off center is definitely misleading. The external carotid artery (ECA) is seen to the right of the distal (DIST) internal carotid but is obscured at a lower level because of the AS and because of the ECA curving out of plane at the origin of the bifurcation. S = skin, M = platysma and sternocleidomastoid muscles, SQ = subcutaneous tissue, F = fascia, PROX = proximal internal carotid artery (bulb), ? = tissue of uncertain composition.

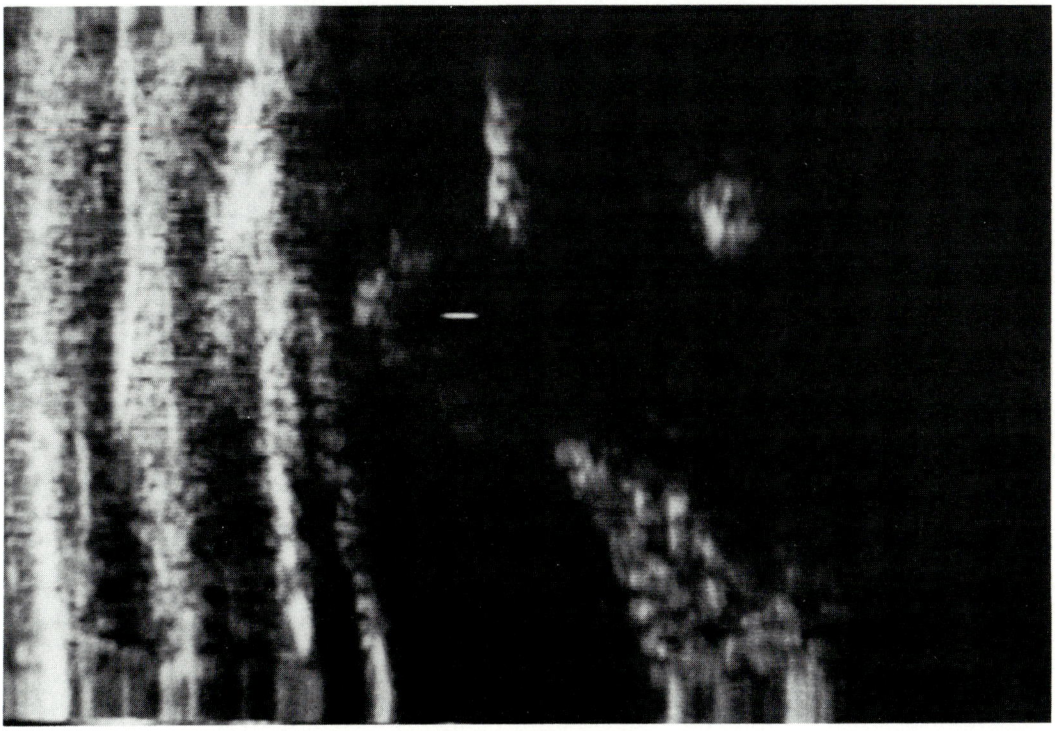
HEAD

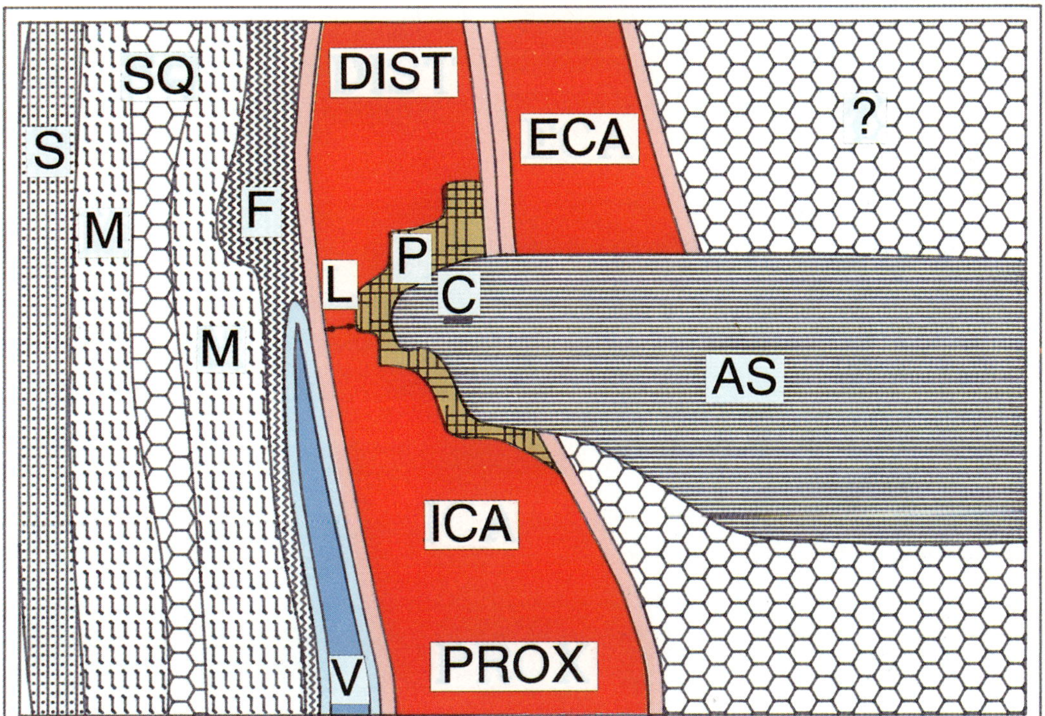
SQ
S
M
F
M
DIST
ECA
?
P
L
C
AS
ICA
V
PROX

CHAPTER 3

PLAQUE COMPOSITION

Figure 41. TYPES OF PLAQUE

Another value of an ultrasound scan in the assessment of plaque is its superiority over an arteriogram in allowing the assessment of composition of a particular plaque. Classification is based upon the echo pattern within the plaque as assessed by two criteria. The first is the degree of echogenicity or brightness of the echo pattern as a whole. This criterion separates examples A and C, which are faintly echogenic, from examples B and D, which are more brightly echogenic. The second criterion is the degree of uniformity of the echo pattern within the plaque, which is called its homogeneity. This criterion subdivides plaque into four different types of composition. A faintly echogenic and homogeneous plaque, as seen in example A, tends to be of lipid composition. A more brightly echogenic but still fairly homogeneous pattern, as seen in example B, is typical of a plaque that has become organized and contains fibrous tissue. A faintly echogenic plaque, which is heterogeneous with a more speckled pattern, is typical of thrombus or of intraplaque hemorrhage as seen in example C. Finally a plaque, as seen in example D, which is brightly echogenic and very heterogeneous is identified as a complex plaque. If there is acoustic shadowing behind the brightly echogenic areas, the plaque is calcified.

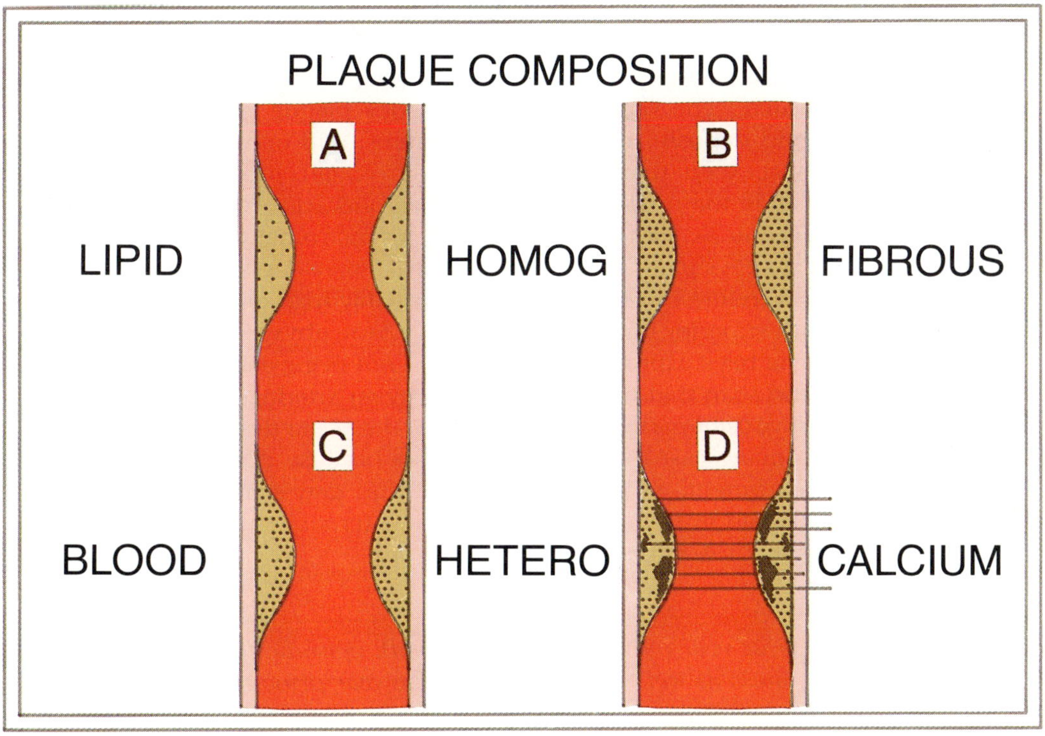
PLAQUE COMPOSITION
A
B
LIPID
HOMOG
FIBROUS
C
D
BLOOD
HETERO
CALCIUM

Figure 42. FAINTLY ECHOGENIC PLAQUE

This is an example of a very faintly echogenic plaque (P) located at the Doppler cursor (not drawn). The very faint homogeneous plaque is characteristic of a nearly pure lipid deposit. It is barely perceptible, and one might mistake this plaque for artifact except that in multiple views it remains present and is attached to the deep wall of the origin of the internal carotid artery (ICA). Obviously, the detection of plaque as faint as this requires an instrument with the ability to distinguish very fine shades of gray. The ability to measure stenosis on a purely visual basis is therefore reliable only in a reasonably high quality scan, using an instrument with superior imaging capabilities. Many physicians who have come to us for training have expressed frustration at not being able to see the plaque in an ultrasound scan that was later revealed by an arteriogram or at operation. This problem is caused partly by a need to train the eye to distinguish fine shades of gray, but in many cases the problem occurs because these physicians have been using instruments with inferior spatial and gray-scale resolution. M = sternocleidomastoid muscle, F = fascia, IJV = internal jugular vein, SQ = subcutaneous tissue, CCA = common carotid artery.

HISTORY *This 62-year-old male presented with episodic left facial and upper extremity numbness as well as dysphasia for the year prior to the scan.*

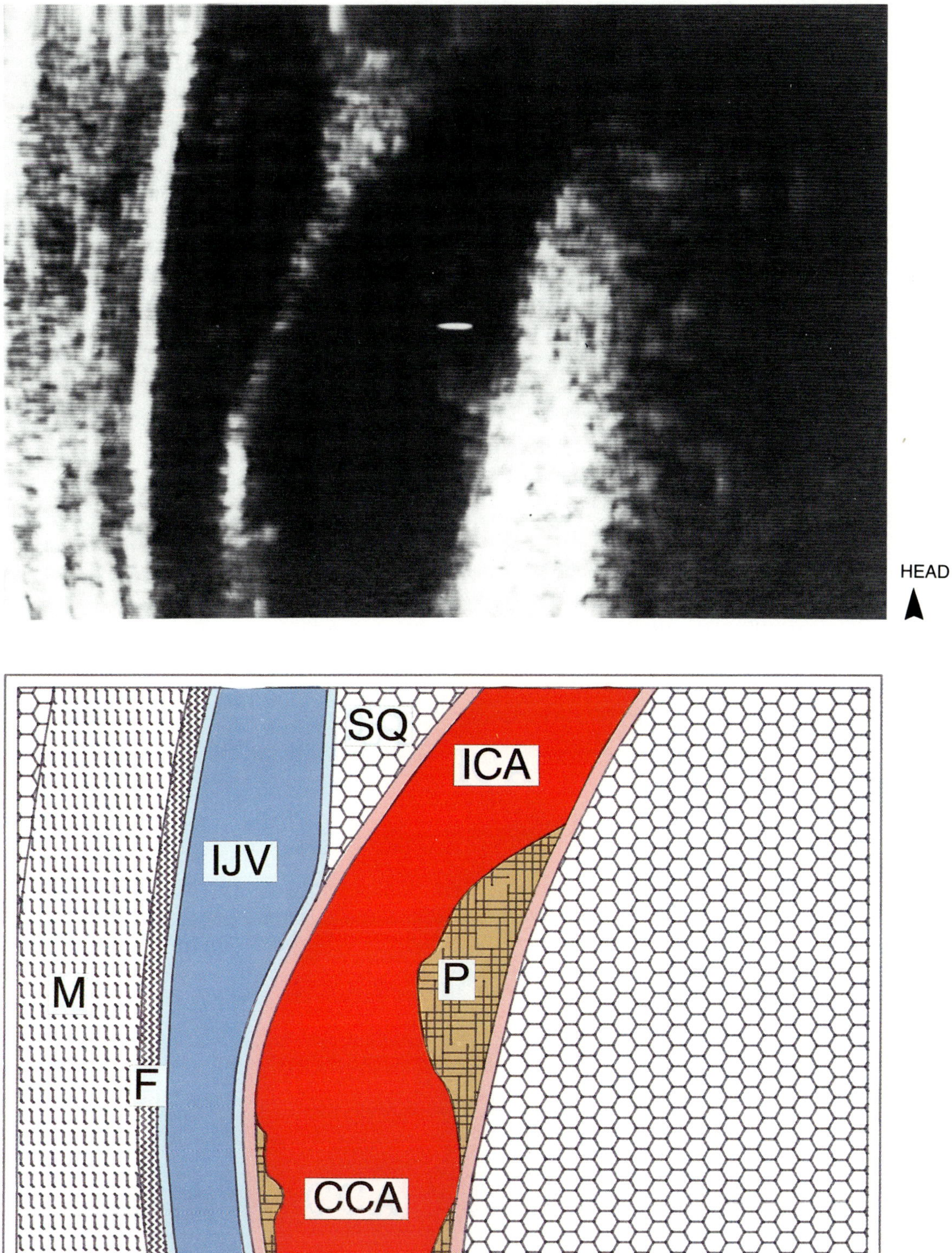
HEAD
SQ
ICA
IJV
M
P
F
CCA

Figure 43. FAINTLY ECHOGENIC PLAQUE

This is another example of a right carotid bifurcation seen in longitudinal view that contains homogeneous, faintly echogenic plaque (P) characteristic of lipid composition. The intimal margins of the external carotid artery (ECA) are particularly well seen. The Doppler cursor (C) is located in the common carotid artery (CCA) just below the origin of the internal carotid artery (ICA) which fades out distally. In this particular view, we would stop to obtain the residual lumen and normal lumen diameters of the ECA as given by dimensions RL1 and RL2, respectively. Likewise, the residual and normal lumens of the ICA would be measured as RL3 and RL4, respectively, staying perpendicular to the long axis of the vessel. The residual lumen of the common carotid artery (CCA) is not drawn but would be measured in a horizontal direction superficial to the letter P. This plaque would be considered to be only mildly irregular with gentle undulations of its surface. S = skin, SQ = subcutaneous tissue (including platsyma muscle), SCM = sternocleidomastoid muscle, F = fascia, ? = tissue of uncertain composition.

HISTORY *This 77-year-old female with a history of hypertension was admitted after an episode of near syncope. Two weeks prior, she had been placed on hydrochlorothiazide. After further evaluation in the hospital it was believed that the syncope was due to volume depletion and labile hypertension. She has remained asymptomatic for the following 8 months.*

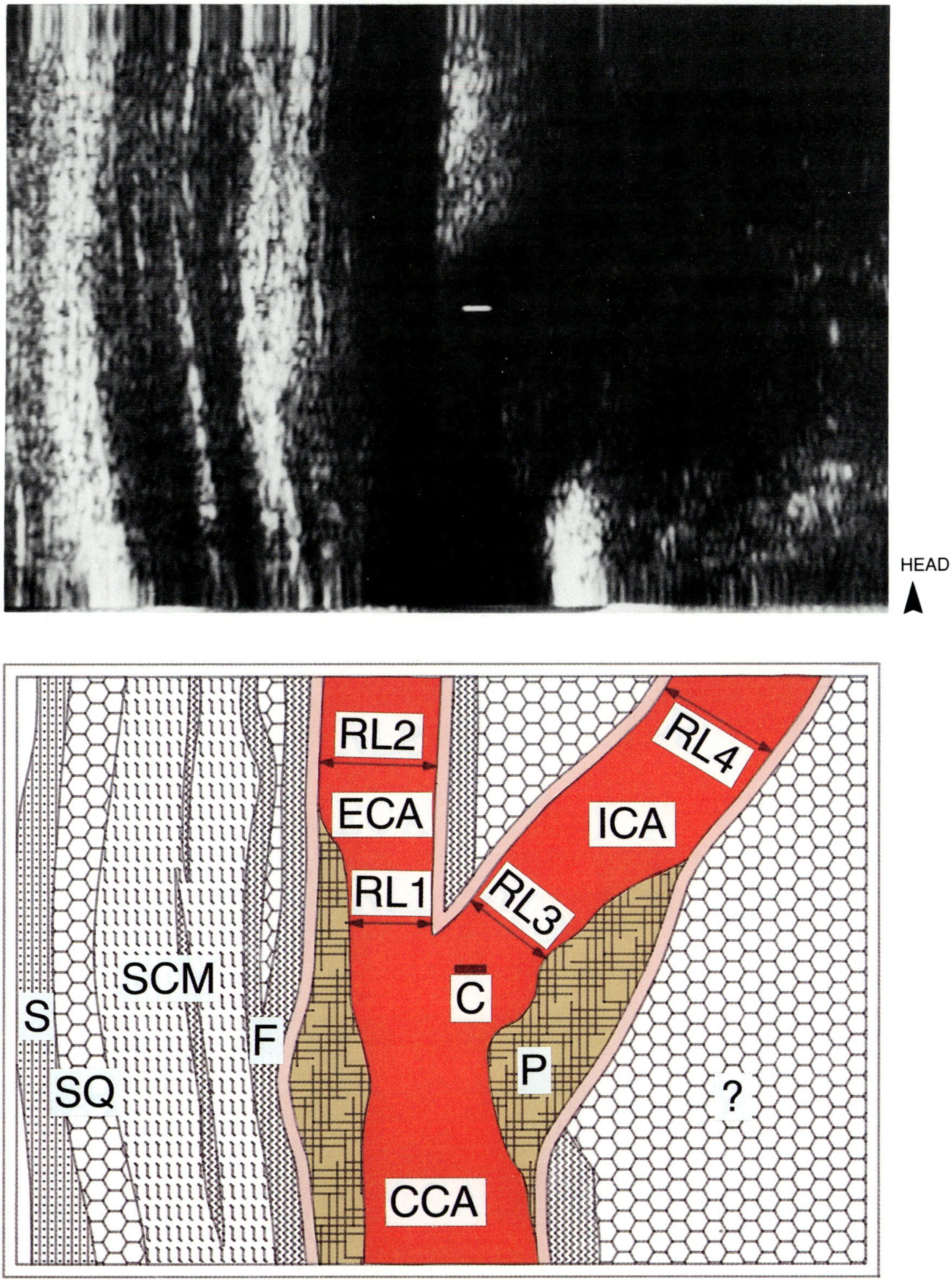
HEAD
RL2
ECA
RL1
RL4
ICA
RL3
C
SCM
S
F
P
SQ
?
CCA

Figure 44. MODERATELY ECHOGENIC PLAQUE

This is a longitudinal view of the right common carotid artery (CCA) at mid neck showing moderately echogenic, homogeneous plaque (P) on the deep wall of the artery. Notice that the brightness of the plaque is approximately equal to the sternocleidomastoid muscle (M) to the left. The surface, which is only minimally irregular, can be clearly distinguished from the open lumen. This appearance is consistent with a stable organized or "fibrous" type plaque. The internal jugular vein (IJV) is seen to the left. The apparent brightness of a plaque is influenced by the gain settings of the probe. Therefore, in order to properly assess echogenicity, it is preferable to compare the brightness of the plaque with surrounding tissue. If the plaque has approximately the same brightness as the surrounding muscle, it is considered moderately echogenic. In like manner, brightly echogenic plaque is similar in brightness to fascia or the brighter portions of subcutaneous tissue. Plaque is considered to be faintly echogenic if it is noticeably more faint than the sternocleidomastoid or surrounding muscle. Faintly echogenic plaque may at times approach the darkness of normal lumen. S = skin, SQ = subcutaneous tissue.

HISTORY *This is of a 68-year-old male who presented with gangrene of the left foot. He underwent a screening carotid study prior to lower extremity bypass and had no cerebrovascular symptoms.*

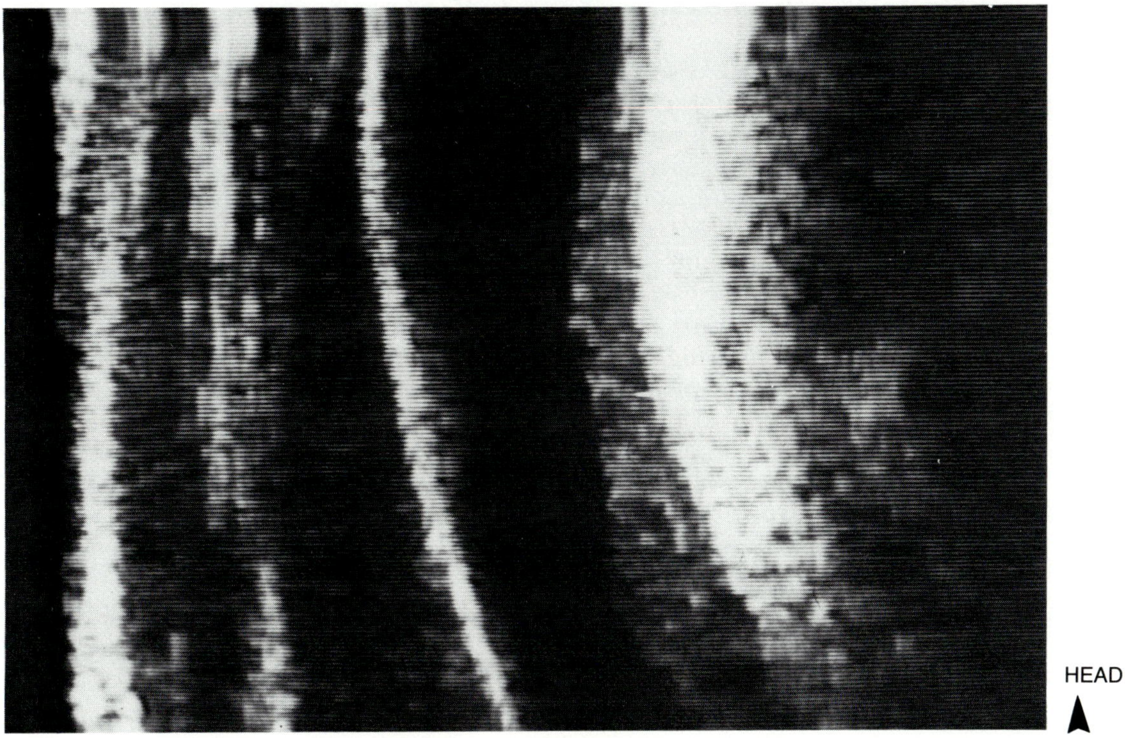
HEAD

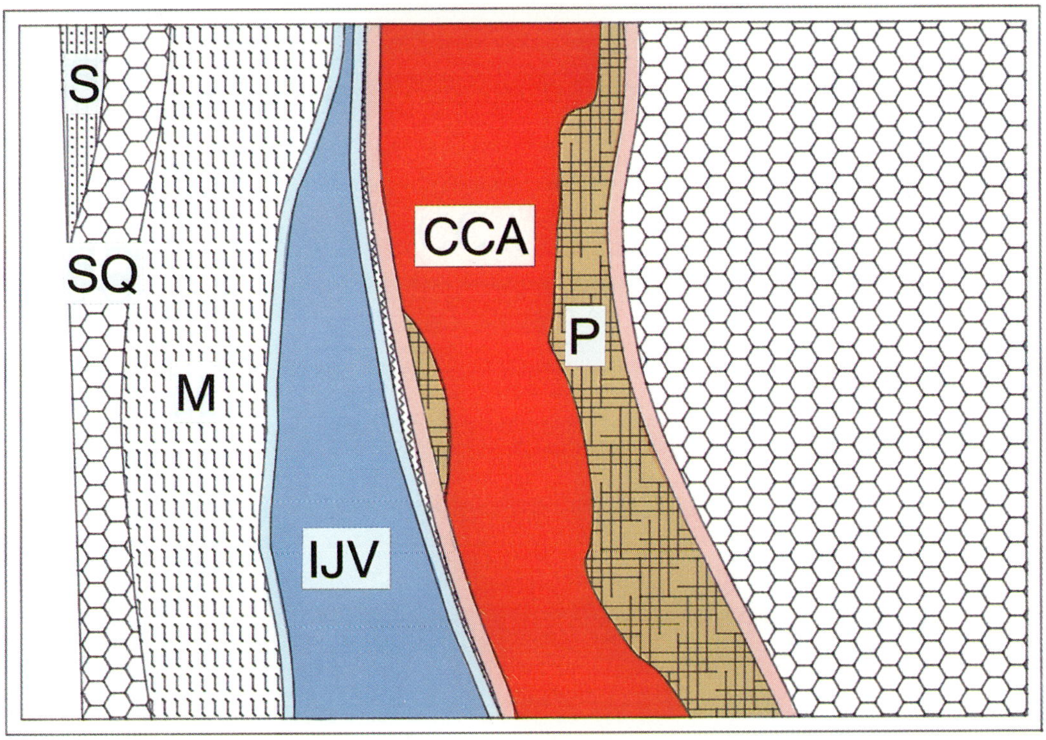
S
SQ
M
IJV
CCA
P

Figure 45. MODERATELY ECHOGENIC PLAQUE

This transverse view of a right carotid bifurcation reveals a fairly tight stenosis caused by a moderately echogenic homogeneous plaque. The view is interesting in that there are two lumens within the plaque, corresponding to the origins of the internal (I) and external (E) carotid arteries, despite the fact that the level of view is still within the common carotid artery that has not yet separated into two branches. This view creates a problem in defining the degree of stenosis. One could combine the two lumens into an "average" lumen and report this value in relation to the common carotid. Alternatively, one could report the degree of stenosis by comparing each lumen separately from the distal arteries. Although the plaque does extend into the common carotid artery at this level, the second option would be preferable because it indicates the relative flow into each artery. The Doppler cursor (C) is slightly smaller than the residual "internal carotid" lumen. Some acoustic shadowing (AS) extending from the bottom wall of the common carotid partially obscures the vagus nerve (VN). G = gel, S = skin, SQ = subcutaneous tissue, SCM = sternocleidomastoid muscle, F = fascia, ? = tissue of uncertain composition.

HISTORY *This 69-year-old male presented with an episode of near syncope but with no complaints related to focal cerebrovascular symptoms.*

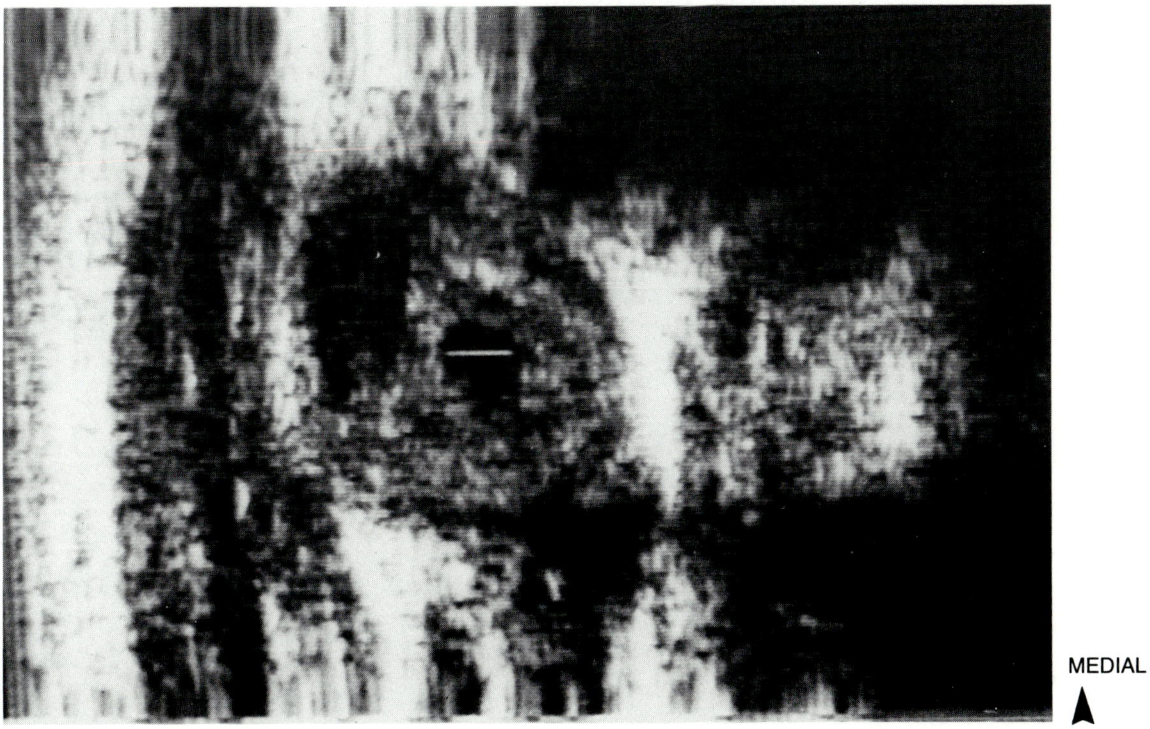
MEDIAL

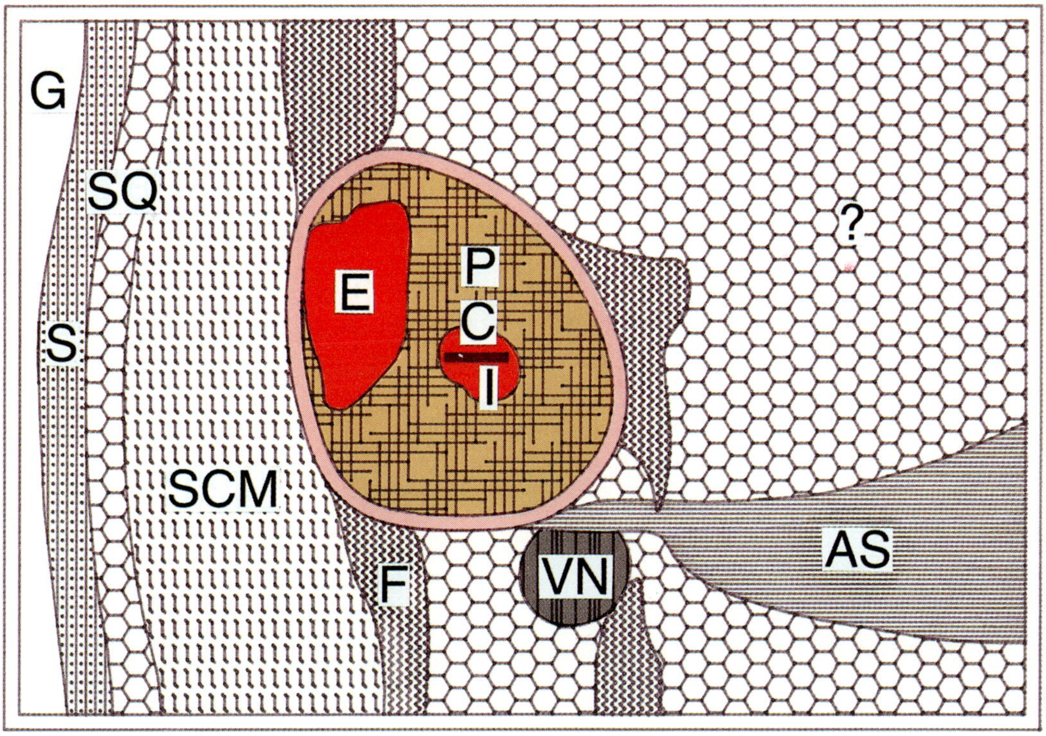
G
SQ
S
SCM
E
P
C
I
?
F
VN
AS

Figure 46. HIGHLY ECHOGENIC PLAQUE

For a moment, ignore the moderately echogenic artifact (AF) in the right third of the artery and note the very high echogenicity of this fairly smooth plaque (P) on the deep wall of the right common carotid artery (CCA). The plaque, particularly at the location of the letter P, is solid white, yet no significant acoustic shadowing extends behind it. The degree of whiteness of this plaque is greater than the surrounding tissue and much greater than that of the sternocleidomastoid muscle (M). It is a highly echogenic plaque, most likely of a mature organized and "fibrous" type composition. The fainter echoes due to artifact could be misconstrued as plaque, but see Figures 162 and 163. S = skin, SQ = subcutaneous tissue, F = fascia, ? = tissue of uncertain composition.

HISTORY *This is of a 67-year-old male who has had no cerebrovascular symptoms and underwent a screening carotid scan prior to lower extremity bypass grafting.*

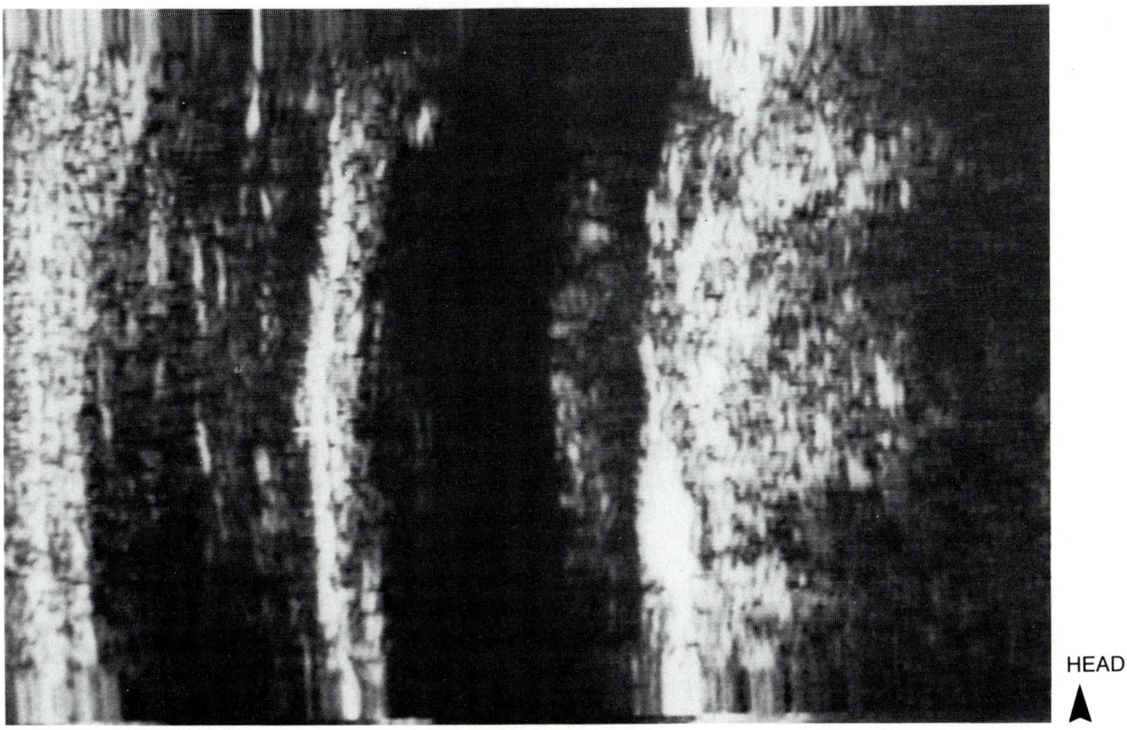
HEAD

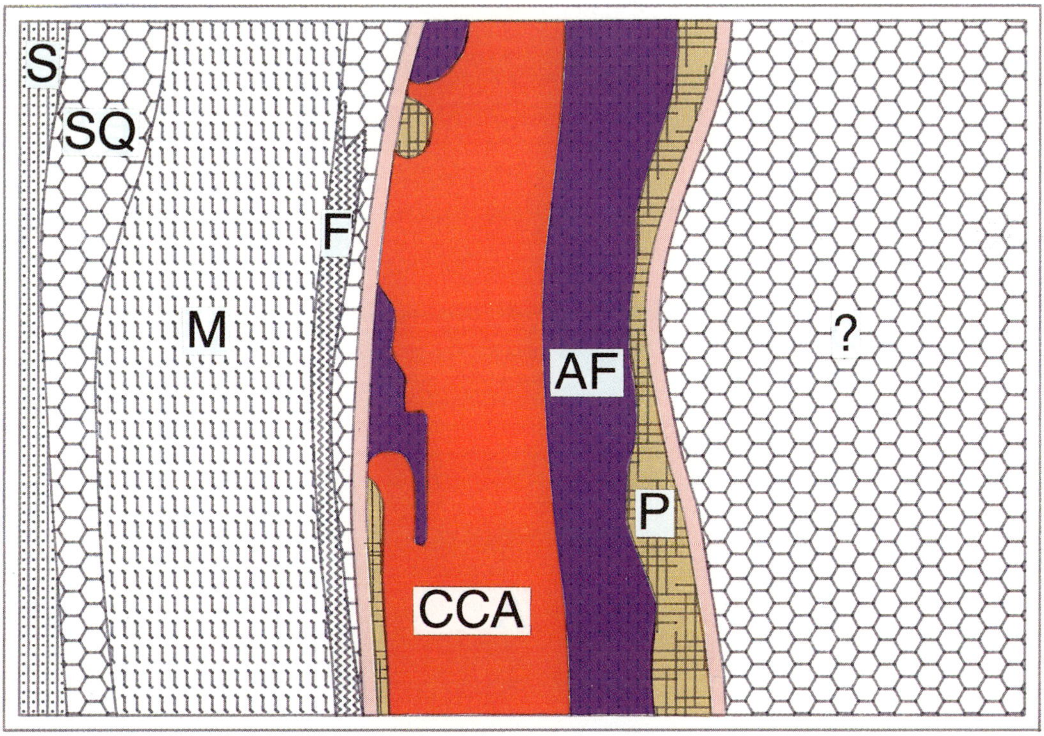
S
SQ
F
M
?
AF
P
CCA

Figure 47. HIGHLY ECHOGENIC PLAQUE

This is a longitudinal view of a left carotid bifurcation with the common carotid artery (CCA) at the top of the scan and the back wall (BW) of the internal carotid artery (ICA) at the bottom of the scan. Most of the ICA is out of plane. The plaque (P) on the deep wall of the bifurcation is classified as highly echogenic. There is a small area of acoustic shadowing (AS) extending from the thickest portion of the plaque, but for the most part the plaque has a fairly homogeneous appearance that is more typical of a chronic organized "fibrous" type atheromatous plaque. The surface is characterized as highly irregular with rather deep indentations suggestive, but not diagnostic, of surface ulceration. There is a very minimal amount of plaque on the superficial wall. Note the contour of this bifurcation with a rather uniform common carotid diameter tapering to an ICA without a clear area of internal carotid dilatation known as a "bulb." The junction of common and internal carotid arteries is approximately at the level of the lower of the two pits in the plaque surface. SCM = sternocleidomastoid muscle, IJV = internal jugular vein, SQ = subcutaneous tissue, ? = tissue of uncertain composition.

HISTORY *This 69-year-old male presented with a 15-month history of episodes of loss of consciousness, confusion, blurred vision, and one episode of right upper extremity paresis. The presence of an irregular calcified plaque was confirmed at operation 3 days later.*

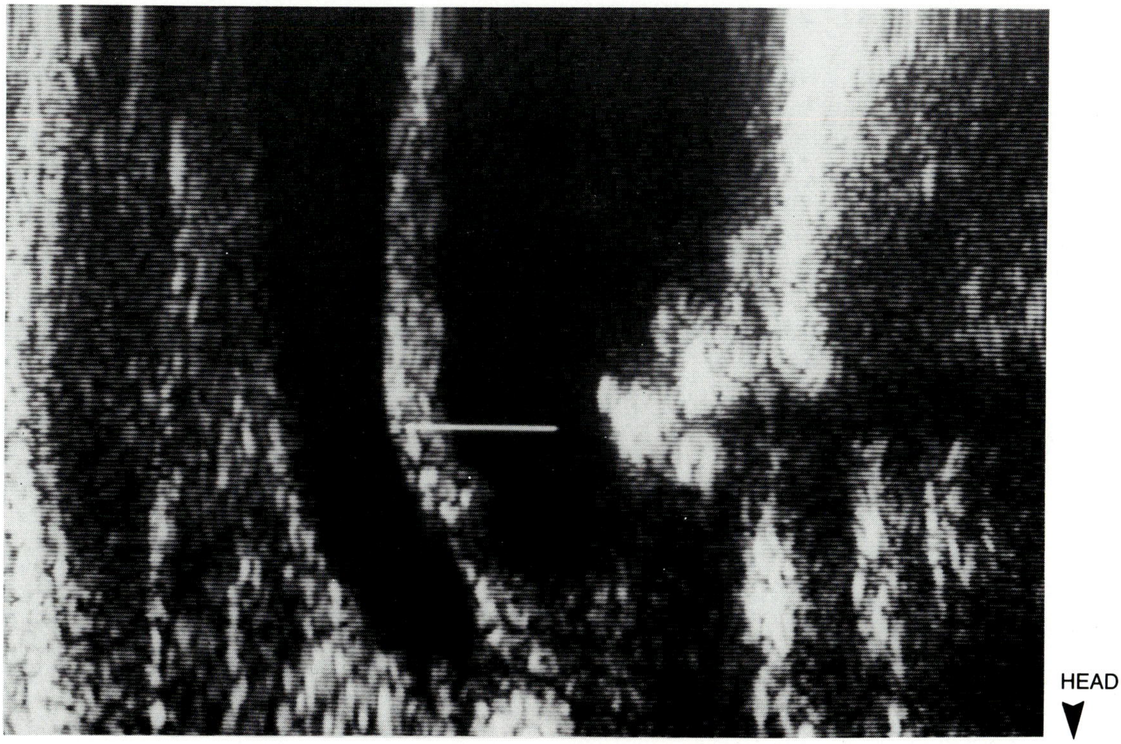
HEAD

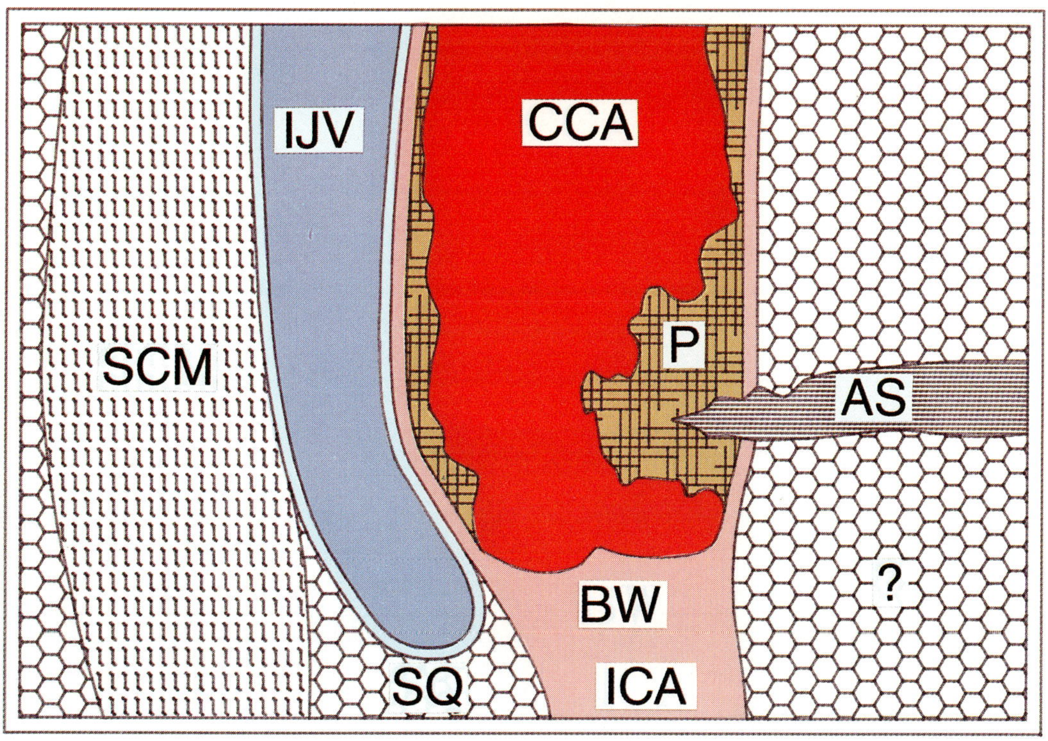
IJV
CCA
P
SCM
AS
BW
?
SQ
ICA

Figure 48. HIGHLY HOMOGENEOUS PLAQUE

This is an example of two plaques (P) that differ in echogenicity. The plaque to the left, causing a 30% stenosis of the origin of the external carotid artery (ECA), is of moderate echogenicity. The plaque lining the deep wall of the common carotid artery (CCA) and the internal carotid artery (ICA) is highly echogenic yet without acoustic shadowing. The dark band to the right of the plaque is the media of the arterial wall and is not due to a change in plaque composition. Each of these plaques, when considered separately, is quite highly homogeneous. Both are characteristic of stable fibrous type plaques, and the one at the origin of the ECA perhaps has a higher lipid content. There is some "snow" artifact within the deep half of the scan, which is not drawn. M = sternocleidomastoid muscle, SQ = subcutaneous tissue.

HISTORY *This 70-year-old female had had a cerebrovascular accident 7 years prior to this scan with a persistent, dense left hemiparesis. She has had no further symptoms for 7 years prior to and 1 year following this scan. An arteriogram 1 month following this ultrasound scan failed to reveal any atherosclerotic plaque in this bifurcation, probably because the plaque is smooth and does not cause significant narrowing relative to the proximal and distal arteries as can be seen in this scan. (Compare with Figure 25.)*

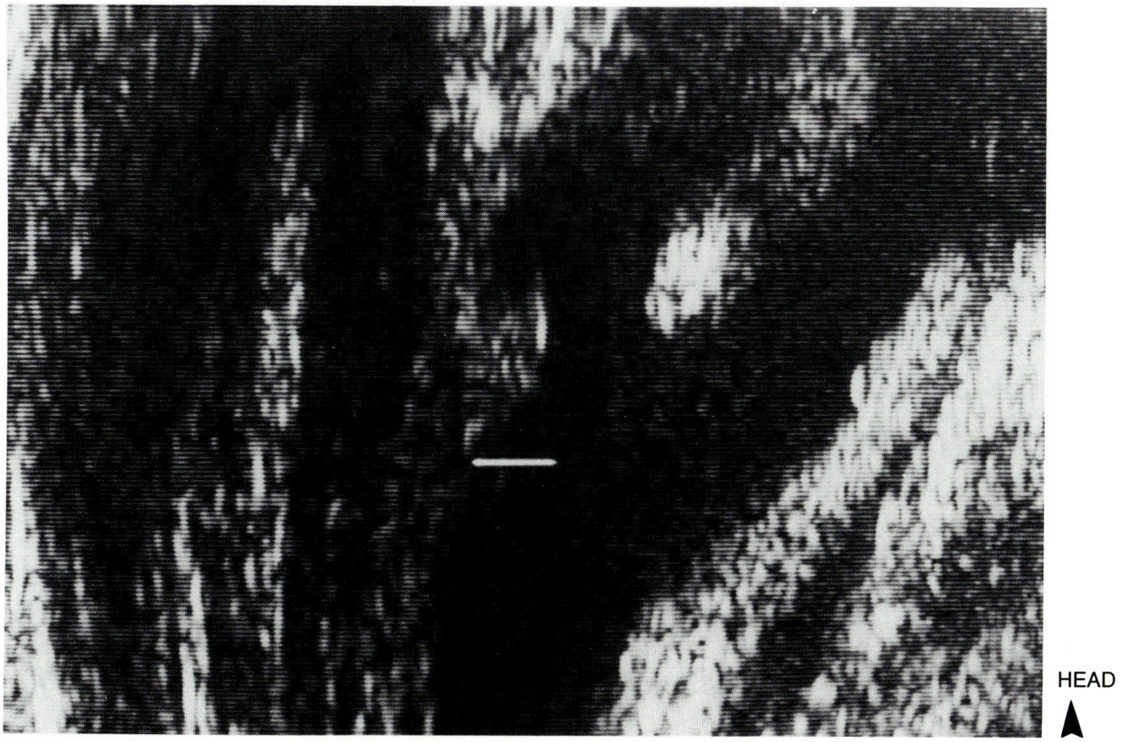
HEAD

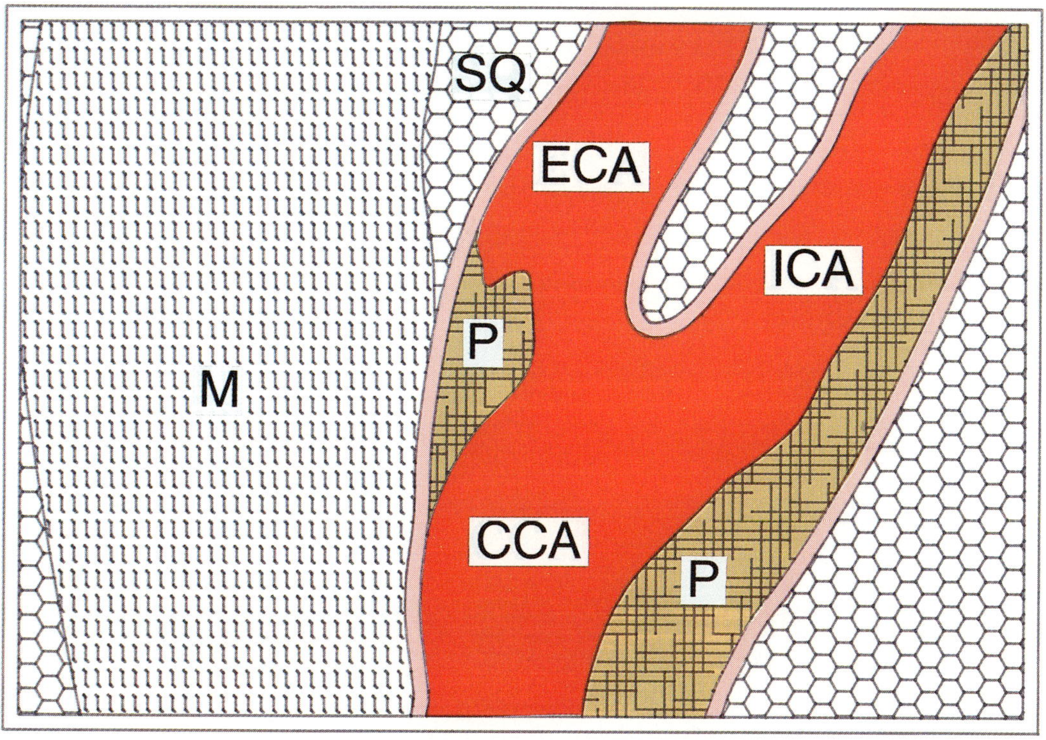
SQ
ECA
ICA
P
M
CCA
P

Figure 49. MODERATELY HETEROGENEOUS PLAQUE

This is a cross-sectional view through the mid section of a left common carotid artery (CCA) showing plaque heterogeneity of moderate degree. The plaque appears to be composed of two types. The fainter plaque (P) surrounding the residual lumen (L) is faint and homogeneous and consistent with a lipid composition. The brighter zone corresponds to some organization and calcification of the plaque along the deep wall (Ca). There is acoustic shadowing (AS), extending from behind the entire vessel, partly due to the "pigtail effect" (see Figure 68) that arises from the top and bottom arterial walls and partly due to the calcified plaque along the deep wall. The Doppler cursor (C) is just slightly off center with respect to the residual lumen but gives a good indication of its transverse diameter, which is equal to 3.2 mm compared with a vertical diameter of 4.6 mm, giving an average residual lumen diameter of 3.9 mm. The common carotid artery at this level has an average diameter of 9.0 mm but was smaller near the base of the neck and measured 7.5 mm at that point. Therefore, this qualifies as 1 − (3.9/7.5) = 48% diameter stenosis, which would be rounded to 50%. (Squaring this, one comes up with a 73% area stenosis.) SQ = subcutaneous tissue, M = sternocleidomastoid muscle, F = fascia.

HISTORY *This 72-year-old male presented with left upper extremity numbness that dated from placement of a transvenous pacemaker through that arm. He was otherwise asymptomatic.*

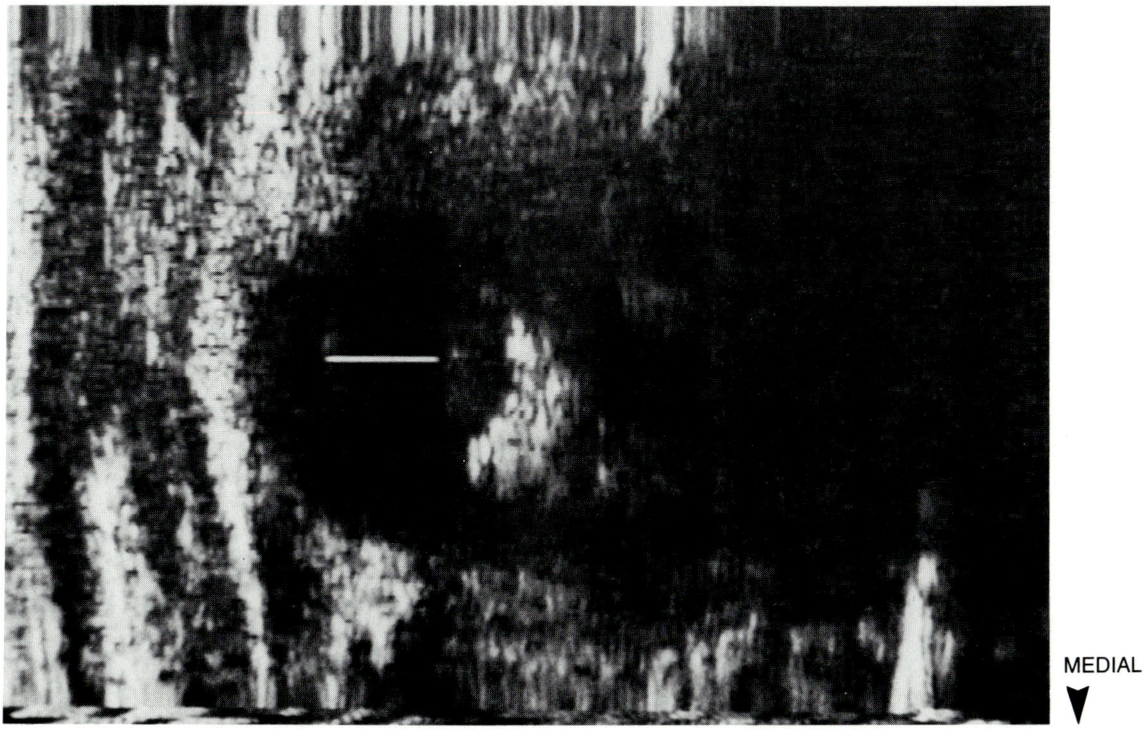
MEDIAL

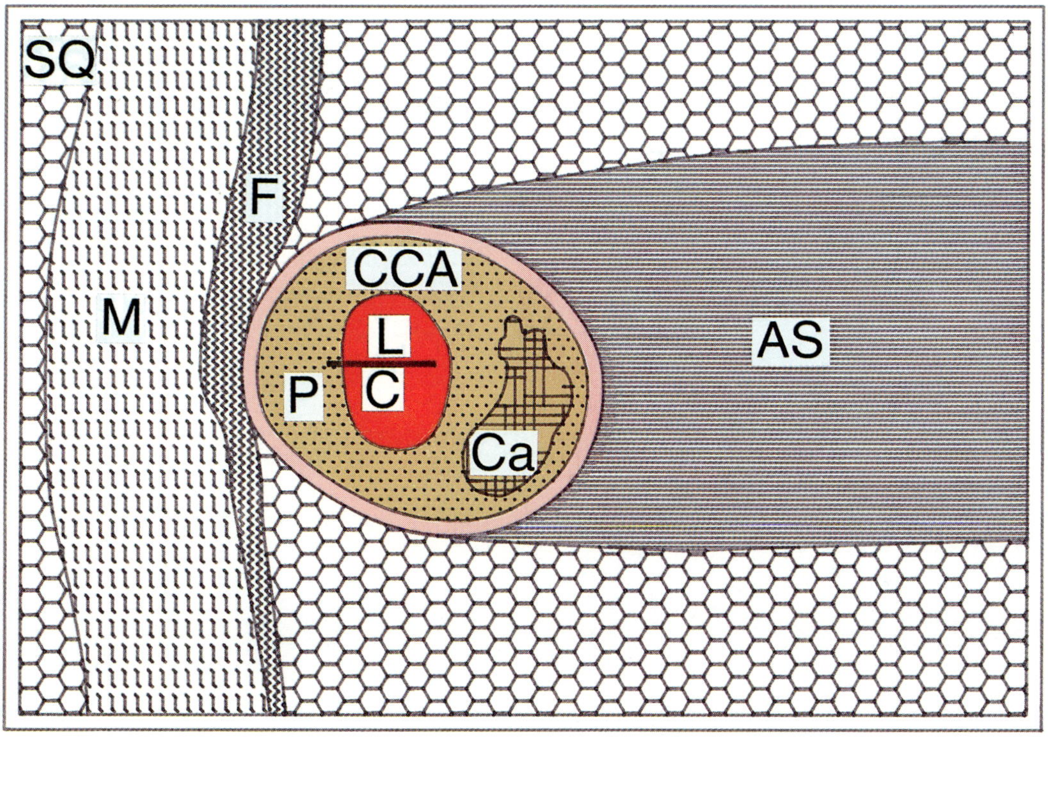
SQ
F
M
CCA
L
C
P
Ca
AS

Figure 50. MODERATELY HETEROGENEOUS PLAQUE

This is a second example of moderately heterogeneous plaque (P) of much smaller extent than the previous example. The greatest degree of narrowing is at the orifice of the internal carotid artery (ICA) with plaque extending along the posterior wall of the internal carotid bulb. The outer surface of this plaque is of brighter echogenicity than the very dark interior. The remainder of the common carotid artery (CCA) and the internal carotid artery as well as the entire external carotid artery (ECA) is free of disease. S = skin, SQ = subcutaneous tissue, M = sternocleidomastoid muscle, F = fascia, V = internal jugular vein (compressed), ? = tissue of uncertain composition.

HISTORY *This is of a 58-year-old female with episodic vertigo, ataxia, and dysphasia over the span of 2 months prior to the scan. She had a right hemispheric cerebrovascular accident 4 years prior.*

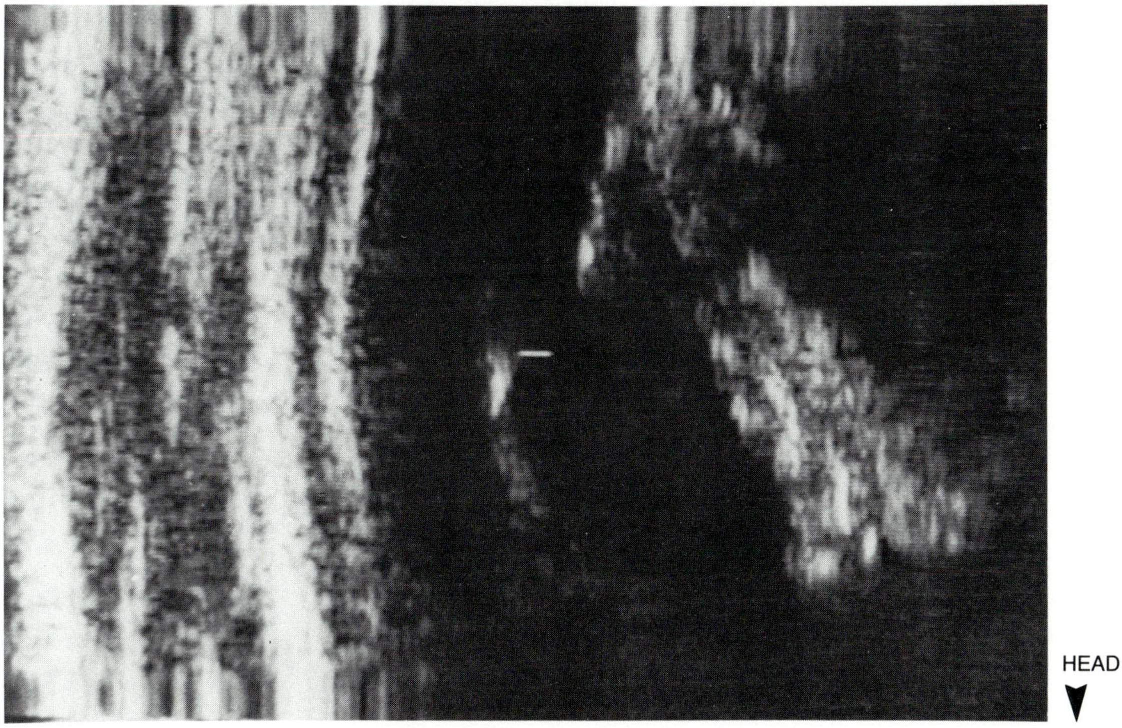
HEAD

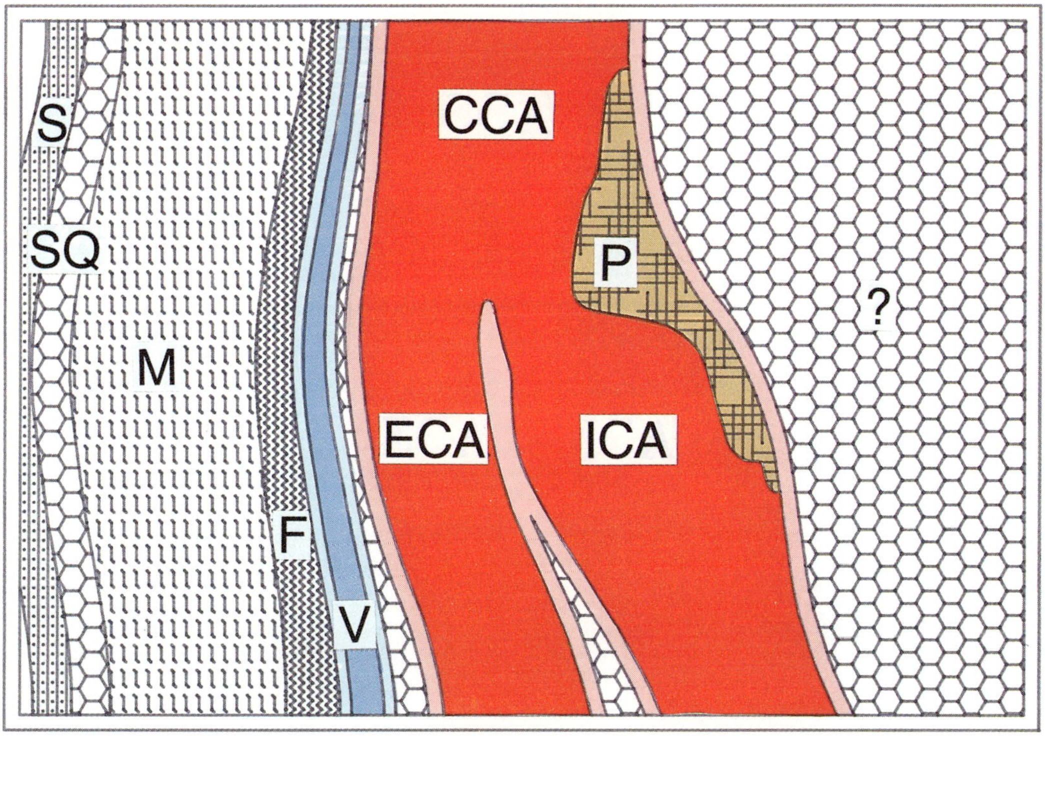
S
SQ
M
F
V
CCA
P
?
ECA
ICA

Figure 51. HIGHLY HETEROGENEOUS PLAQUE

The plaque (P) within this distal right internal carotid artery (ICA) is highly heterogeneous. Overall the echogenicity is moderate, but there are some very bright areas, some medium gray areas, and some very dark areas within the same plaque along the superficial wall of the artery. The plaque is also highly irregular in contour yet without any discrete defects that are easily classified as an ulcer. G = gel, S = skin, SQ = subcutaneous tissue, M = sternocleidomastoid muscle, F = fascia, ? = tissue of uncertain composition.

HISTORY *This 62-year-old female presented with amaurosis fugax of the right eye which lasted 6½ hours and occurred 5 weeks prior to the ultrasound scan. Because of a history of allergy to contrast agents, a right carotid endarterectomy was performed without pre-operative arteriography. At operation, an elongated irregular plaque was found. No large ulcer was present.*

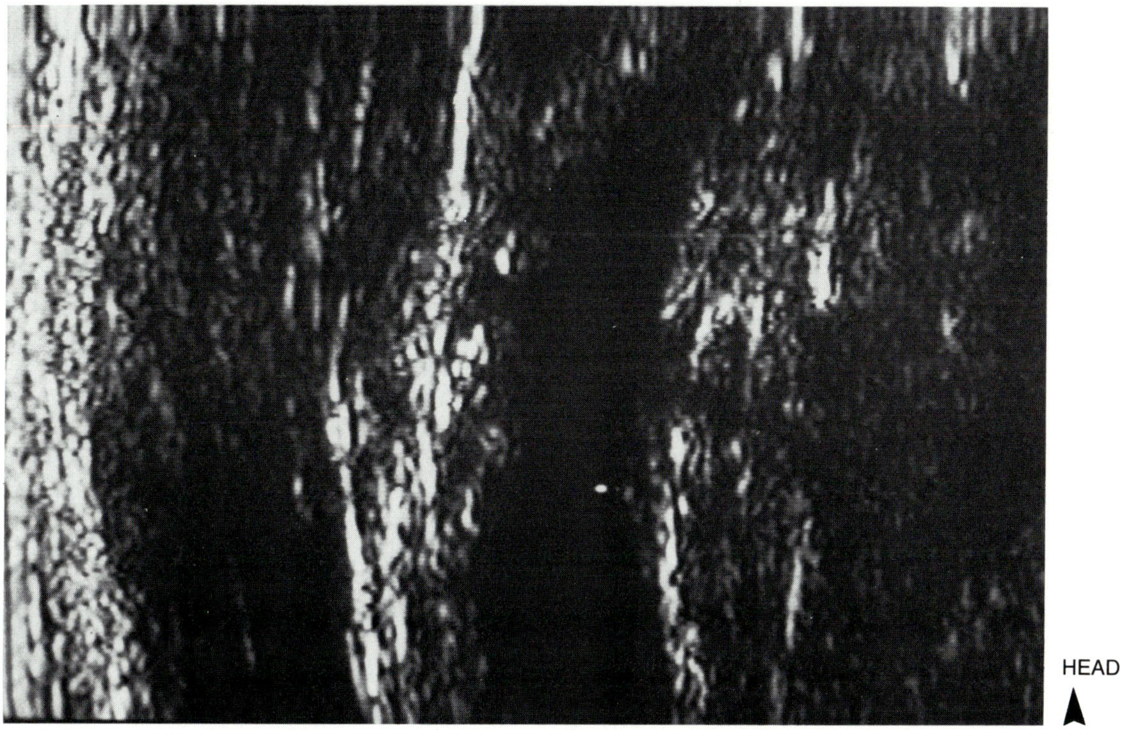
HEAD

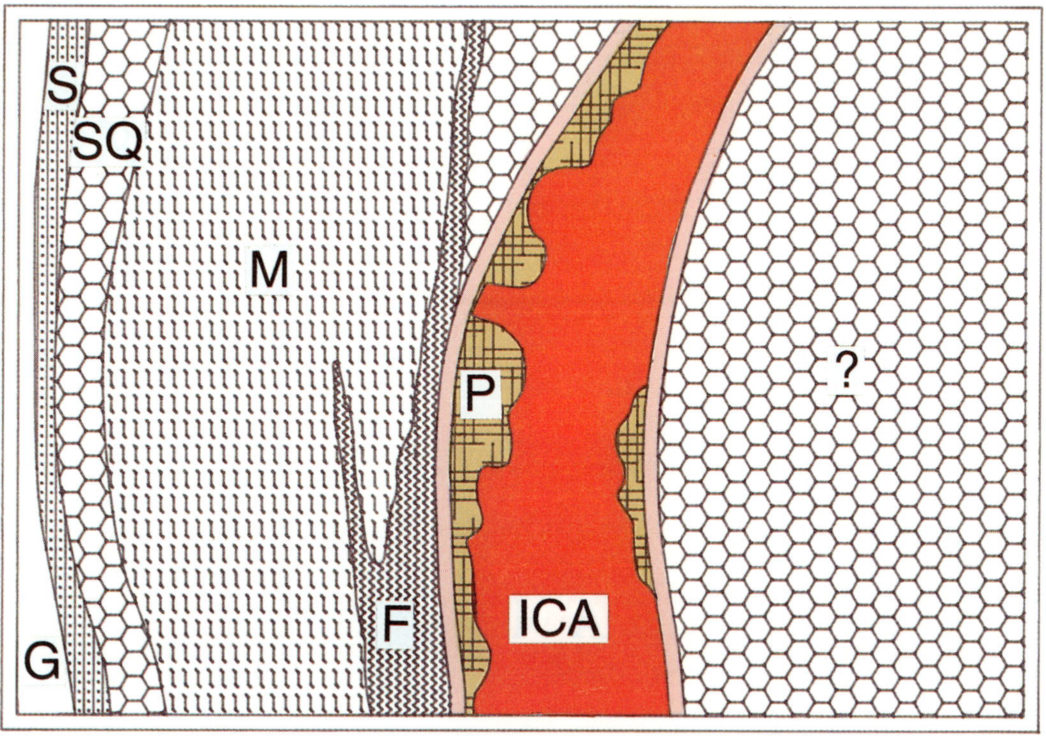
S
SQ
M
F
P
ICA
?
G

Figure 52. HIGHLY HETEROGENEOUS PLAQUE

This is an example of highly heterogeneous plaque with areas of high (H), medium (M), and low (L) echogenicity scattered within the same plaque (P) along both the superficial and deep walls of the external carotid artery (ECA). The common carotid (CCA) is seen below. The internal carotid artery arises out of plane. Some of the areas of high echogenicity are associated with acoustic shadowing (AS). S = skin, PM = platysma muscle, SCM = sternocleidomastoid muscle, F = fascia, V = facial vein, ? = tissue of uncertain composition.

HISTORY *This is of a 65-year-old male who presented with episodes of bilateral amaurosis fugax over 2 months prior to the ultrasound scan. He underwent a thromboendarterectomy on the opposite side for an acute total occlusion that was found during this ultrasound scan. Six months later the opposite side was still patent following the thromboendarterectomy, and he had no further symptoms involving this right carotid bifurcation.*

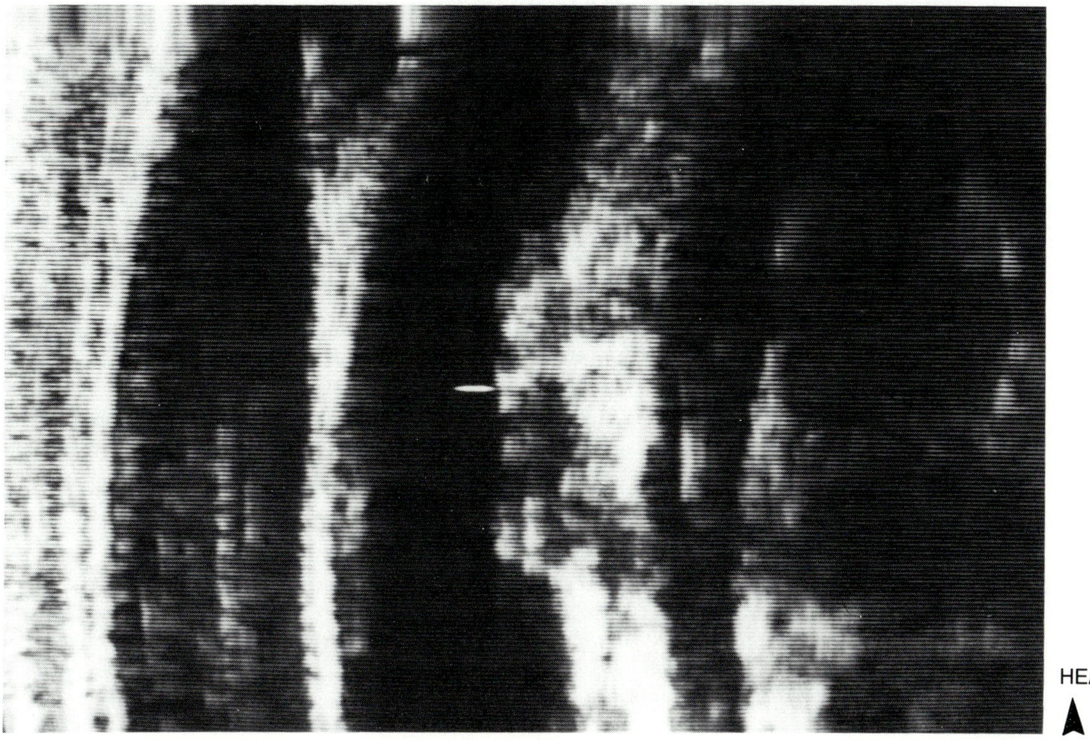
HEAD

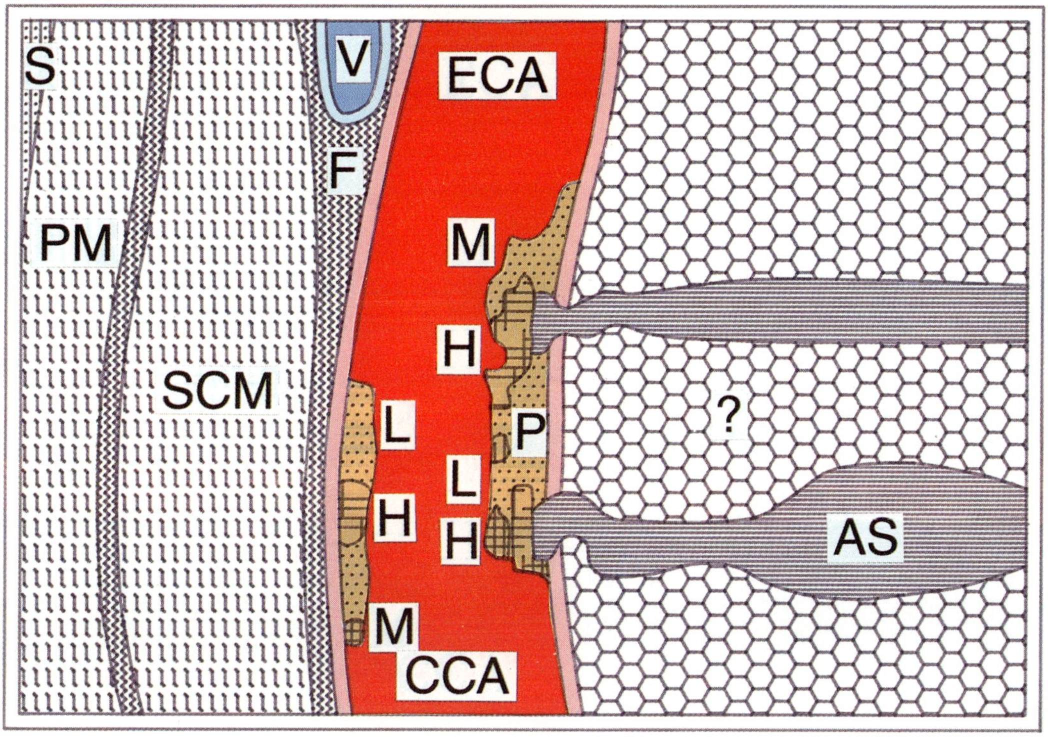
S
V
ECA
F
PM
M
H
SCM
L
P
?
L
H
H
AS
M
CCA

Figure 53. SUPERFICIAL WALL PLAQUE CALCIFICATION

This is an example of calcified plaque (P) on the superficial wall of the bifurcation causing acoustic shadowing (AS) that obscures the deep wall of the internal carotid artery (ICA) and common carotid artery (CCA). With such acoustic shadowing it is not possible to measure accurately a residual lumen, since the extension of plaque from the deep wall cannot be seen. Fortunately, this situation is not common. Most plaque within the carotid bifurcation tends to develop on the deep wall, and shadowing from the deep wall is of no consequence as long as the superficial wall plaque can be clearly seen. Moreover, even if there is plaque on the superficial wall, as in this case, it is often possible to approach the bifurcation with the probe directed from a more medial or lateral point of contact on the neck. Thus, to some extent, one is able to see into the arteries around the sides of the superficial wall plaque. The plaque that is seen is highly heterogeneous with bright and dark areas and is markedly irregular. By other views there was a possibility that this central area in front of the shadowing was an ulcer crater. S = skin, M = muscle (platysma and sternocleidomastoid), F = fascia, SQ = subcutaneous tissue.

HISTORY *This is of an 89-year-old female presenting with left hemiparesis for the week prior to the ultrasound scan. In other views we were able to measure the stenosis of the ICA as 30%.*

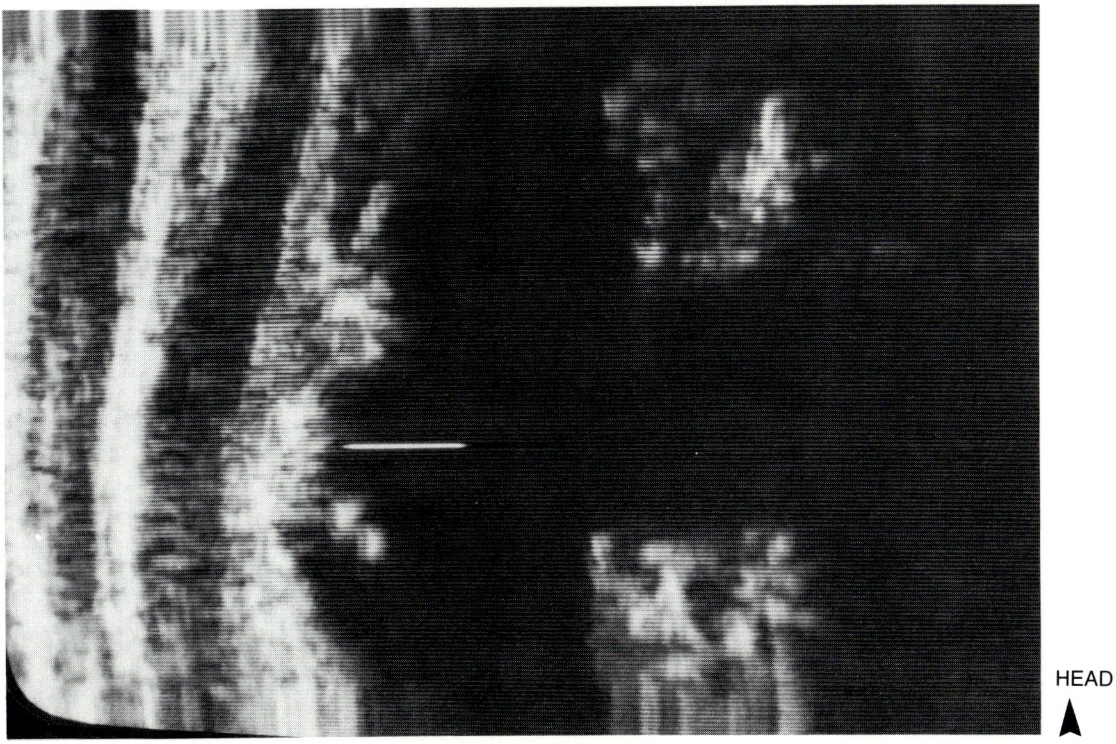
HEAD

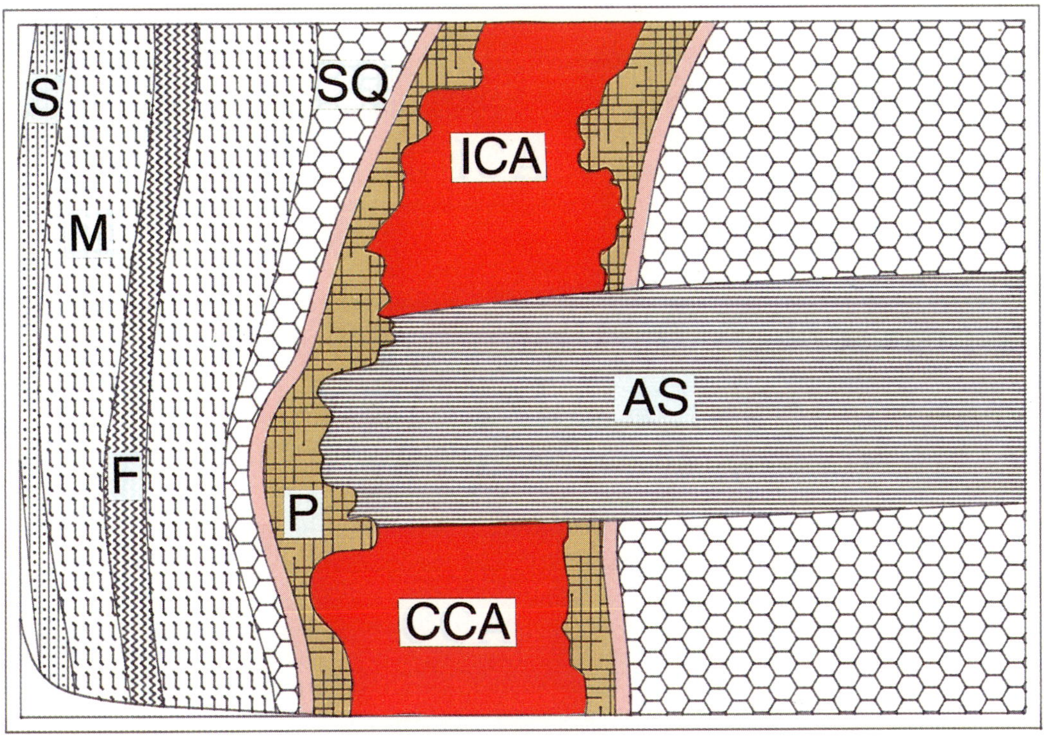
S
SQ
ICA
M
AS
F
P
CCA

Figure 54. CALCIFIED DEEP WALL PLAQUE

Note the very prominent acoustic shadowing (AS) extending behind this calcified plaque (P) within the right internal carotid artery (ICA). Because this plaque is on the deep wall it does not interfere with visualization of the residual lumen which has a clear-cut, half-pie type of shape. The plaque occupies slightly more than 50% of the cross-sectional area of the ICA. In keeping with the previously mentioned principles of reporting stenosis by average residual diameter, this would qualify as a 30% diameter stenosis (compare with Figure 20). The external carotid artery (ECA) is seen above and to the left and is free of disease at this level. M = sternocleidomastoid muscle, F = fascia.

HISTORY *This 68-year-old male was admitted with a left hemispheric cerebrovascular accident and had right upper extremity paresis. The plaque present on this right side caused no symptoms.*

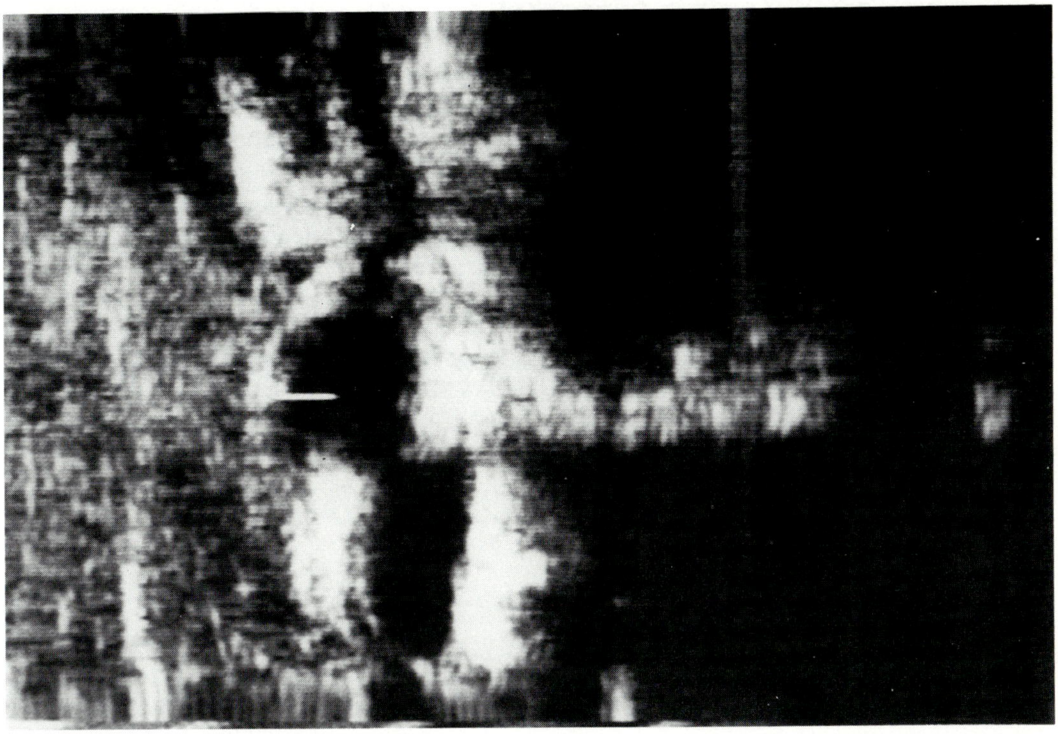

MEDIAL

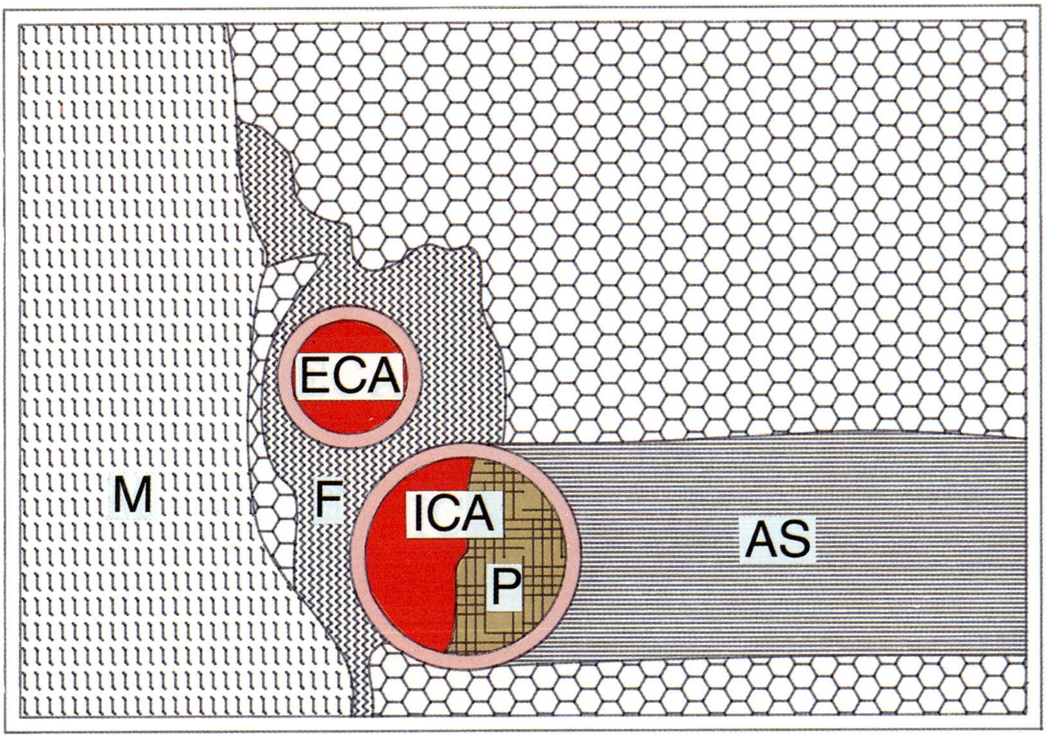

Figure 55. CALCIFIED DEEP WALL PLAQUE

This is another view of the calcified plaque (P) on the deep wall of the same right internal carotid artery (ICA) as was seen in the transverse view of Figure 54. Note the very prominent acoustic shadowing (AS) extending from two areas in the plaque. In this view the plaque appears to cause only about a 40% diameter stenosis, not counting the artifact (AF) immediately superficial to the bottom half of this plaque. In the previous ultrasound scan, the plaque was seen as a half-pie type of lesion within the artery. The reason for the apparent lesser degree of stenosis seen in this view, therefore, is passage of the ultrasound beam in an oblique fashion, slightly off center, so as to maximize the appearance of the residual lumen. This example emphasizes the value of transverse views in assessing the overall degree of stenosis; misleading impressions of the degree of stenosis are frequently obtained from single longitudinal planes. S = skin, SQ = subcutaneous tissue, M = sternocleidomastoid muscle, ? = tissue of uncertain composition.

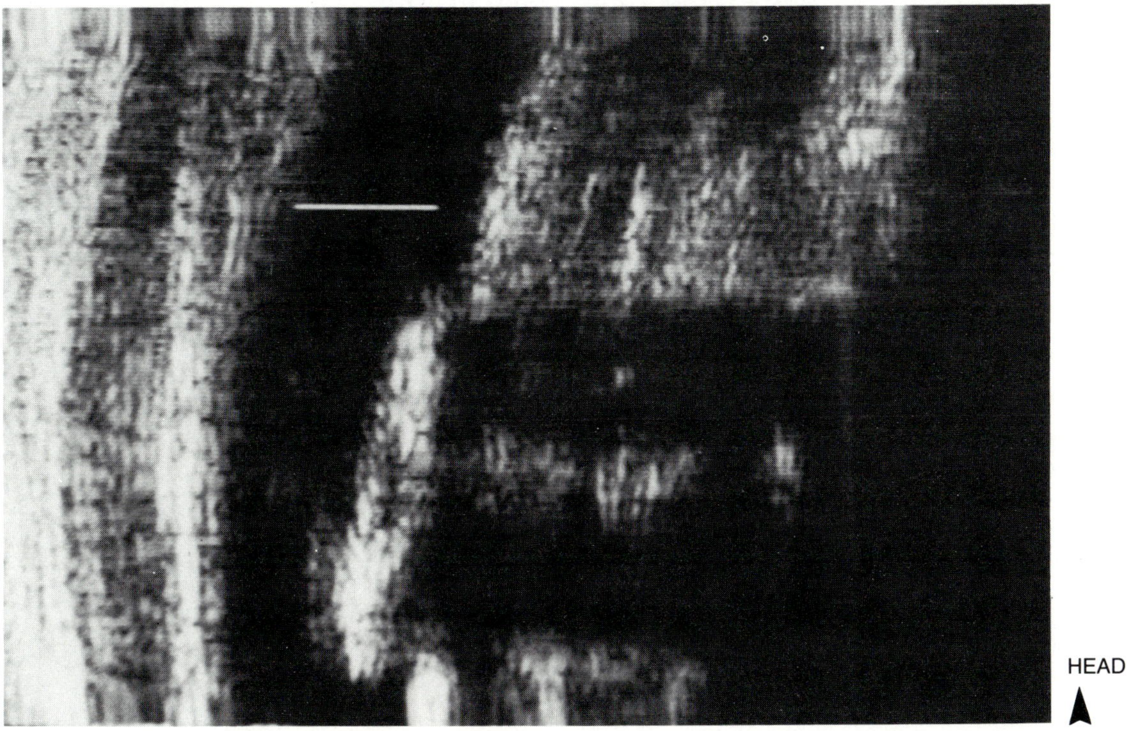
HEAD

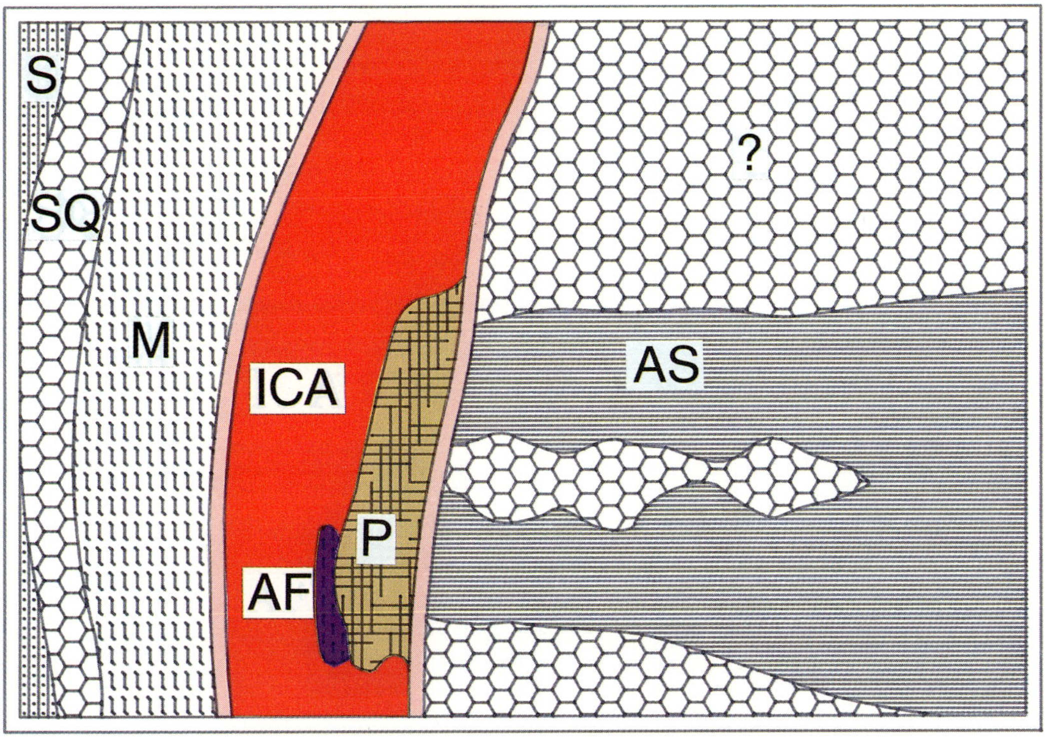
S
SQ
M
ICA
P
AF
AS
?

Figure 56. CALCIFIED DEEP WALL PLAQUE

This is an example of a quite small plaque (P) on the deep wall of the common carotid artery (CCA) just before the origin of the external carotid artery (ECA). There is acoustic shadowing (AS) extending from the middle of this plaque. This ultrasound scan is included to illustrate the fact that plaques do not have to be extensive in length or thickness in order to have calcification. Some faintly visible echos at the top and bottom of the ultrasound scan within the CCA and ECA are due to artifact. The internal carotid artery (ICA) is widely patent, and for the most part normal "intimal stripes" can be seen. S = skin, M = platysma muscle, SQ = subcutaneous tissue, SCM = sternocleidomastoid muscle, F = fascia, IJV = internal jugular vein, ? = tissue of uncertain composition.

HISTORY *This is of a 46-year-old female with sudden onset of tunnel vision that lasted for 15 minutes on one occasion 3 days prior to the ultrasound scan. She was screened for carotid disease and has been otherwise asymptomatic.*

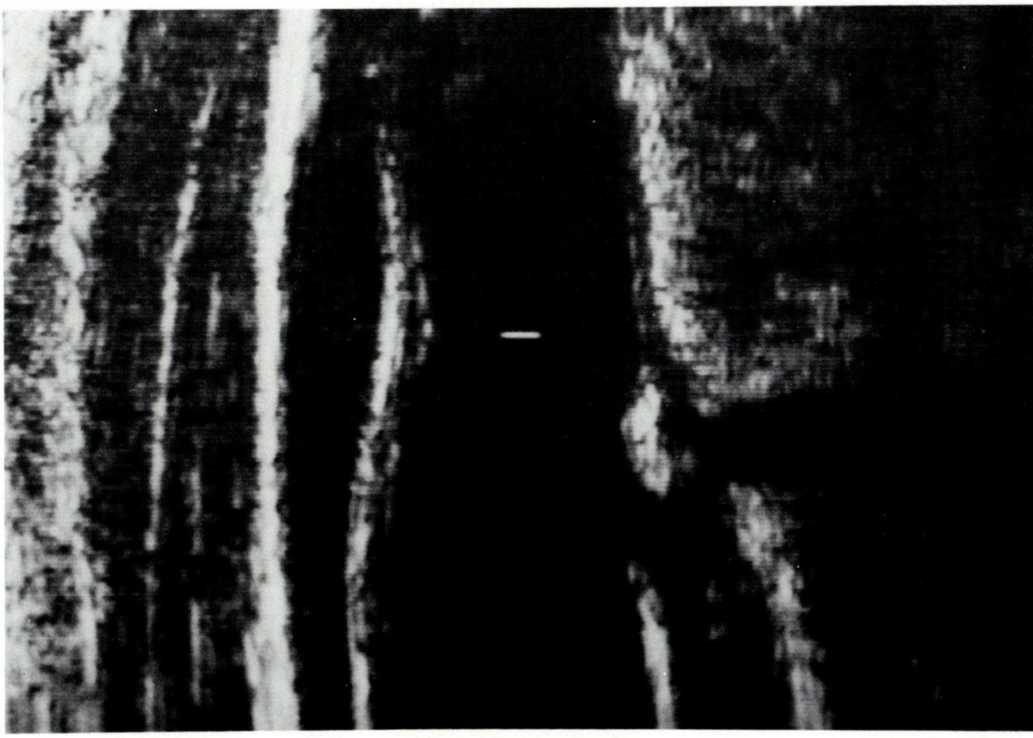

HEAD

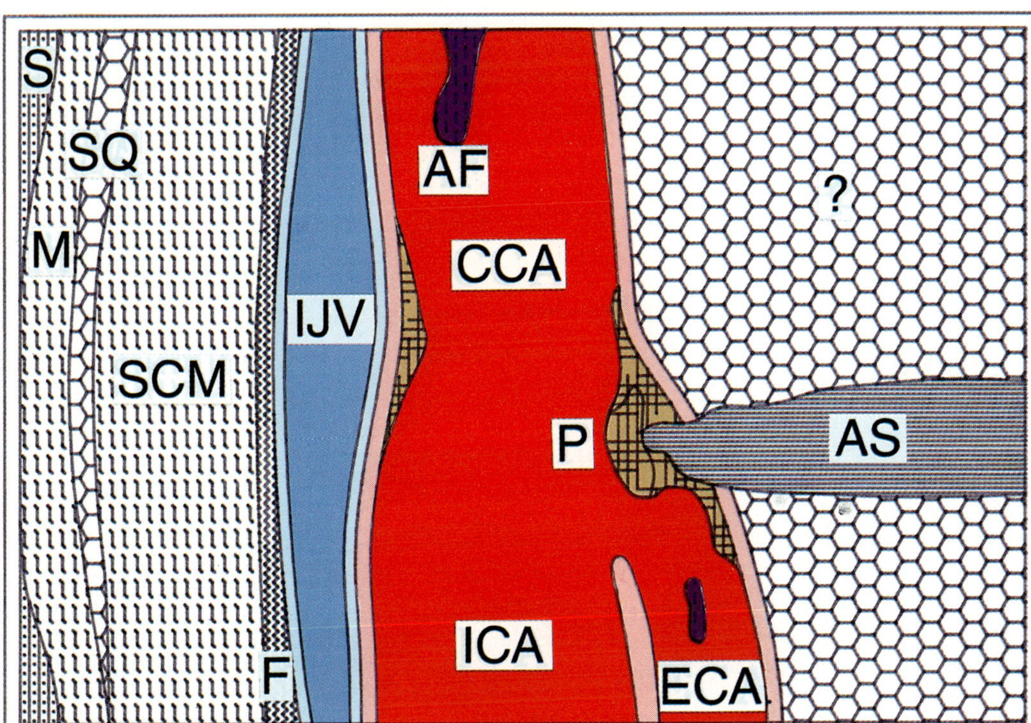

Figure 57. CALCIFIED DEEP WALL PLAQUE

Note how clearly the residual lumen (RL) is seen in this example of a calcified plaque (P) on the deep wall of this distal right internal carotid artery (ICA). The appearance of plaque calcification is not synonymous with a poor quality scan. Note, however, how completely the acoustic shadowing (AS) obliterates all detail behind the plaque surface. It is not correct to say that this plaque is highly heterogeneous, because the deeper portions of the plaque might be highly echogenic, if the ultrasound beam were able to penetrate the surface. In this sense, one does not consider all calcified plaques as being highly heterogeneous simply because of AS. Rather, the term is used to imply differences in echodensity of the portions of the plaque that can be properly assessed. That portion of the plaque hidden by AS cannot be assessed. The plaque in this particular example is heterogeneous. However, it is heterogeneous by comparison with adjacent areas and not by comparison with the surface brightness with the AS behind it. This plaque is mildly irregular with shallow undulations. S = skin, M = platsyma muscle, F = fascia, SCM = sternocleidomastoid muscle, ? = tissue of uncertain composition.

HISTORY *This 72-year-old male with no cerebrovascular symptoms underwent a screening carotid study.*

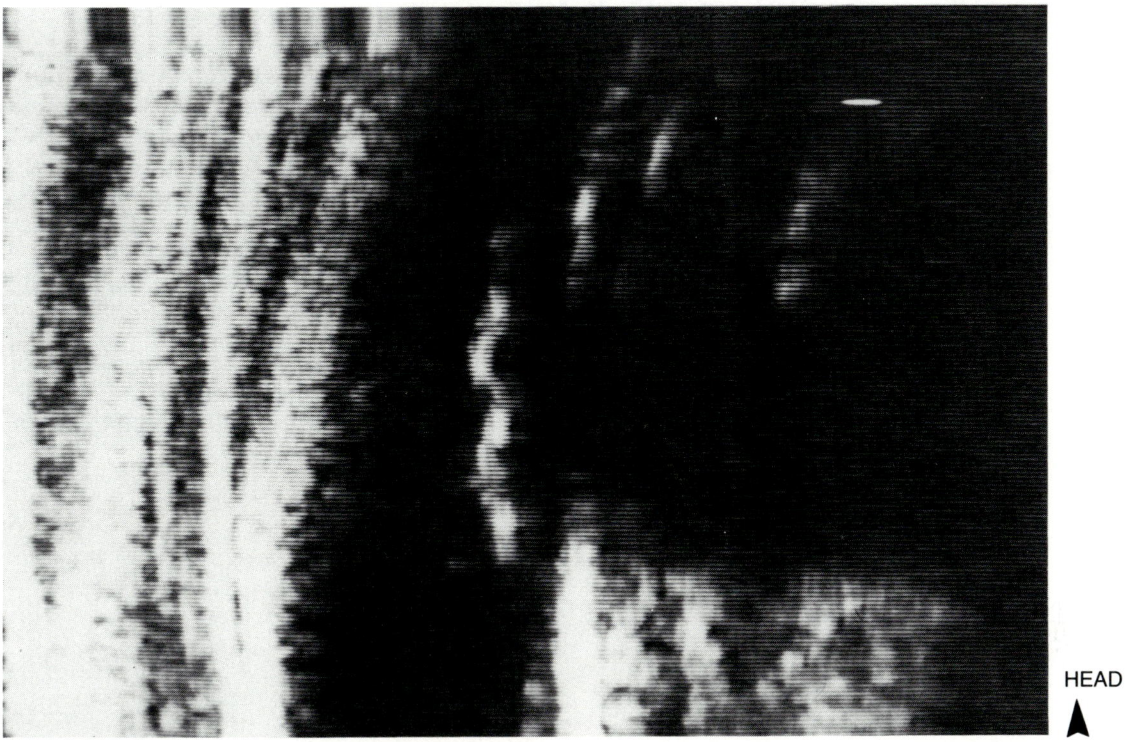
HEAD

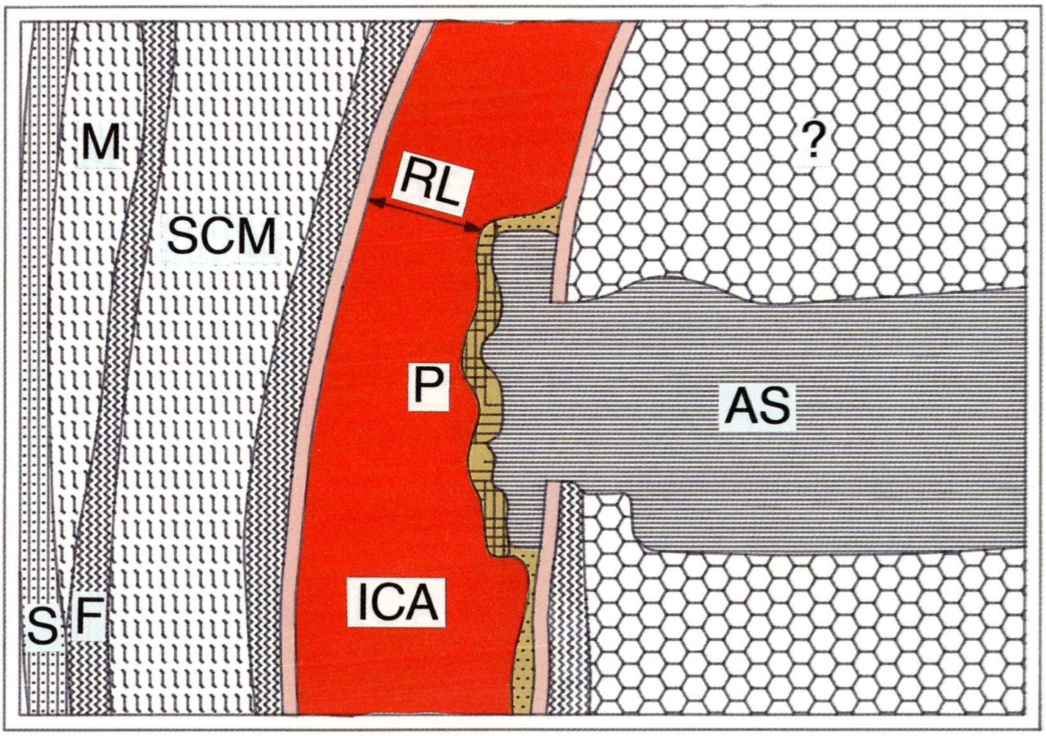
M
SCM
RL
?
P
AS
ICA
S F

Figure 58. INTRAPLAQUE HEMORRHAGE

This is a transverse view of the left internal carotid artery (ICA) above the bifurcation, showing a thin rim of plaque (P) that has been separated from the arterial wall by a dark crescent of intraplaque hemorrhage (H) along the superficial wall of the artery. Although the dissection is faintly visible, the residual lumen is not clearly seen because of echogenic artifact appearing as "snow" within the central lumen. The internal jugular vein (IJV) is located to the left of the artery. SQ = subcutaneous tissue, M = sternocleidomastoid muscle, F = fascia.

HISTORY *This 82-year-old male had a corresponding history of right upper extremity paresis and vertigo prior to this ultrasound scan. Intraplaque hemorrhage was not present on a scan performed 15 months earlier but was still present on a repeat scan shortly thereafter.*

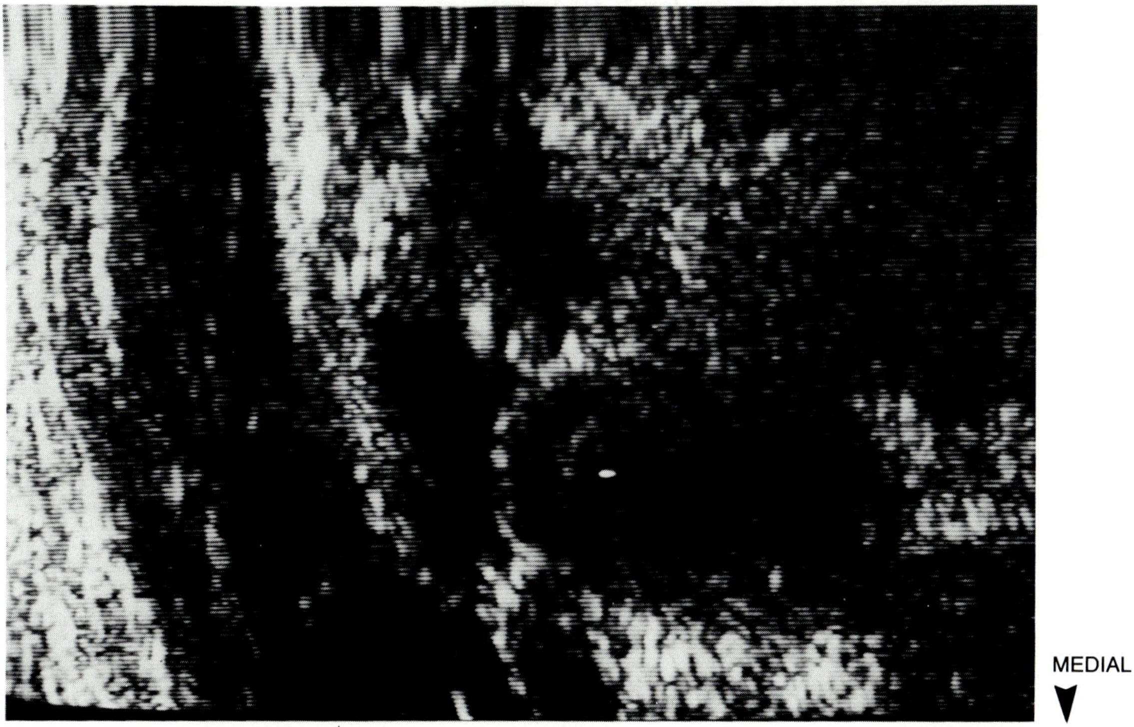
MEDIAL

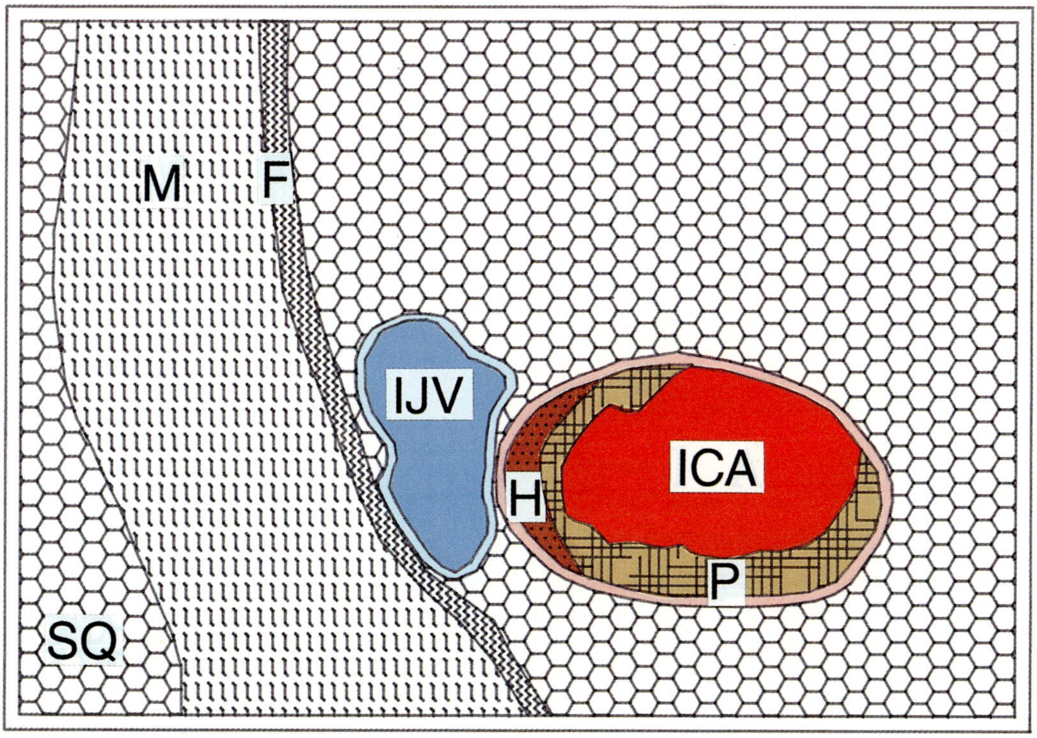
M
F
IJV
ICA
H
P
SQ

Figure 59. INTRAPLAQUE HEMORRHAGE

Note how much better the separation of the plaque (P) from the arterial wall is seen in this longitudinal view. Actually, this view is not quite longitudinal, since the internal carotid artery (ICA) passes obliquely out of plane at the bottom of the picture. The intraplaque hemorrhage (H), to the left of the plaque, is almost indistinguishable from flowing blood, to the right of the plaque. The internal jugular vein (V) is seen to the left of the artery. Longitudinal views are best for assessing plaque contour and composition. Transverse views are best for assessing the exact dimensions of the residual lumen. SQ = subcutaneous tissue, M = sternocleidomastoid muscle, F = fascia.

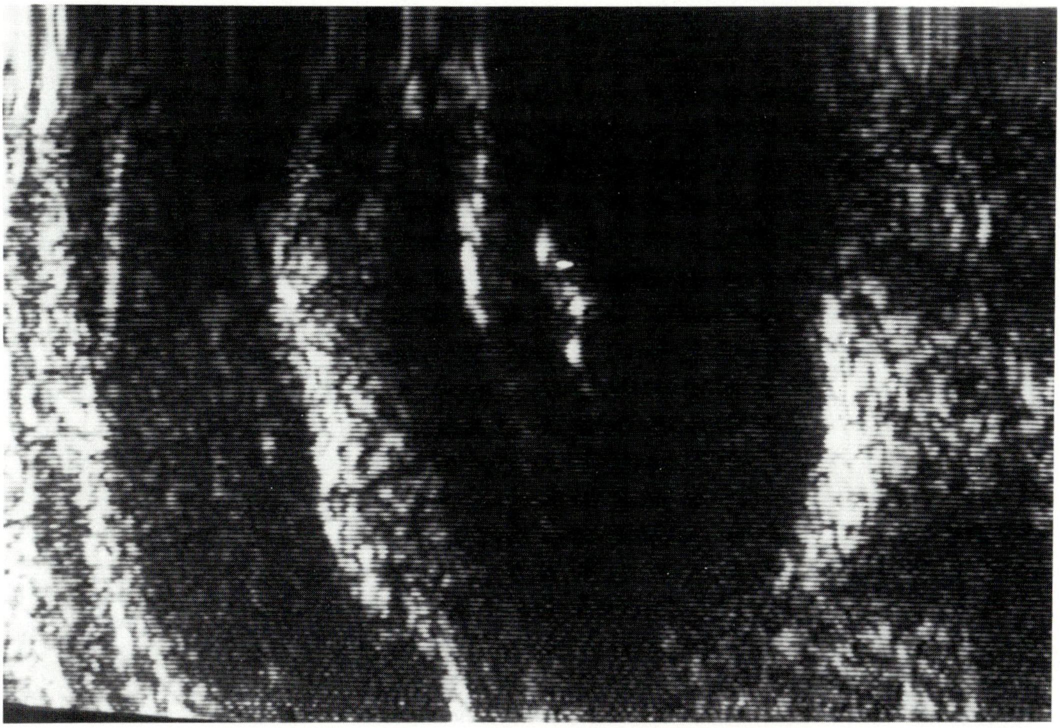

HEAD

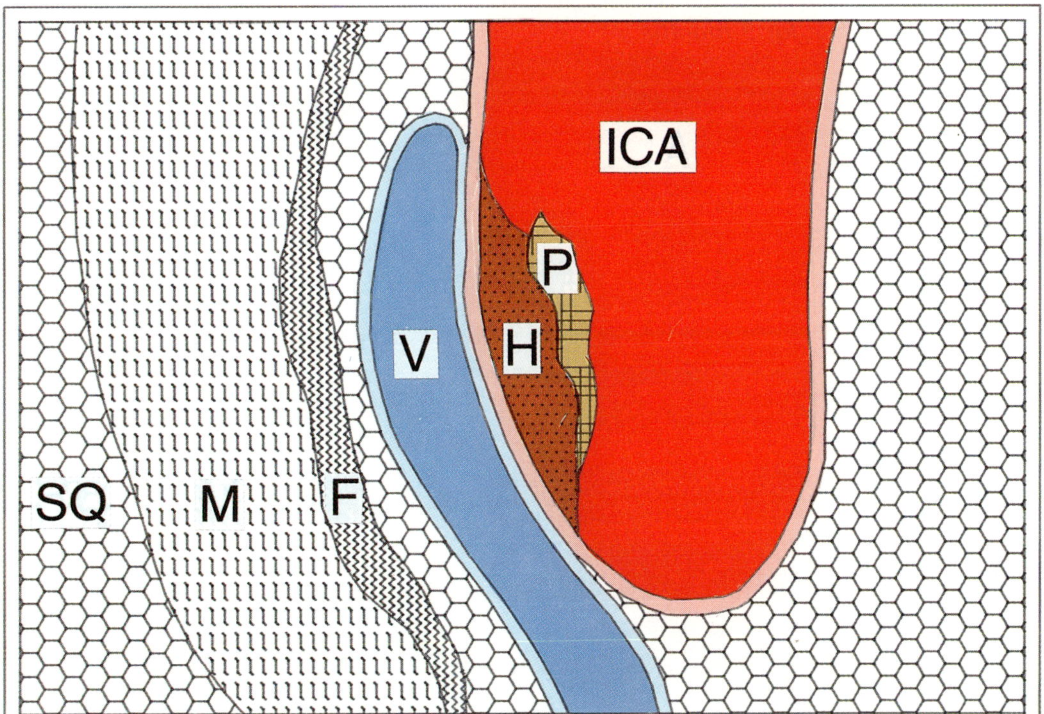

Figure 60. INTRAPLAQUE HEMORRHAGE

This is a transverse view of a right internal carotid artery (ICA) and external carotid artery (ECA) just above the bifurcation. The internal carotid bulb is mostly filled with moderately echogenic thrombus (T). Along the superficial and deep walls of the artery is some more brightly echogenic plaque (P) with a few isolated pieces of plaque along the surface of the residual lumen (L). This residual lumen measures 4.5 mm by 3.0 mm, and the Doppler cursor measures 3.5 mm in length. The residual lumen does not have a well-defined surface with a discrete surface echo as can be seen in most stable plaques. The appearance of the surface as shown here is characteristic of thrombus. The superficial third of the external carotid artery contains some echoes due to artifact (AF), arising from re-echoing of more superficial tissues. There is, however, a thin crescent of intimal thickening on the deep wall of the external carotid artery. Note again the acoustic shadowing extending deep from the top and bottom walls of the ICA. S = skin, M = platsyma muscle, SQ = subcutaneous tissue, SCM = sternocleidomastoid muscle, ? = tissue of uncertain composition.

HISTORY *This 64-year-old male presented with right-sided amaurosis fugax. Following this scan he developed crescendo transient ischemic attacks with left hemiparesis increasing in frequency despite continuous intravenous heparin. He underwent endarterectomy 6 days following the ultrasound scan. At operation he was found to have a large ulcerated plaque with "almost complete stenosis." Most of the stenosis was due to overlying thrombus. He has subsequently remained asymptomatic for 9 months.*

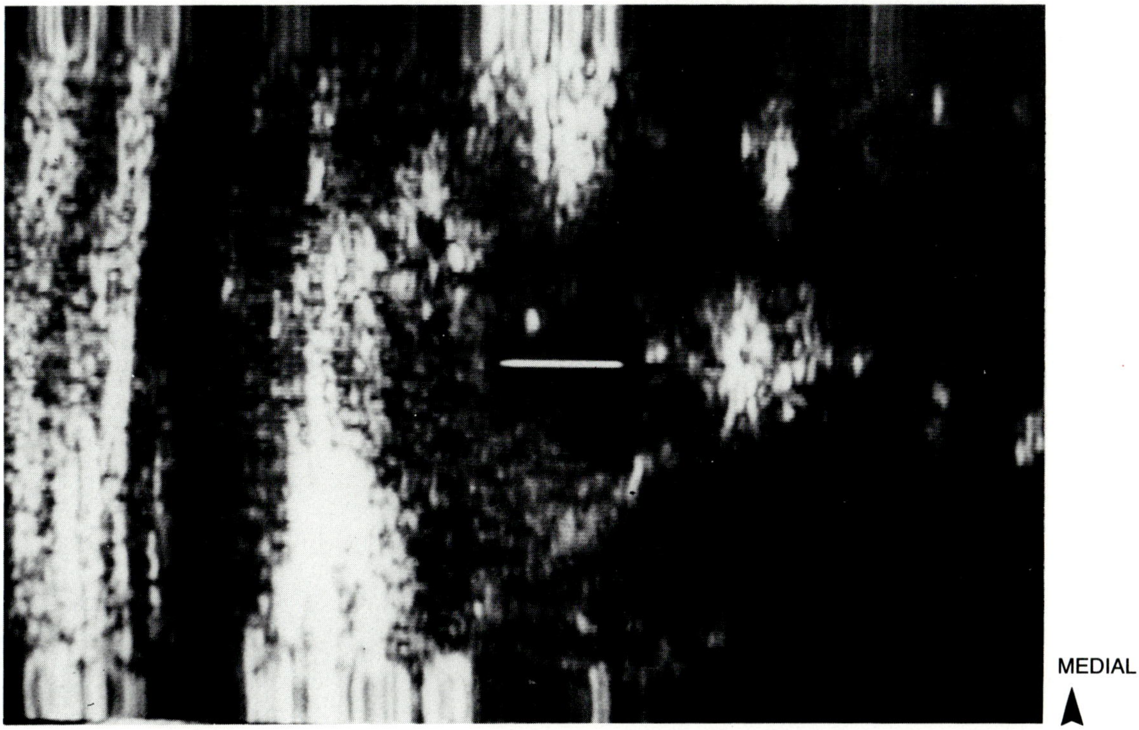
MEDIAL

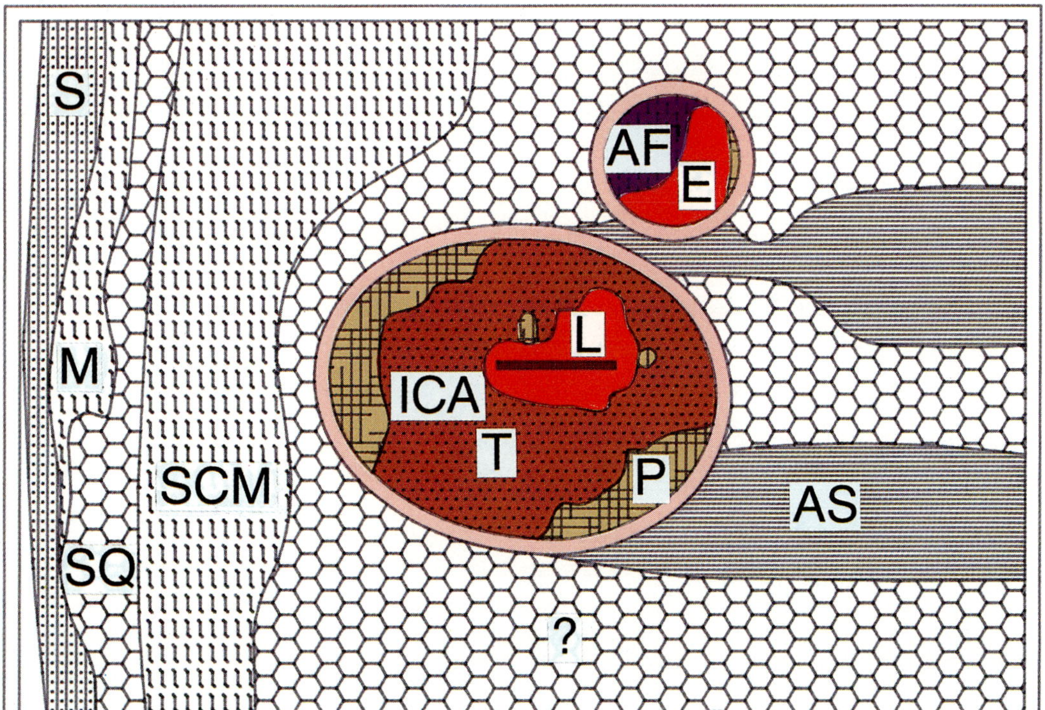
S
M
SQ
SCM
AF
E
L
ICA
T
P
AS
?

Figure 61. INTRAPLAQUE HEMORRHAGE

At a slightly higher level, before the distal tapering of the internal carotid artery (ICA), the thrombus (T) is still present. Note the irregular, ill-defined surface of the residual lumen (L). Again, there is some brightly echogenic plaque (P) against the deep wall of the artery. The external carotid artery (ECA) is now quite clearly seen as a separate vessel. S = skin, F = fascia, M = platysma muscle, SQ = subcutaneous tissue, SCM = sternocleidomastoid muscle, V = internal jugular vein (mostly compressed), C = Doppler cursor, AS = acoustic shadowing (from the edges of the internal carotid artery).

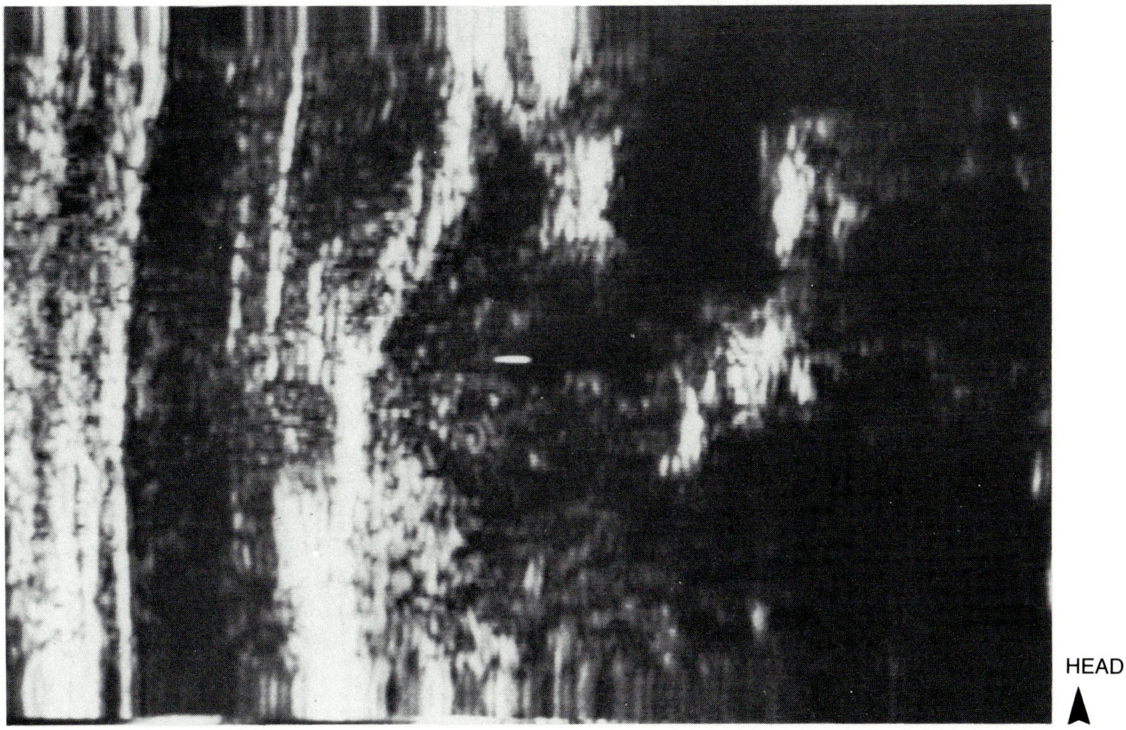
HEAD

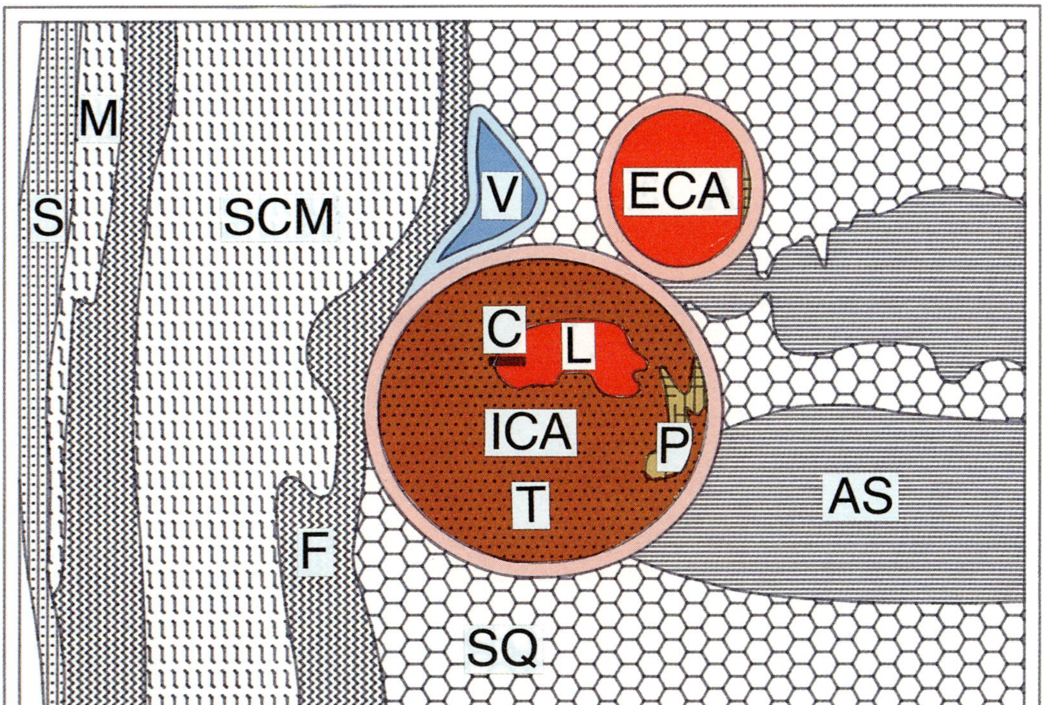
M
S
SCM
V
ECA
C
L
ICA
P
T
AS
F
SQ

Figure 62. INTRAPLAQUE HEMORRHAGE

This is a transverse view above the left carotid bifurcation revealing moderately echogenic plaque (P) on the superficial wall of the internal carotid artery (ICA) and also occupying approximately three fourths the circumference of the external carotid artery (ECA). The residual lumens are mildly irregular and are fairly well defined in the ECA. However, near the location of the Doppler cursor the upper margin of the residual lumen in the ICA is poorly defined with faintly echogenic homogeneous material extending superiorly, which is characteristic of thrombus (T) from intraplaque hemorrhage. There is approximately a 40% stenosis of the ICA with a 3.3-mm diameter residual lumen compared with a 5.5-mm diameter ICA. This lesion is located in the mid ICA, which has tapered to a uniform size. Therefore, measurements can be taken of both the residual and normal lumens at the same level. S = skin, F = fascia, SQ = subcutaneous tissue, M = sternocleidomastoid muscle, ? = tissue of uncertain composition.

HISTORY *This 56-year-old male underwent carotid endarterectomy 2 weeks after this ultrasound scan. At the time of operation, the residual lumen was nearly totally obliterated by fresh thrombus, which had filled a plane of dissection under the plaque extending nearly 2 cm above the bifurcation. This intraplaque hemorrhage had been asymptomatic.*

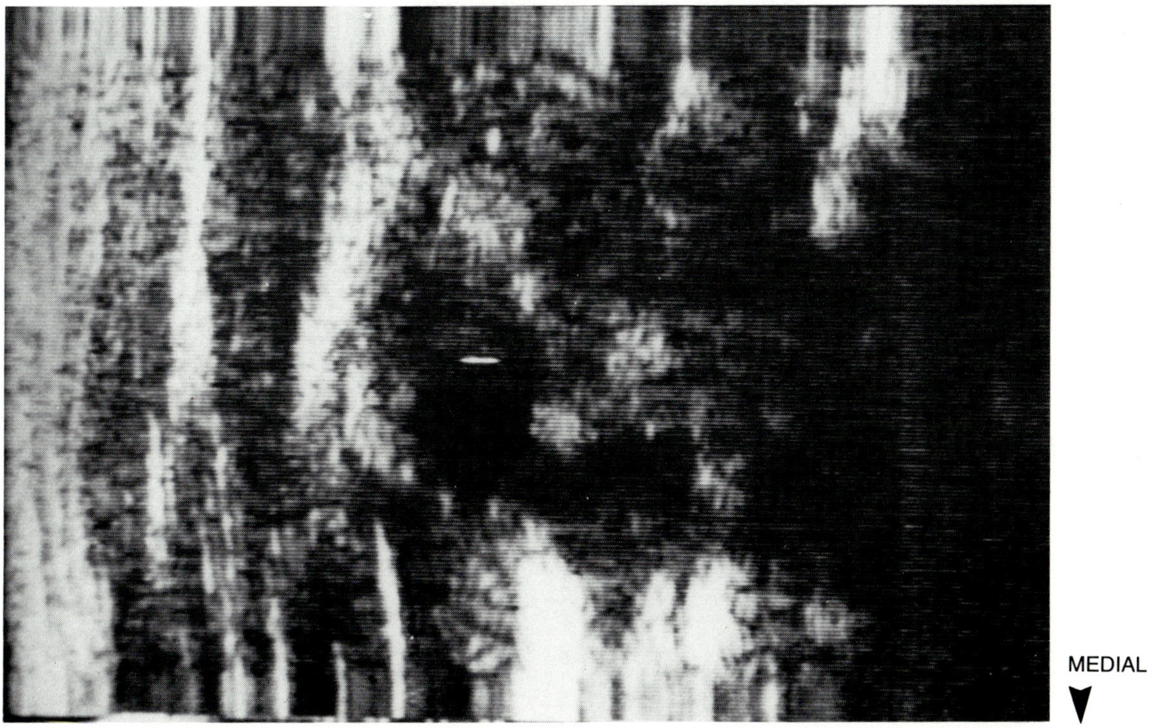
MEDIAL

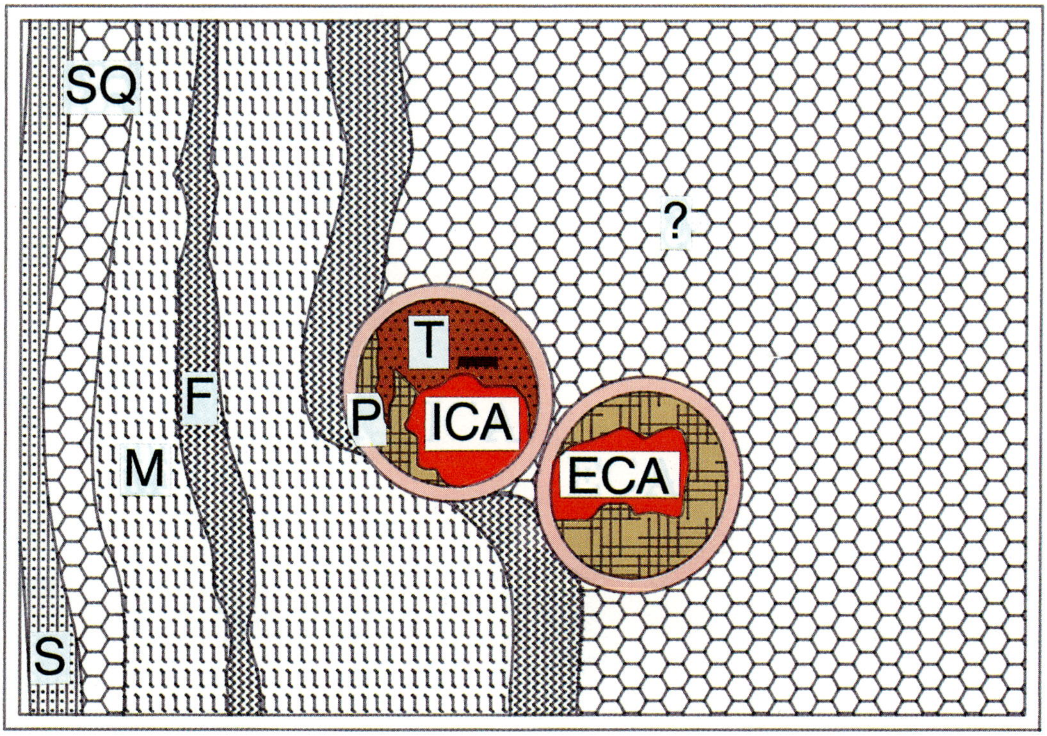
SQ
?
T
F
P
ICA
M
ECA
S

Figure 63. INTRAPLAQUE HEMORRHAGE

This is a transverse view of the right internal carotid artery (ICA) just above the bifurcation showing faintly echogenic plaque (P) in the midst of which is some intraplaque hemorrhage with thrombus (T), giving the appearance of a double lumen. The external carotid artery is at the very top of the ultrasound scan and is only partially seen and not drawn. S = skin, SQ = subcutaneous tissue (including platysmal muscle), M = sternocleidomastoid muscle, F = fascia.

HISTORY *This 71-year-old male presented with dizziness 4 years after bilateral carotid endarterectomies. An arteriogram 1 month after this ultrasound scan showed that this lesion had become a total occlusion.*

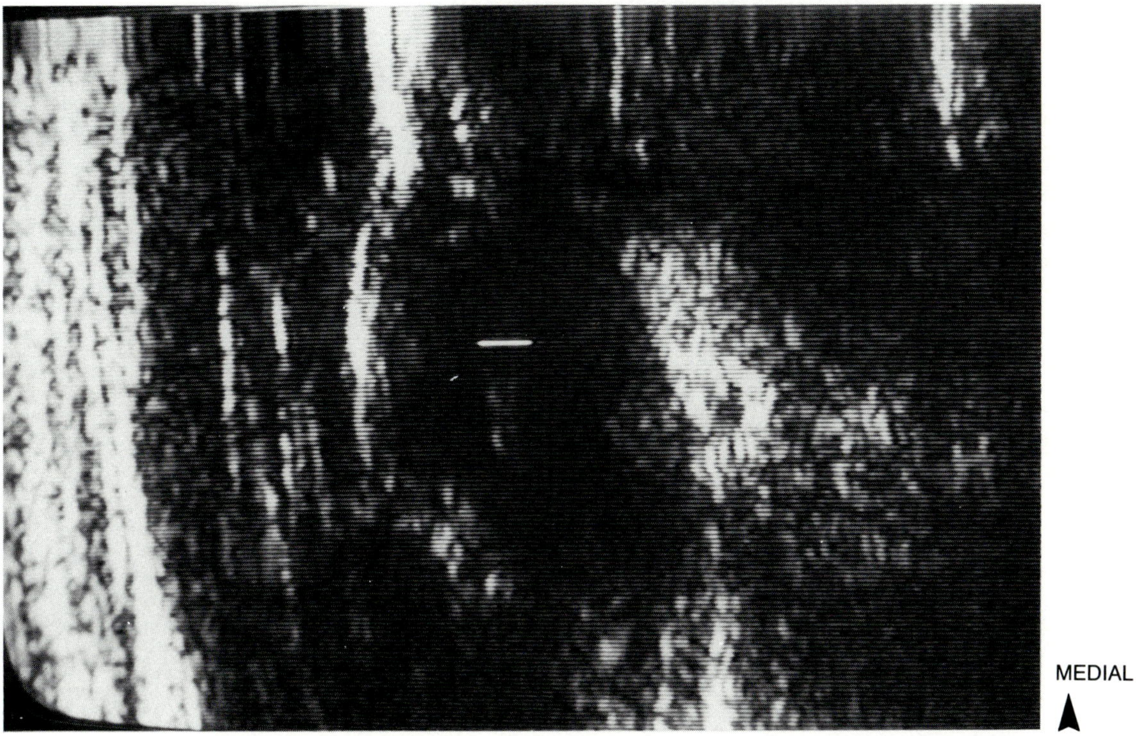
MEDIAL

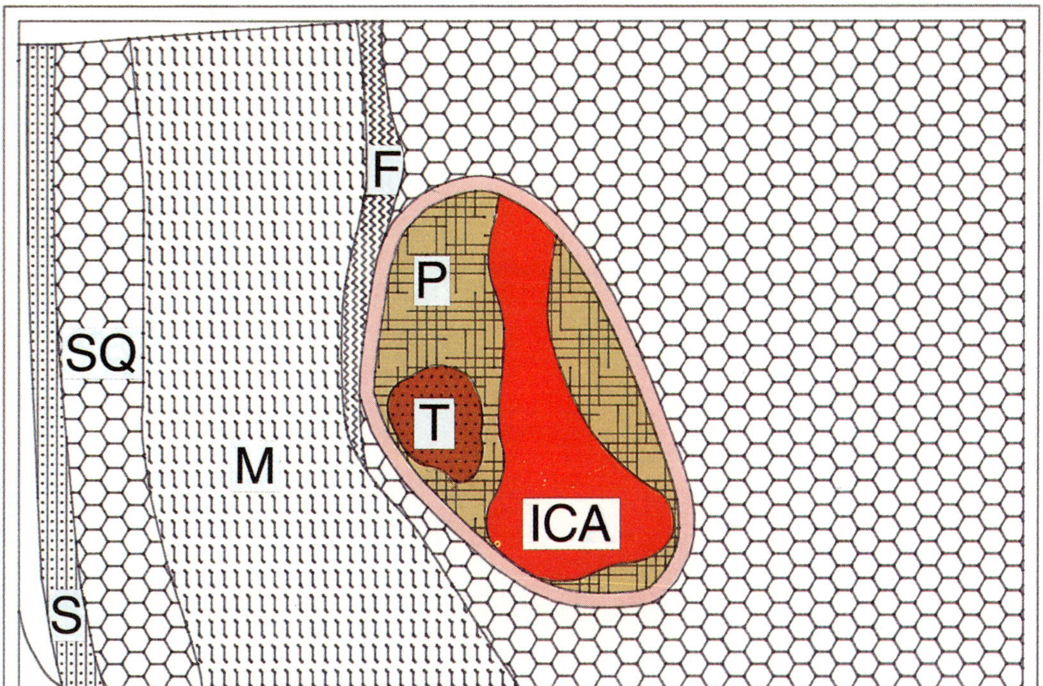
F
P
SQ
T
M
ICA
S

Figure 64. INTRAPLAQUE HEMORRHAGE

This is an oblique view that is nearly longitudinal through the same internal carotid artery (ICA), as in Figure 63 showing a much better visualized contour of the plaque (P) on the superficial wall containing an area of thrombus (T). This appearance of a double lumen cannot be distinguished from an open ulcer seen face on, except for the fact that a Doppler signal is absent within the apparent lumen. SQ = subcutaneous tissue (including skin and platysma muscle), M = sternocleidomastoid muscle.

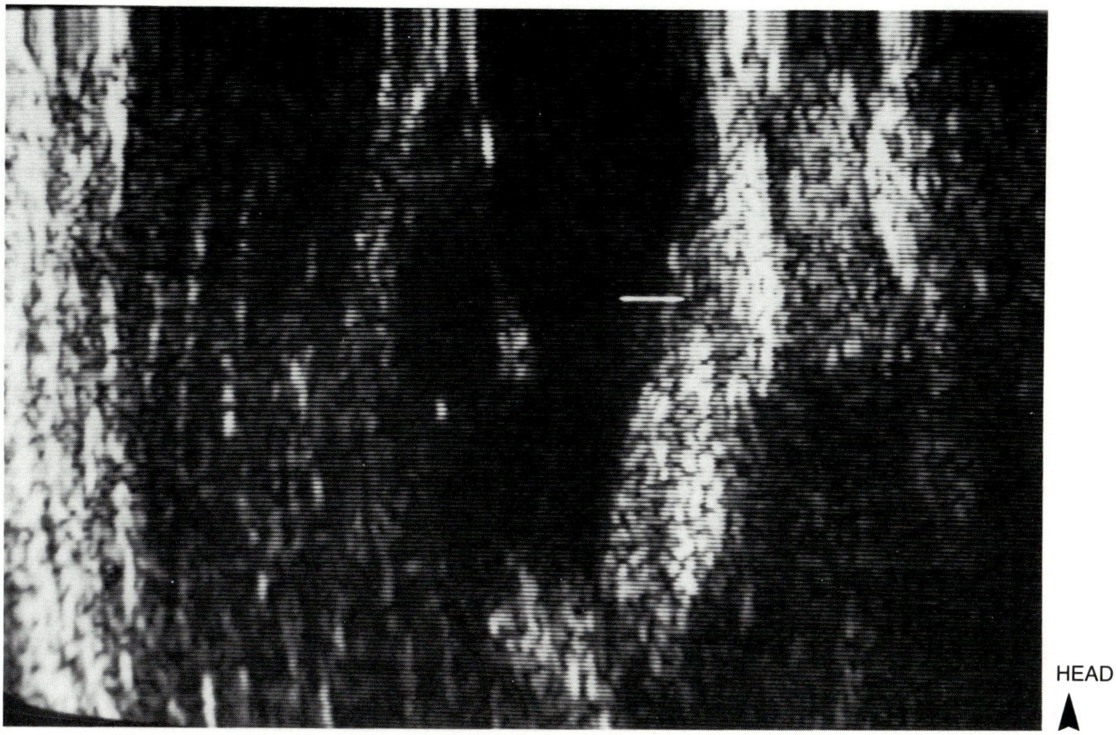
HEAD

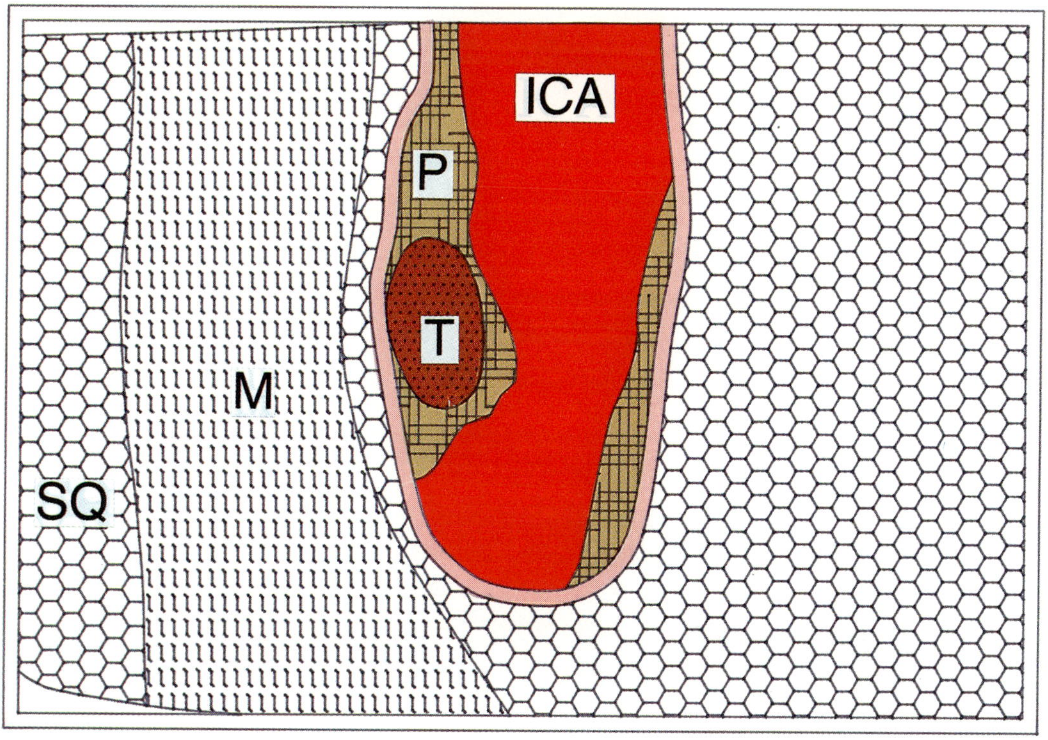
ICA
P
T
M
SQ

Figure 65. INTRAPLAQUE HEMORRHAGE

This is a transverse view of the left internal artery (ICA) and the external carotid artery (ECA) at a level just above the bifurcation. This is another example of intraplaque hemorrhage (H) where the true arterial lumen (3.0 mm in diameter) with a strong Doppler signal is located in the left half of the artery, and the dark zone within the right half of the artery is consistent with H that has separated the plaque (P) from the deep wall. There is no Doppler signal obtainable within this deeper right half of the artery. Note how faintly echogenic clotted blood can sometimes be. S = skin, SQ = subcutaneous tissue (including platysma muscle), F = fascia, M = sternocleidomastoid muscle.

HISTORY *This 82-year-old female had one episode of syncope 2 years prior and has been followed for asymptomatic stenosis, estimated at 30%, with ultrasound scans every 6 months showing no change in the severity of stenosis.*

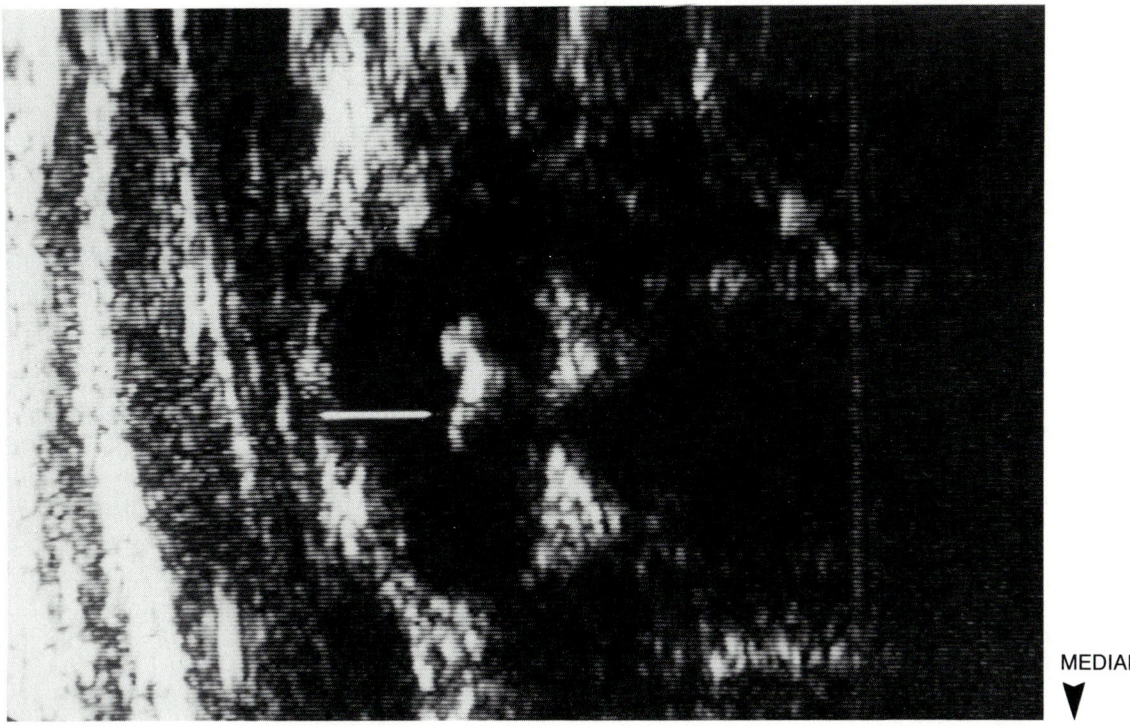
MEDIAL

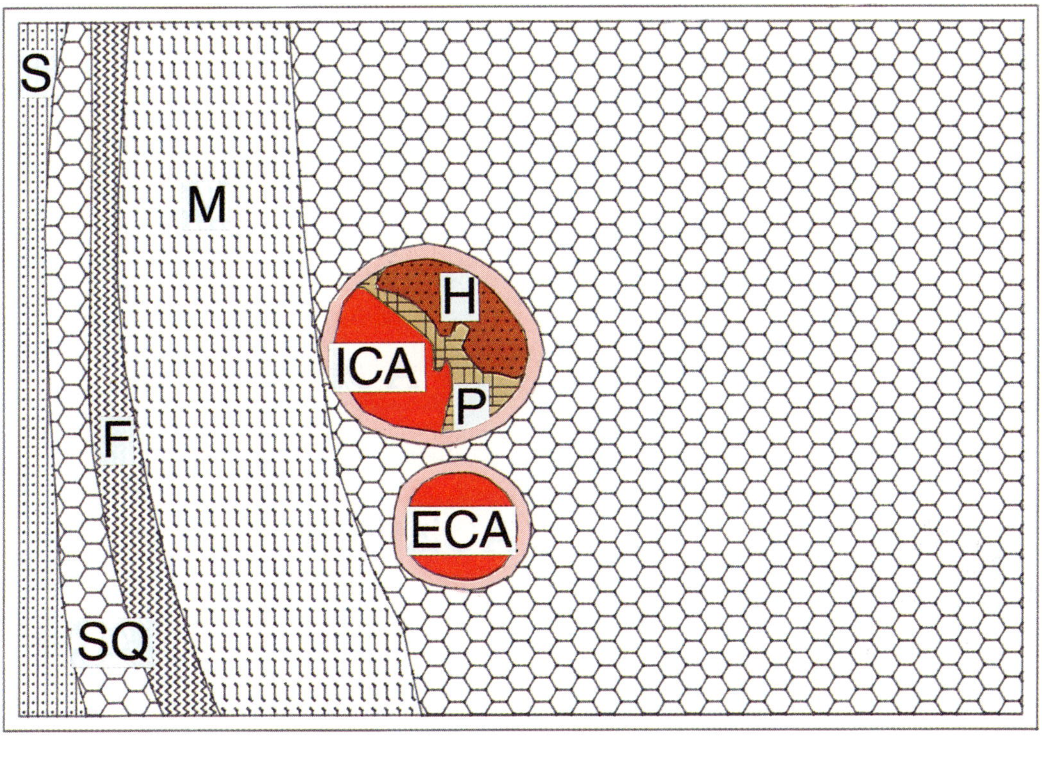
S
M
H
ICA
P
F
ECA
SQ

Figure 66. TYPES OF SURFACE CHARACTER

It is believed that the degree of irregularity of the plaque surface carries some prognostic significance. For this purpose, we report plaque as having four degrees of irregularity. Example A shows a smooth plaque. There are no surface indentations. Example B shows a plaque that is mildly irregular. The surface is gently undulating but without discrete defects. Example C illustrates a moderately irregular plaque. There appear to be discrete surface defects best described as scalloping. However, the indentations do not have sloping walls at angles approaching 90 degrees to the surface as a whole. In example D, the left-hand side of the plaque is highly irregular. There are clefts that have edges indented at angles approaching 90 degrees to the surface as a whole.

What follows is largely based on opinion with selected confirmation by endarterectomy specimens. On the right side of example D there is a discrete ulcer. This is seen as a pocket in the midst of the plaque containing a base larger than its orifice with overhanging edges. This type of finding is consistently confirmed to be an ulcer at operation. On pathological examination, many of the highly irregular plaques as illustrated in the left-hand side of example D, and quite a few of the moderately irregular plaques as seen in example C, will in fact contain areas of ulceration. It does not seem possible to separate those moderately and highly irregular plaques which contain ulcers from those which do not, unless a discrete crater is present. This factor leads to under-reporting the true incidence of ulceration. However, this under-reporting is preferable to over-diagnosing ulceration. In questionable cases, it is better to describe the plaque as being moderately or highly irregular. These descriptive terms are more acceptable than the word "ulceration," which might not be present. If one is overzealous in diagnosing ulcers, the referring physician may be forced wrongly into a course of action solely on the basis of a duplex scan.

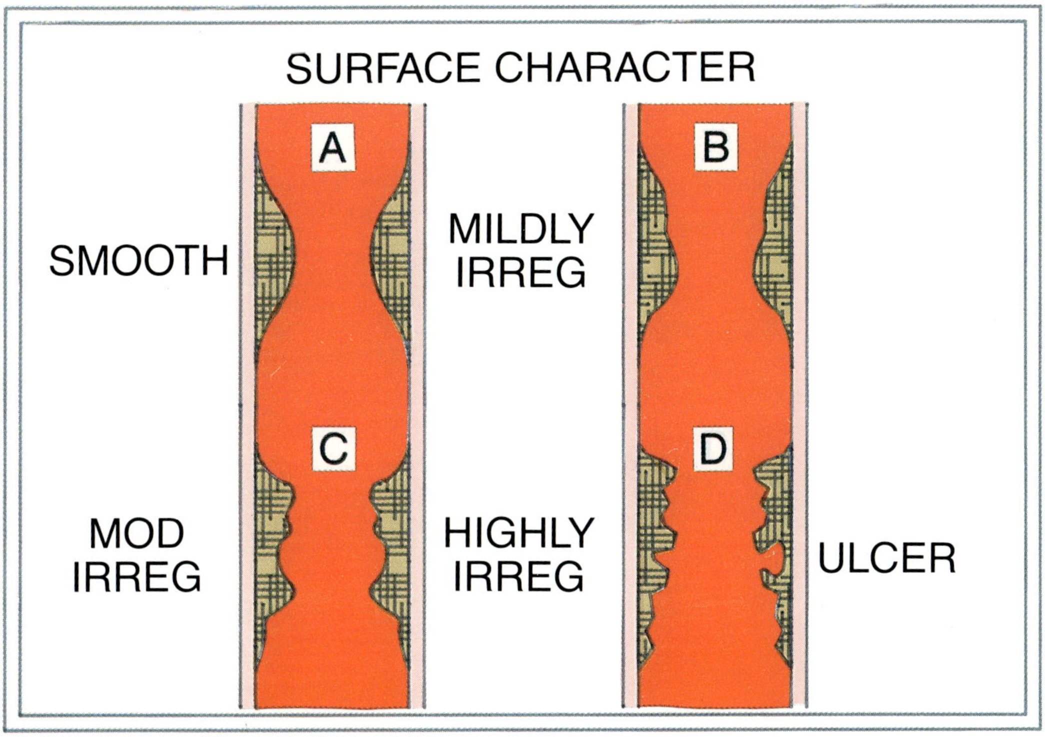
SURFACE CHARACTER
A
B
SMOOTH
MILDLY
IRREG
C
D
MOD
IRREG
HIGHLY
IRREG
ULCER

CHAPTER 4

SURFACE CHARACTER

Figure 67. SMOOTH CAROTID PLAQUE

This is an example of a plaque (P) with a smooth surface containing no indentations. Note also that the plaque is of moderate echogenicity, approximately equal in brightness to the surrounding tissue and quite homogeneous in echo distribution. It has the appearance of a stable, organized plaque and appears to cause about a 60% diameter stenosis in this single longitudinal view. The common carotid artery (CCA) is smaller in diameter at the base of the neck toward the bottom of the scan, and thus the normal lumen in this case is smaller in diameter than one would measure at the level of the plaque. The light and dark bands at the left edge of the screen are artifact from the probe's surface and obscure the surface of the underlying skin. SQ = subcutaneous tissue, M = sternocleidomastoid muscle.

HISTORY *This is of an 82-year-old male who presented with syncope. The ultrasound scan was obtained to rule out significant carotid disease, although the patient had a history of atrial fibrillation and congestive heart failure with mitral regurgitation and an ejection fraction of 14%. He has remained asymptomatic over the following 5 months.*

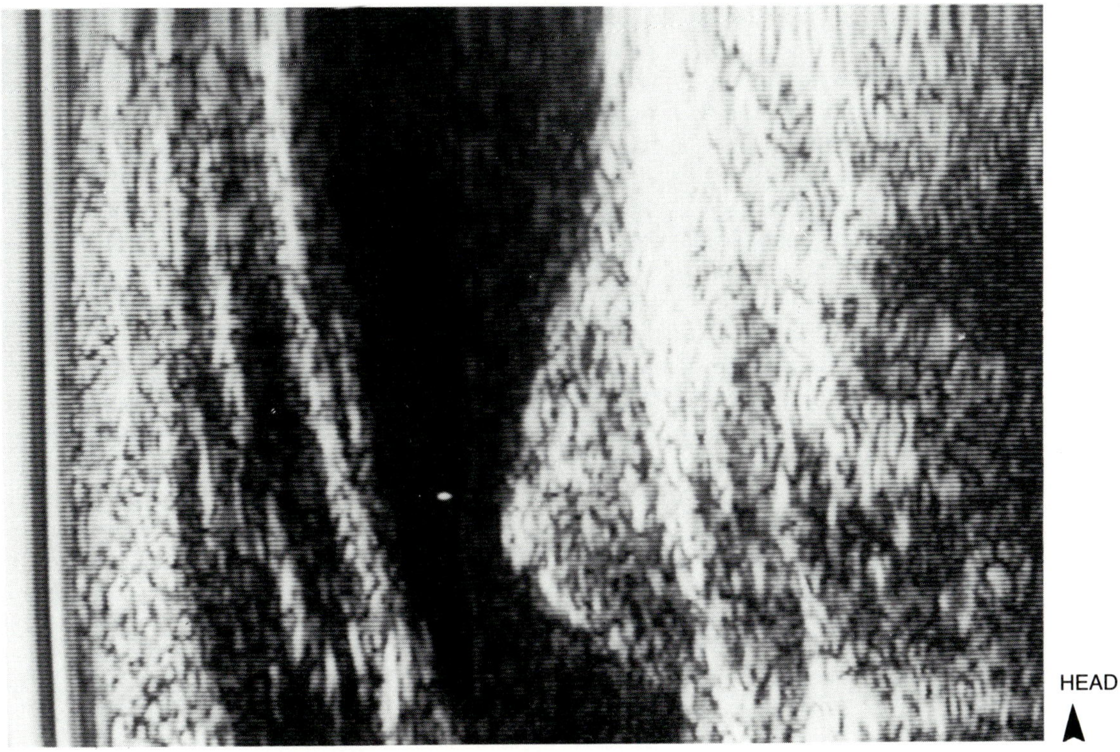
HEAD

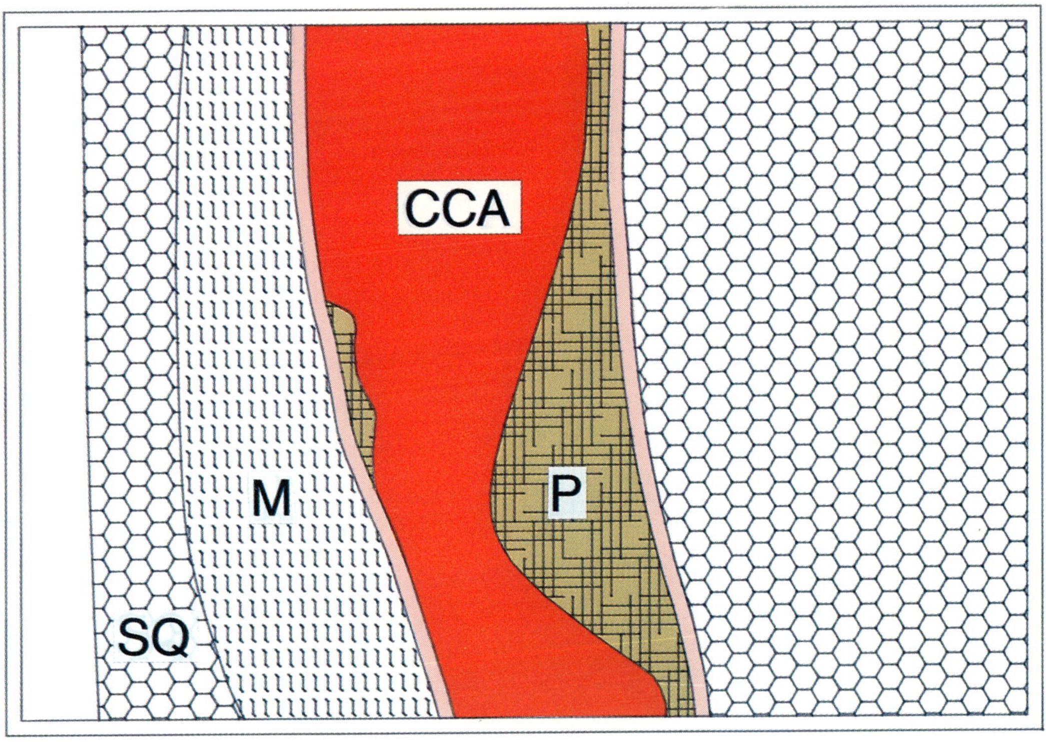
CCA
M
P
SQ

Figure 68. SMOOTH CAROTID PLAQUE

In this transverse view of the same artery as in Figure 67 at the level of greatest stenosis, one can see that the residual lumen (L) is, in fact, not round, but elliptical and measures 2.5 by 4.5 mm. The common carotid artery (CCA) has a smallest normal arterial diameter of 7.0 mm and, thus, is equal to a 50% stenosis. Also, note the "double pig-tail effect" of dark streaks extending to the right of the top and bottom "back" walls of the artery. This effect, which is somewhat pronounced in this particular ultrasound scan, occurs as a result of refraction of the ultrasound beam. That portion of the ultrasound beam that passes tangentially through the top and bottom walls of the artery is refracted toward the center deep wall of the artery. This convergence of the ultrasound beam gives rise to two effects. The first is the dark "pig-tails" themselves. This is a result of attenuation of the beam in these areas. The second effect is the bright spot on the deep wall resulting from convergence of the beam. This bright spot is not calcified tissue. If it were, there would be shadowing behind it. The same effect is seen if one shines light transversely through a cylindrical glass rod and notices the concentration of brightness on a piece of paper behind it. Both effects are caused by refraction. SQ = subcutaneous tissue, M = sternocleidomastoid muscle, CCA = common carotid artery, P = plaque.

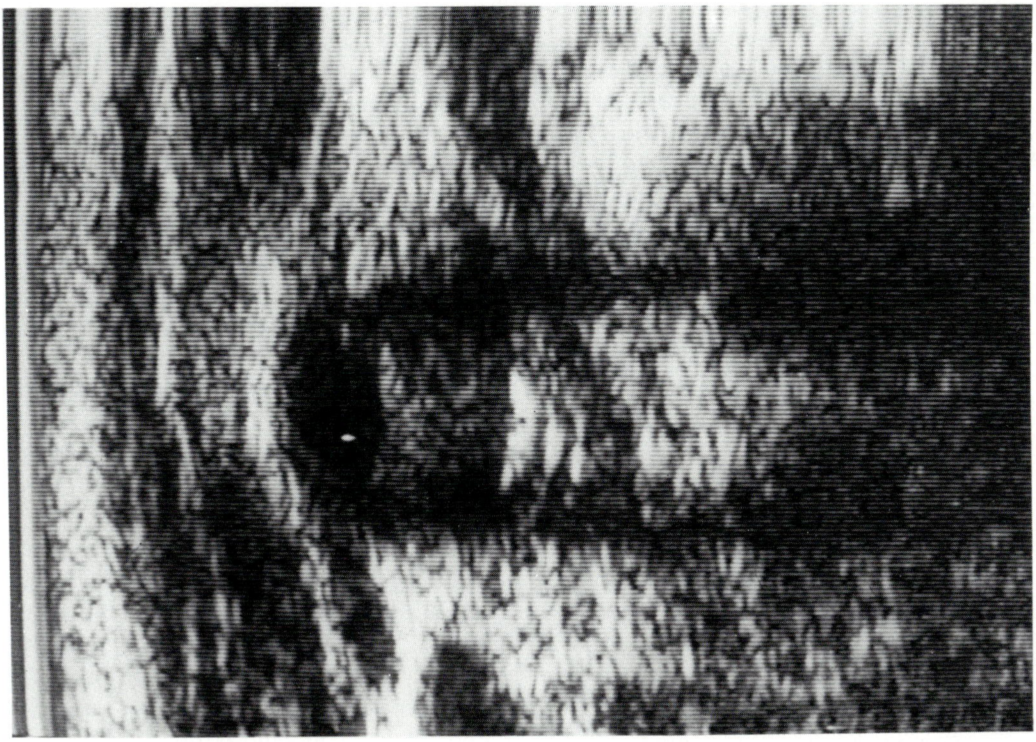

MEDIAL

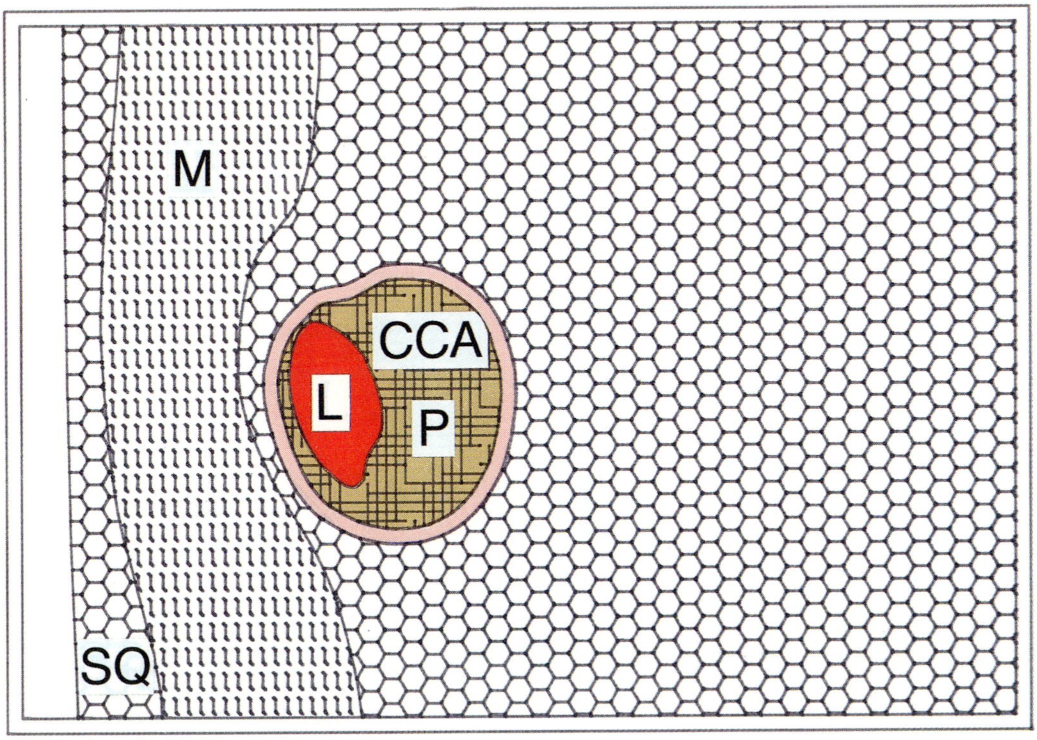

Figure 69. MILDLY IRREGULAR PLAQUE

This is an example of a mildly irregular plaque (P) causing a rather severe stenosis with a residual lumen equal to dimension 2. Notice the overall contour of the plaque that has gradual undulations without any discrete defects, thus qualifying as mildly irregular. The plaque is moderately heterogeneous with fainter echogenicity at the bottom of the ultrasound scan characteristic of lipid composition. The protuberant portion of the plaque may be thrombus (see History that follows). The residual lumen (2) measuring 0.8 mm causes a 75% stenosis by diameter in comparison with the distal arterial diameter (RL1) of 3.2 mm. Obviously, a much greater degree of stenosis (90%) could be calculated in relation to the arterial diameter at the level of plaque (RL3) that measures 7.8 mm. The degree of stenosis in other views was not as severe as in this particular view, and the overall percent stenosis was calculated at 60%. S = skin, SQ = subcutaneous tissue, M = sternocleidomastoid muscle, F = fascia, ICA = internal carotid artery, ? = tissue of uncertain composition.

HISTORY *This is the last of four ultrasound scans of this 64-year-old male who initially presented with vertigo and was found to have a 60% right internal carotid stenosis. The second scan 6 months later showed no change, but the third scan 6 months after the second showed ulceration of the plaque with a reduction in the percent stenosis to 50%. For several months coincident with the third scan the patient had multiple transient ischemic attacks involving left hemiparesis. He was treated with aspirin and dipyridamole. The ultrasound scan shown here was taken 6 months after the third and showed a progression of stenosis again to 60%. The ulcer is no longer present, having been filled in by the protuberant portion of the plaque seen in this scan, and may well be thrombus. However, in the 9 months since this ultrasound scan the patient has had no further transient ischemic attacks.*

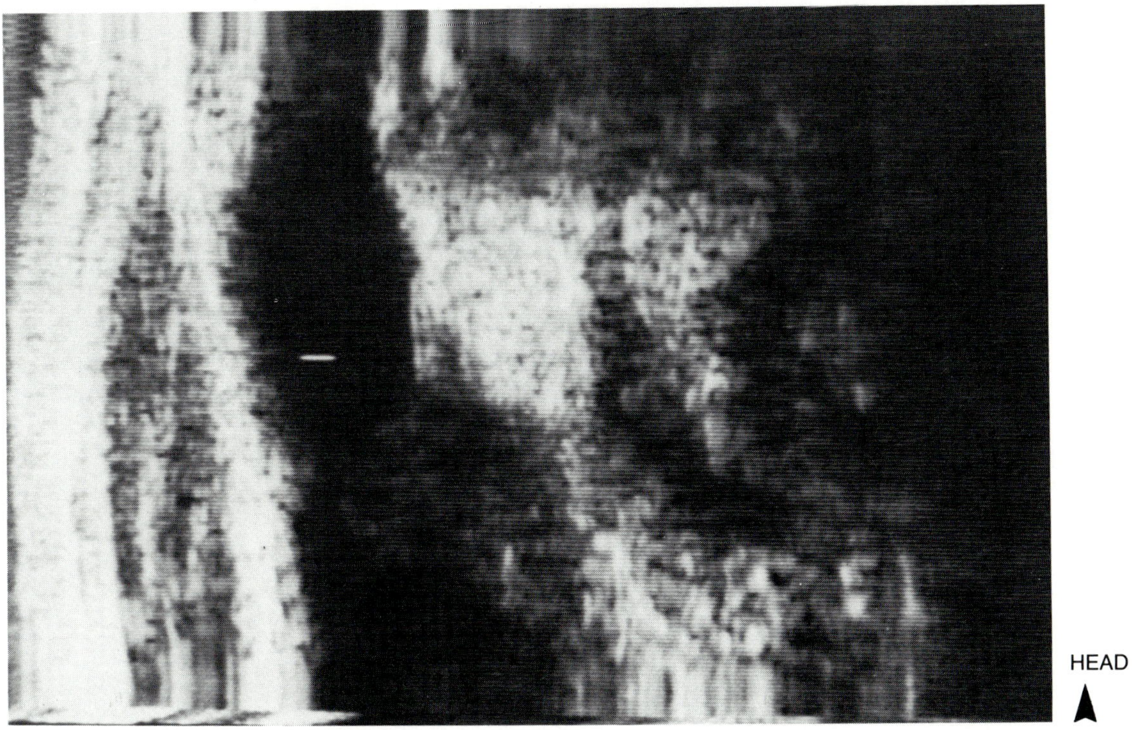
HEAD

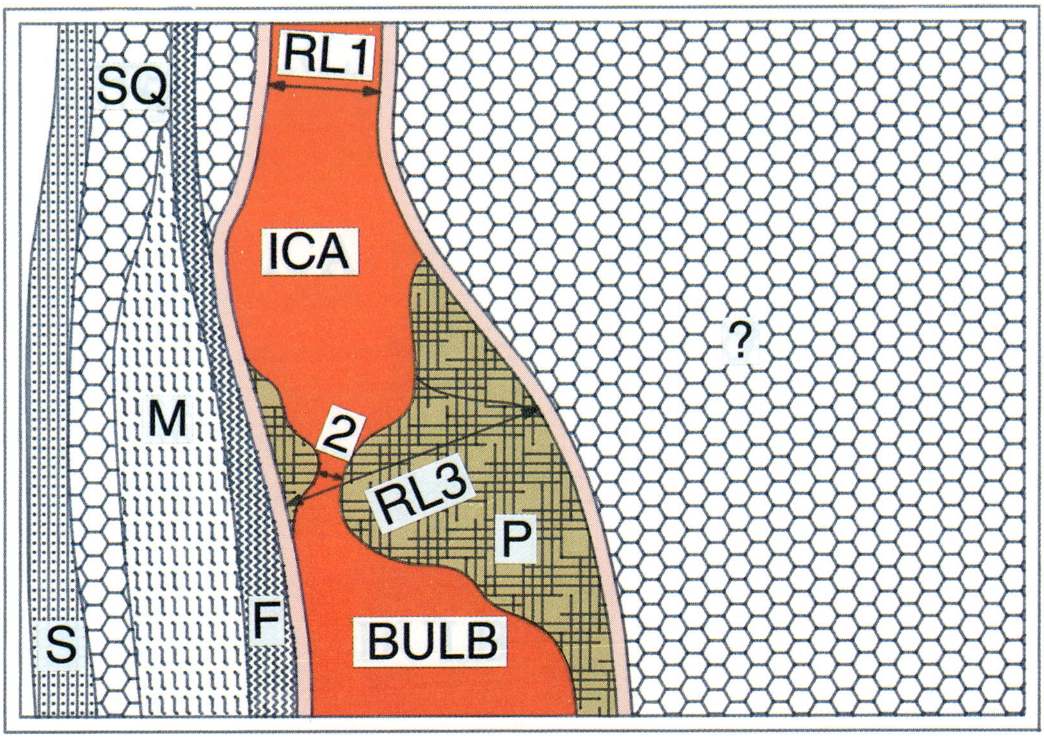
RL1
SQ
ICA
?
M
2
RL3
P
F
S
BULB

Figure 70. MODERATELY IRREGULAR PLAQUE

This is an example of moderately irregular plaque. The severe stenosis caused by the plaque (P) within the bulb of this left internal carotid artery (ICA) has a surface with rather sharp yet shallow indentations. Thus, the surface is intermediate between being highly irregular and mildly irregular. The plaque is moderately echogenic and moderately homogeneous. M = sternocleidomastoid muscle, IJV = internal jugular vein, F = fascia, VN = vagus nerve.

HISTORY *This is a 54-year-old male who underwent ultrasound scanning because of an asymptomatic right bruit. His vascular surgeon has elected to follow this lesion. The patient has remained asymptomatic over the subsequent 5 months; repeat studies have not been done.*

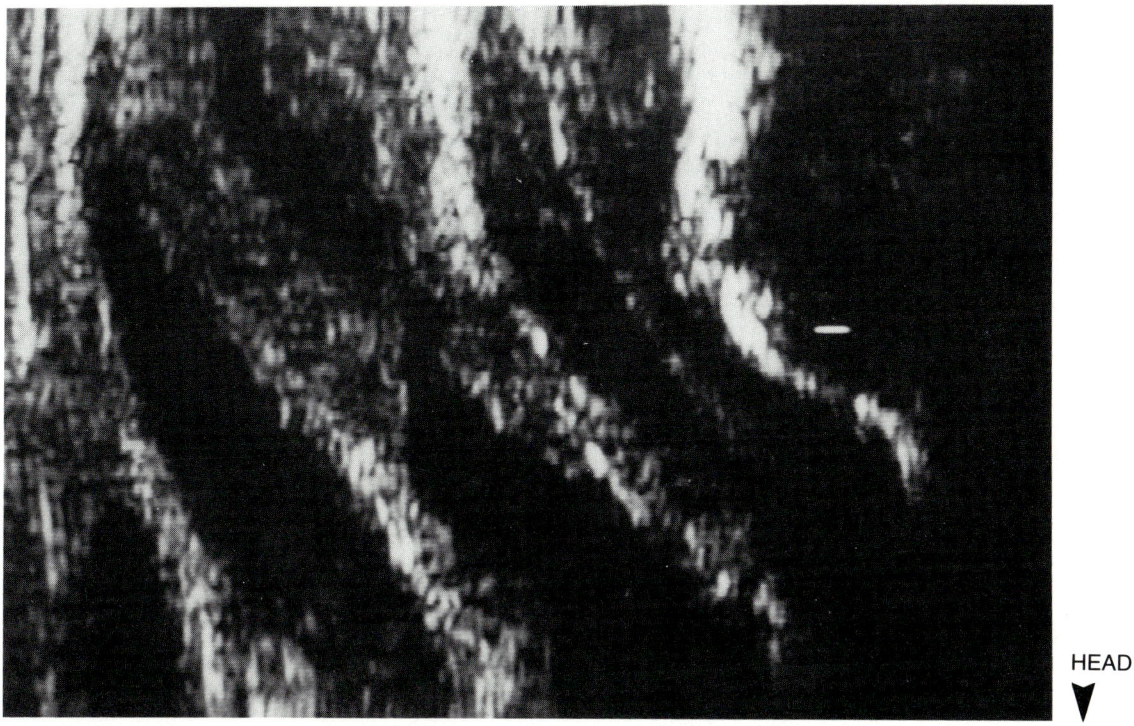
HEAD

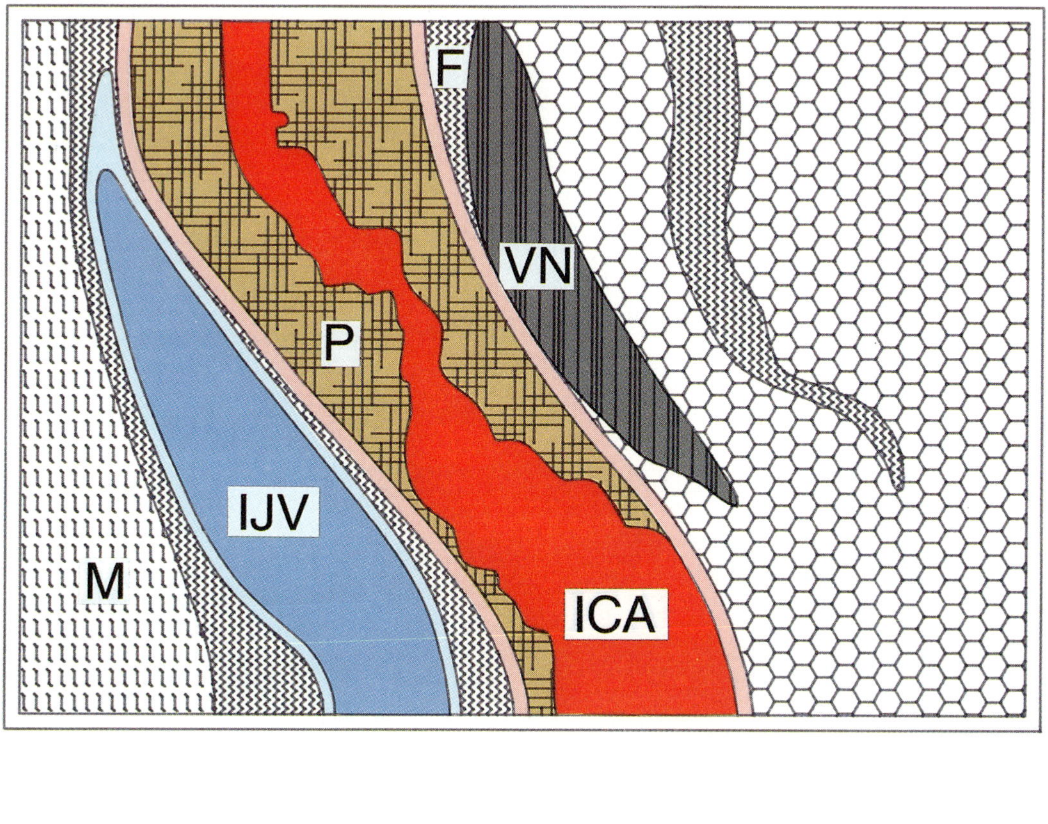
F
VN
P
IJV
M
ICA

Figure 71. HIGHLY IRREGULAR PLAQUE

The plaque (P) on the deep wall of this carotid bifurcation is best described as highly irregular. The surface has abrupt peaks and valleys. None of the valleys appears deep enough with overhanging edges to qualify as a discrete ulcer. Nevertheless, on microscopical examination, many plaques with this surface appearance have been found to be ulcerated. This plaque is faintly echogenic. The crotch of the arterial bifurcation separating the external carotid artery (ECA) and internal carotid artery (ICA) is barely visible. SQ = subcutaneous tissue, M = sternocleidomastoid muscle, CCA = common carotid artery, F = fascia.

HISTORY *This patient is a 35-year-old female who had a left hemispheric cerebrovascular accident 8 years ago. She complained of bilateral upper and lower extremity numbness and tingling at the time of this ultrasound scan.*

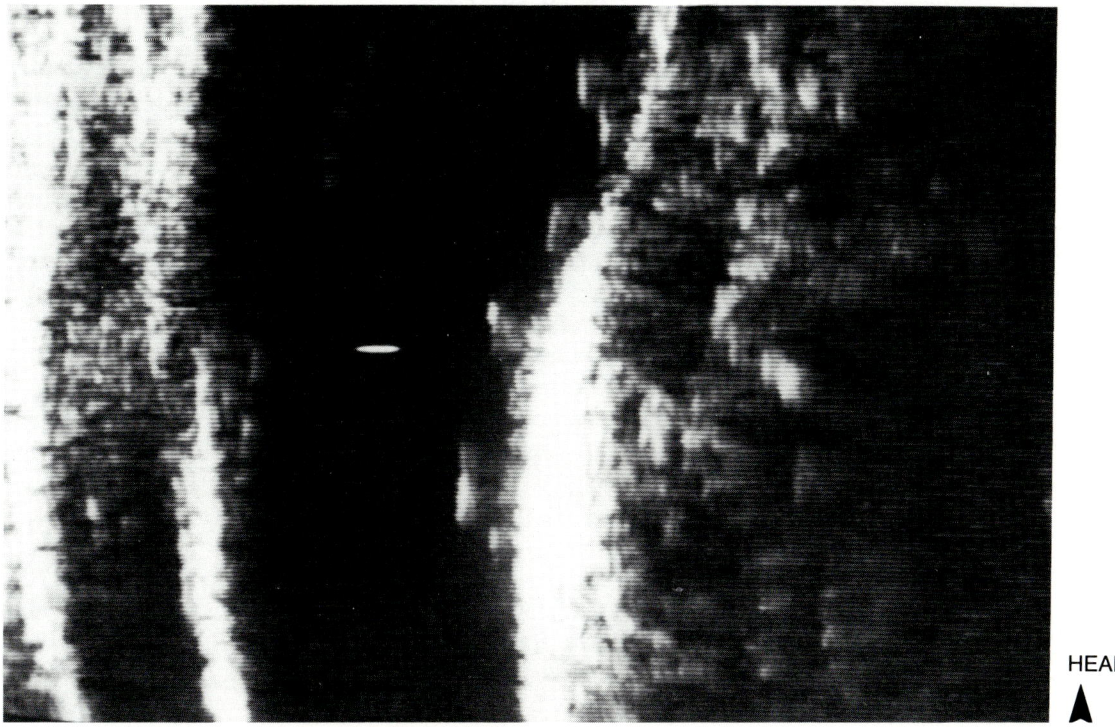
HEAD

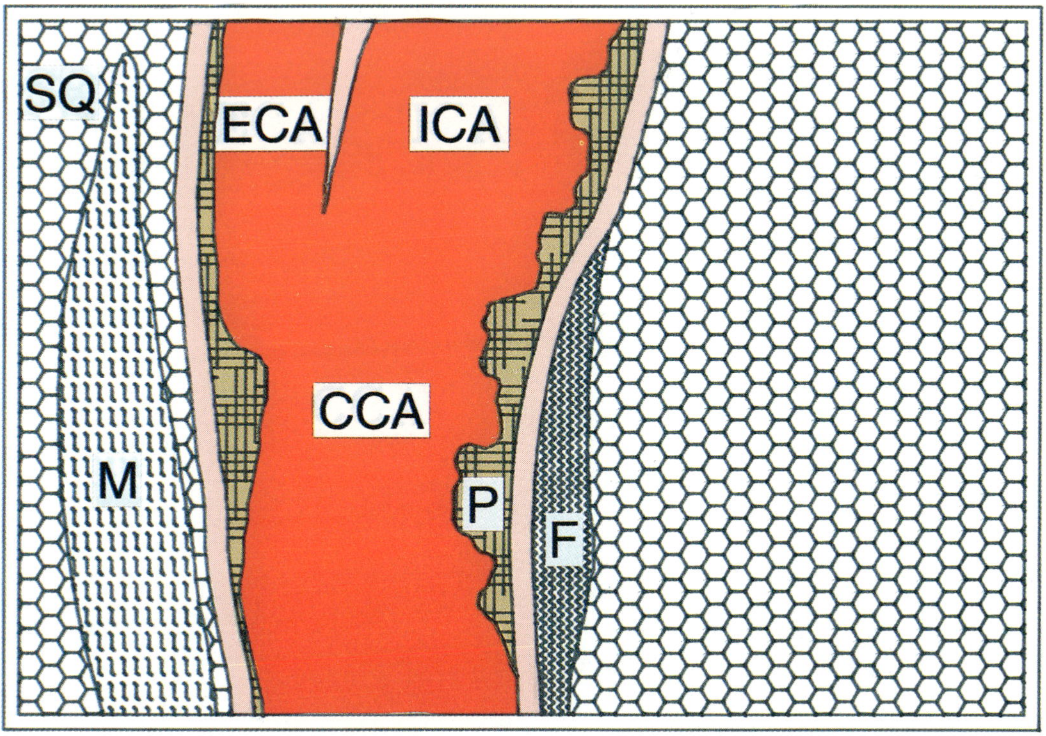
SQ
ECA
ICA
CCA
M
P
F

Figure 72. HIGHLY IRREGULAR PLAQUE

The plaque (P) seen in this longitudinal view of a right carotid bifurcation is classified as highly irregular. Again there are abrupt "step-offs" without discrete ulcer craters. The plaque is also calcified with acoustic shadowing (AS) obscuring the deeper portions. Nevertheless, the plaque is moderately heterogeneous with light and dark areas. It is located on the deep wall of the common carotid artery (CCA) just before the bifurcation and appears to cause a 55% stenosis of the origin of the internal carotid artery (ICA) with a 2.0 mm residual lumen compared with a 4.5 mm diameter artery distally. In this view there is a 2.0-mm residual lumen compared with a 6.0-mm diameter CCA proximally. These measurements of stenosis, however, are calculated from a single view and must be corrected according to other views. The external carotid artery (ECA) is free of disease. There is some artifact (AF) with an appearance similar to plaque on the superficial wall of the ICA. AF cannot be distinguished from plaque in this single view but was not present in other views. SCM = sternocleidomastoid muscle, F = fascia, SQ = subcutaneous tissue, ? = tissue of uncertain composition.

HISTORY *This 77-year-old female was admitted with complaints of ataxia and several falls within 2 weeks prior to the ultrasound scan. A neurological consultant believes that her symptoms were due to multiple medications.*

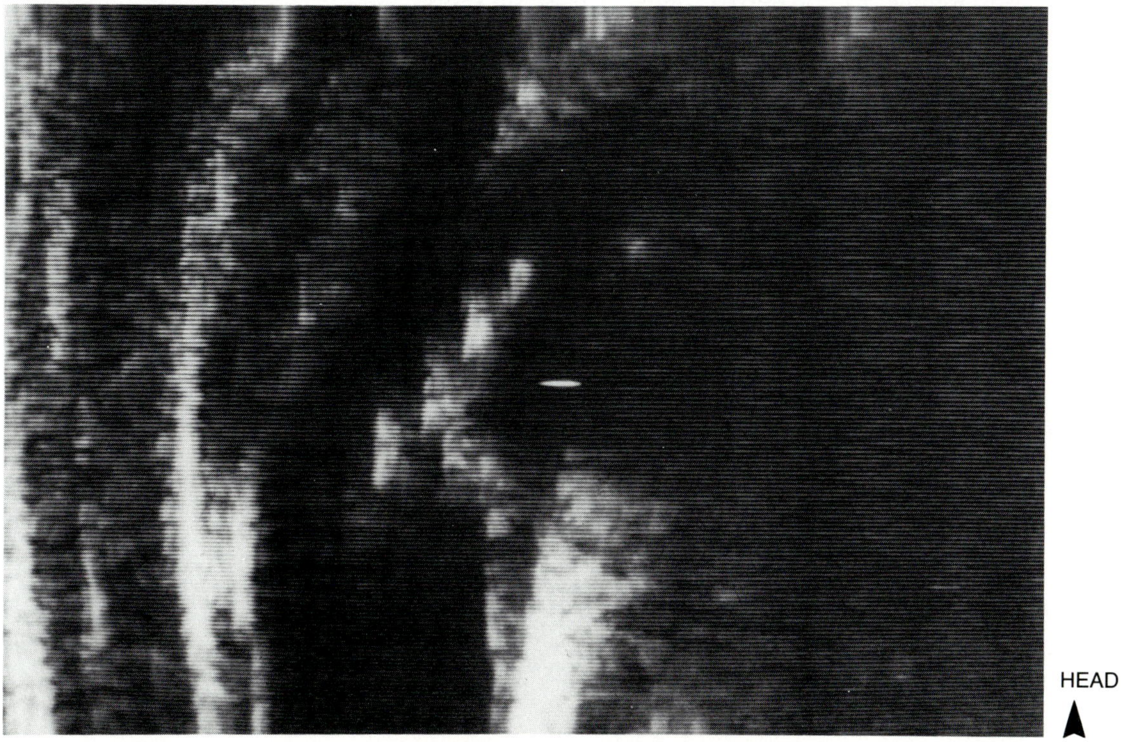
HEAD

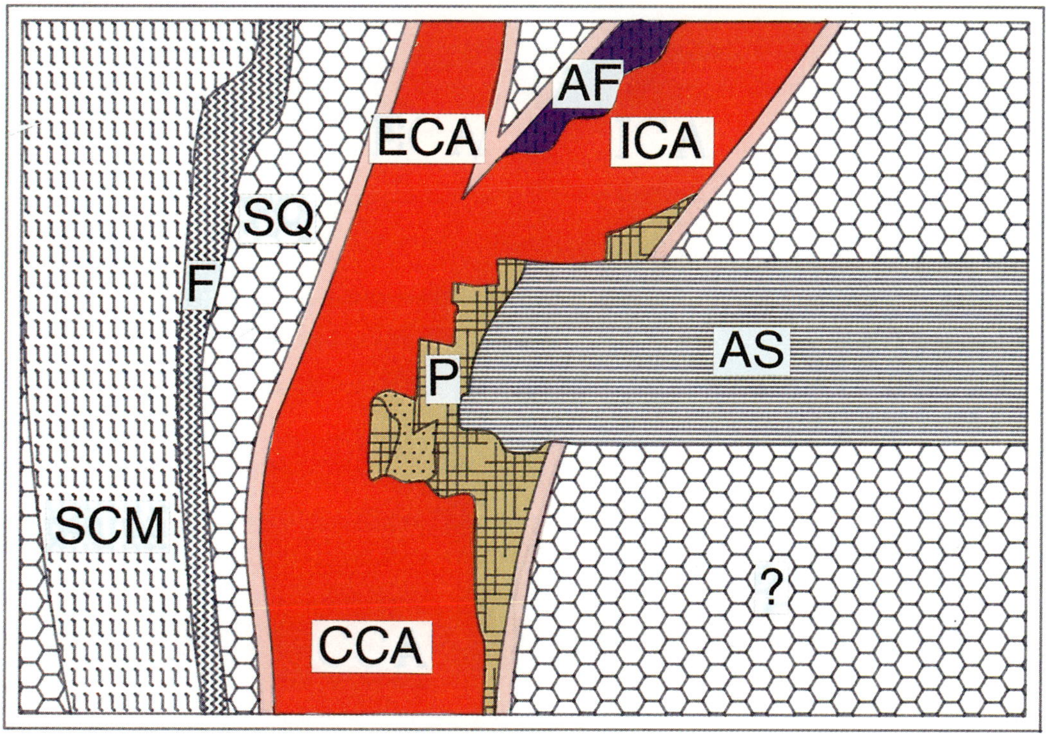
AF
ECA
ICA
SQ
F
AS
P
SCM
?
CCA

Figure 73. HIGHLY IRREGULAR PLAQUE

This is another example of highly irregular plaque (P) that is difficult to call a discrete ulcer. The plaque is moderately heterogeneous with bright and dark areas at different points in the longitudinal view of this left common carotid artery (CCA). The rather homogeneous thyroid gland (THYROID) is seen to the right. G = gel, S = skin, M = platysma muscle, SCM = sternocleidomastoid muscle, IJV = internal jugular vein, V = facial vein, SQ = subcutaneous tissue, C = Doppler cursor.

HISTORY *This 80-year-old female experienced a central visual field defect that persisted over the 5 days prior to the ultrasound scan. She was subsequently placed on aspirin and dipyridamole and has had no further symptoms over the following 3 months.*

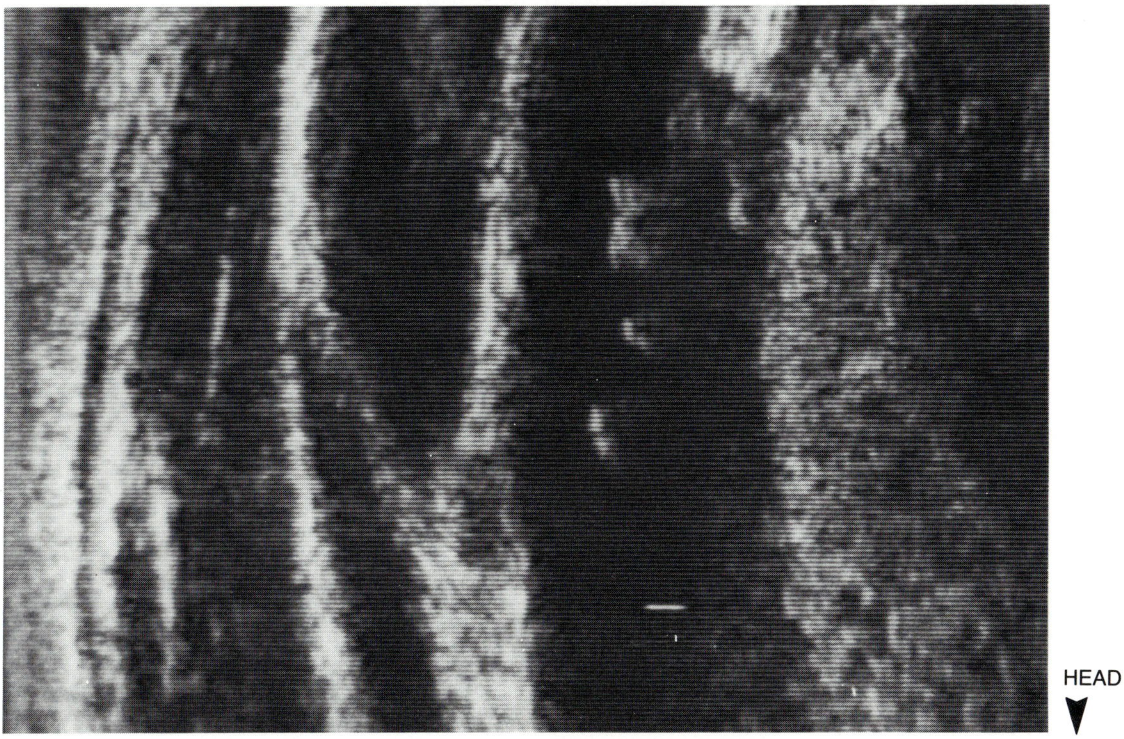
HEAD

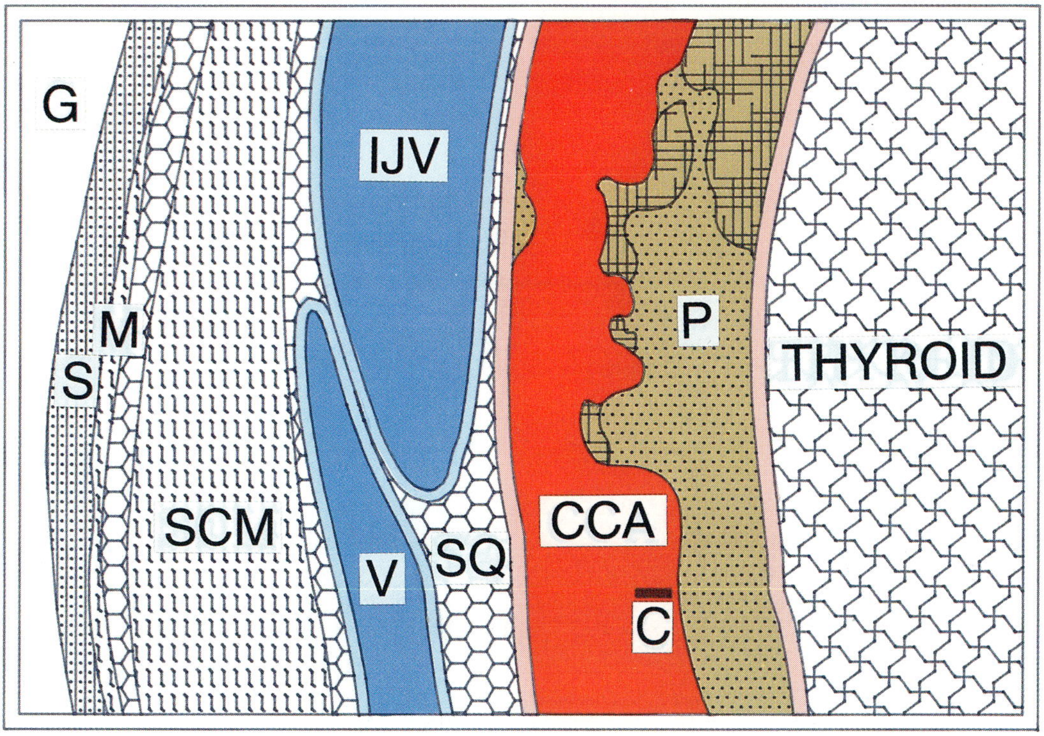
G
IJV
M
S
P
THYROID
SCM
V
SQ
CCA
C

Figure 74. HIGHLY IRREGULAR PLAQUE

This longitudinal view of highly irregular plaque (P) on the deep wall of the left carotid bifurcation was obtained by a slightly more posterior rocking of the probe compared with Figure 47. Note the surface contour of this plaque with indentations and sharp projections suggestive but not diagnostic of ulceration. Sometimes plaque can appear to be more irregular than it really is. This often occurs when the ultrasound beam is directed off center through the artery, and one begins to see portions of the plaque wrapped around the "back wall." These portions of the plaque that are seen at a very glancing angle give highly exaggerated projections, sometimes appearing as isolated "islands" of plaque in the center of the artery. Such is not the case here, however. This plaque had the appearance of surface irregularities regardless of rocking the probe (compare with Figure 47). Note also the "hard line" (HL) artifact in the darker portion of the deep field, which is totally obscured by the more echogenic tissues above. G = gel, S = skin, SQ = subcutaneous tissue, SCM = sternocleidomastoid muscle, F = fascia, CCA = common carotid artery, ICA = internal carotid artery, ? = tissue of uncertain composition, AS = acoustic shadowing.

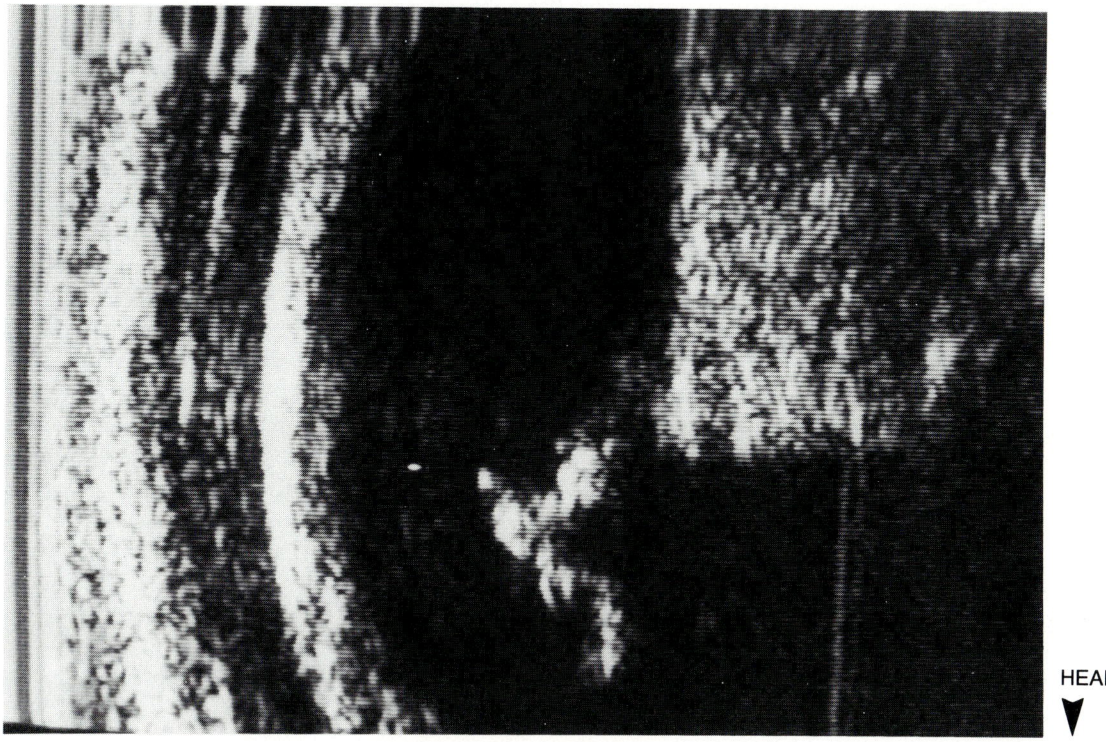
HEAD

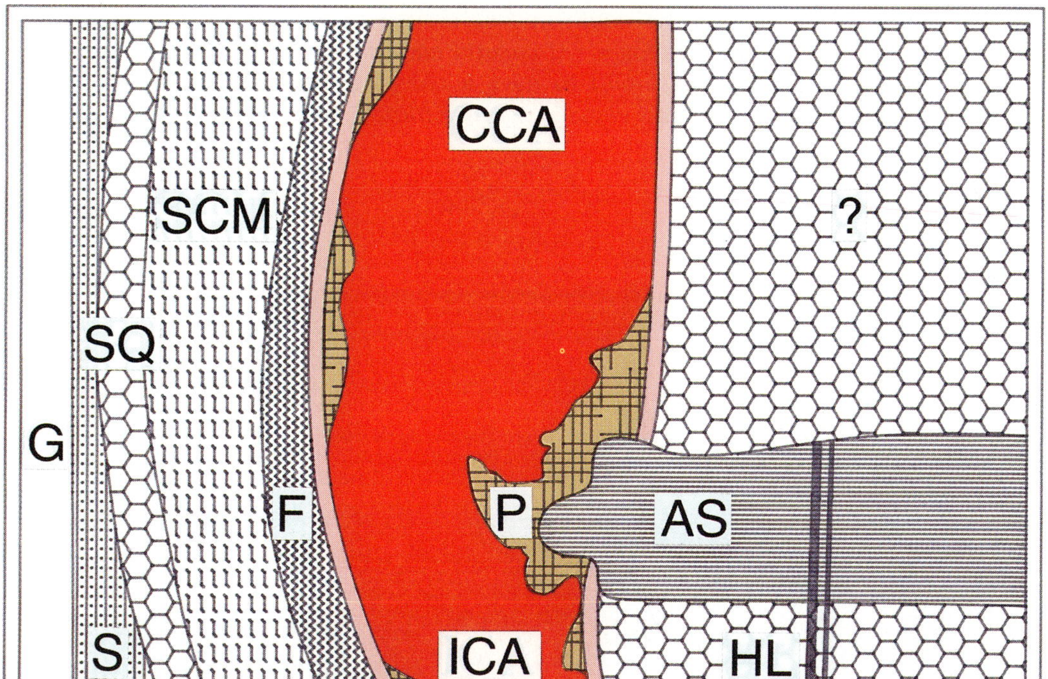
CCA
SCM
?
SQ
G
F
P
AS
S
ICA
HL

Figure 75. IRREGULAR RESIDUAL LUMEN

This is a transverse view of a right common carotid artery (CCA) demonstrating a highly irregular residual lumen as seen in transverse view. The plaque (P) is moderately echogenic but also moderately heterogeneous with bright and dark areas. In particular, there is a defect in the surface contour near the top of the artery that could be either an ulcer crater or a plaque of extremely faint echogenicity, which is not imaged in this particular view. Confirmation of this defect as truly representing an ulcer crater would depend upon the appearance in longitudinal views, preferably by applying the probe from a posterior approach on the neck (at the lower left corner of this transverse image) and angling the beam through the artery so as to pass to the upper right corner of this scan. By obtaining a longitudinal view in this manner, this portion of the plaque would be seen squarely on the deep aspect of the longitudinal view, which would improve the image quality of plaque in this area to the greatest degree. It is best to confirm the presence of actual ulceration by means of more than one view prior to diagnosis. G = gel, S = skin, SQ = subcutaneous tissue, SCM = sternocleidomastoid muscle, F = fascia, C = Doppler cursor, AS = acoustic shadowing, ? = tissue of uncertain composition.

HISTORY *This is of a 72-year-old male who experienced right-sided amaurosis fugax on three occasions in the week prior to the ultrasound scan. He had had progression of disease by ultrasound scanning to a 70% stenosis in the internal carotid artery above the level of this view compared with a 50% stenosis 16 months prior. These findings were confirmed by a subsequent arteriogram revealing a "90% internal carotid stenosis." At carotid endarterectomy 1 week following the ultrasound scan he was found to have a calcified irregular "thick and deeply penetrating plaque." He has remained asymptomatic over the following 5 months.*

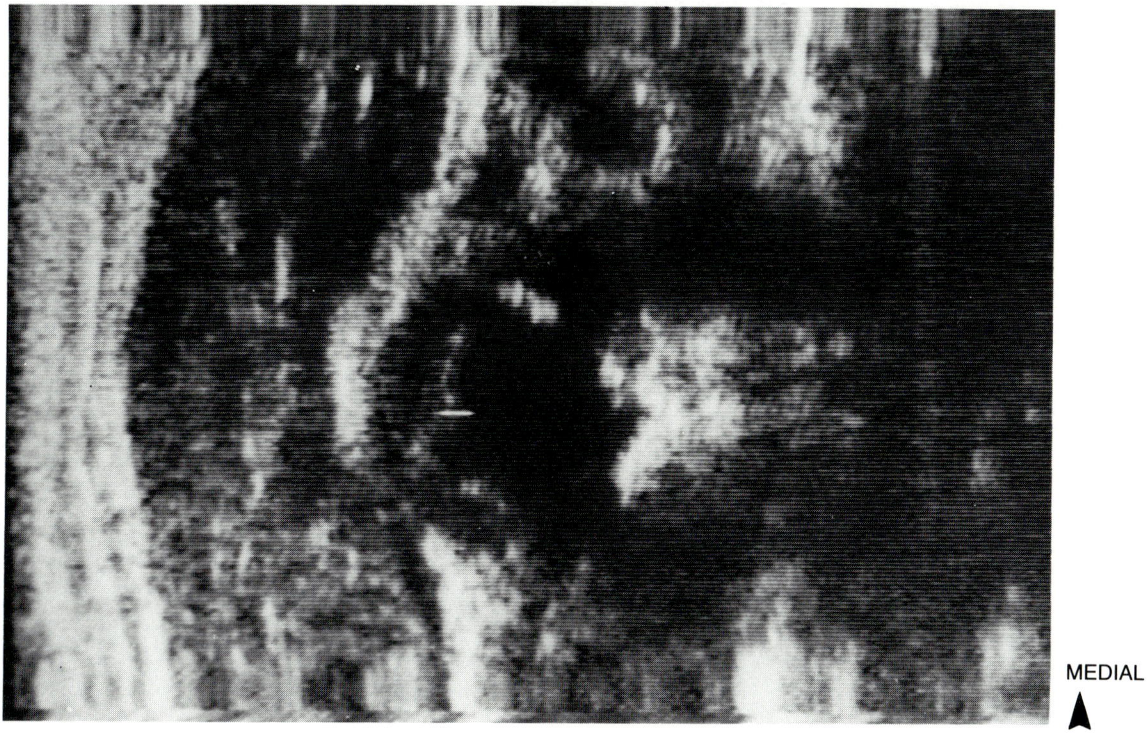
MEDIAL

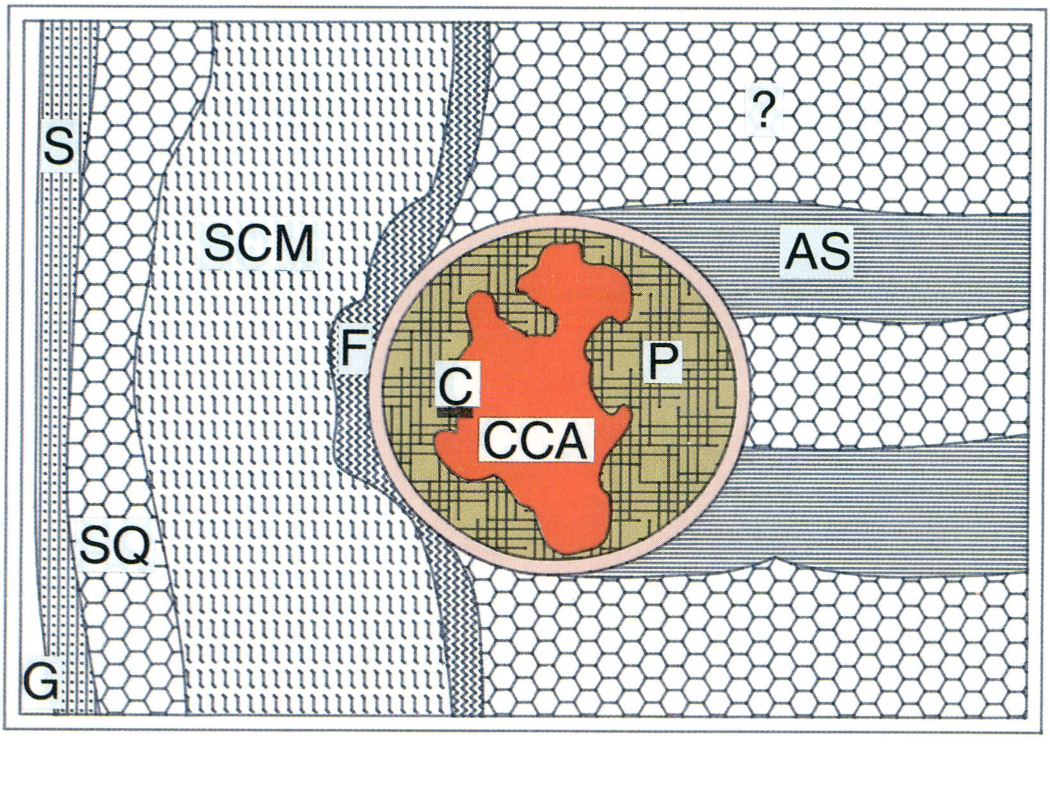
S
SCM
?
AS
F
C
P
CCA
SQ
G

Figure 76. IRREGULAR RESIDUAL LUMEN

This is an example of highly irregular plaque as seen in a transverse view just above the right carotid bifurcation. This irregular residual lumen is difficult to quantitate in terms of percent stenosis. The internal carotid bulb at this level measures 11.0 mm in diameter. The crossbar of the H-shaped lumen measures 2.0 mm in width; the width of the residual lumen from left to right measures 6.0 mm; and the maximum luminal diameter from lower left to upper right measures 9.5 mm in width. These larger and smaller diameters have a mean luminal diameter of approximately 6.0 mm. However, the distal internal carotid artery (ICA) above the plane of this scan is only 5.5 mm in diameter, and so by comparison with the distal artery this plaque effectively has a 0% stenosis. (From the vessel wall, the plaque is not calcified.) G = gel, S = skin, SQ = subcutaneous tissue, M = muscle, F = fascia, V = internal jugular vein, ECA = external carotid artery, ICA = internal carotid artery, P = plaque, AS = acoustical shadowing.

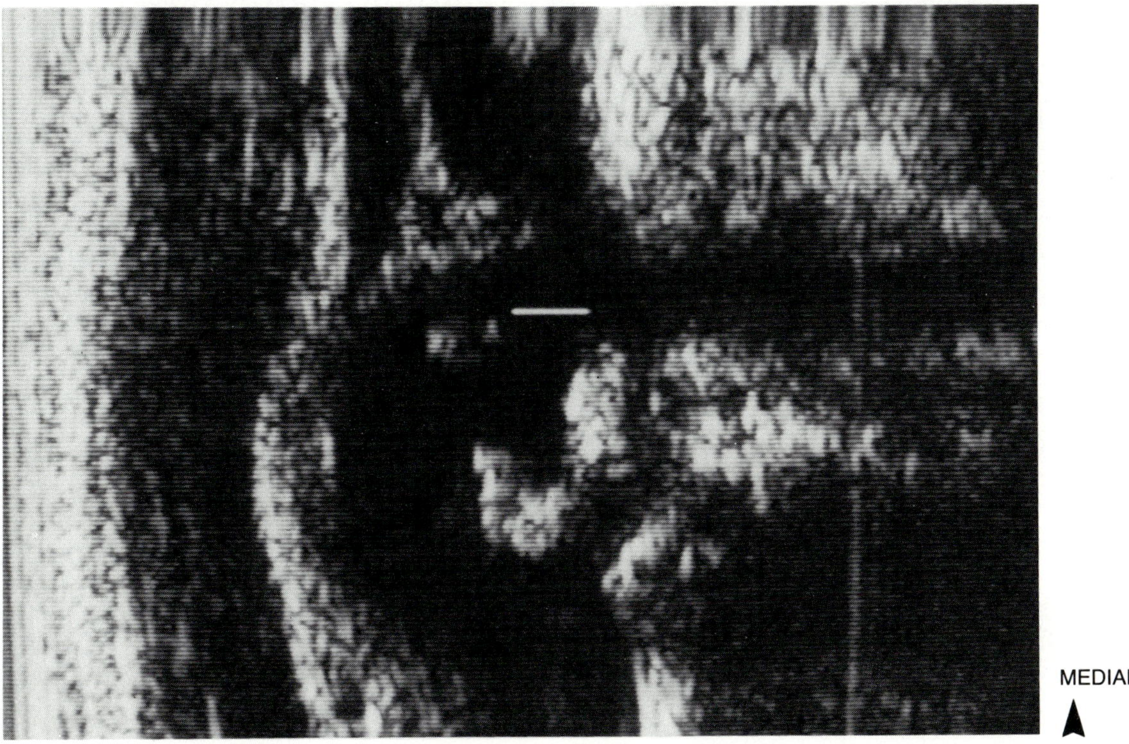
MEDIAL

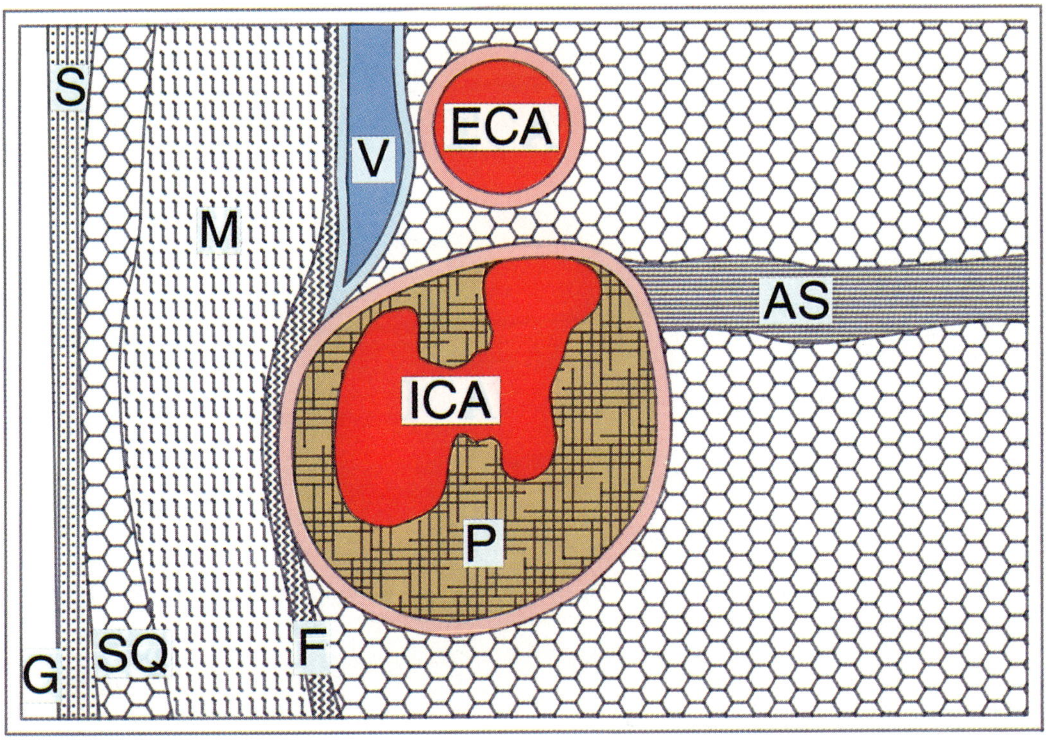
S
ECA
V
M
AS
ICA
P
G
SQ
F

Figure 77. ULCERATED PLAQUE—COMMON CAROTID ARTERY

This is a longitudinal view of the common carotid artery (CCA) below the bifurcation demonstrating an ulcer that measures 1.0 mm in depth and 3.5 mm in width. It is located within moderately echogenic and slightly heterogeneous plaque on the deep wall of the artery. Note the slightly overhanging upper edge of the ulcer crater that has a clearly punched-out appearance. Except for the presence of this ulcer, the plaque on the deep wall would be described as only mildly irregular. Note also the variation in composition of plaque. The plaque on the superficial wall to the left has an extremely faintly echogenic and homogeneous appearance characteristic of lipid plaque. The plaque on the right is more brightly echogenic and characteristic of an organized fibrous plaque with a small area at its upper end that may be of lipid composition. The vagus nerve is seen deep to the artery and has the typical appearance of a small vessel filled with faintly echogenic material. Large nerves may look like thrombosed veins; the anatomical location becomes important in distinguishing between them. Deep to the vagus nerve is the thyroid gland that has a typical, moderately echogenic appearance with coarse heterogeneity, probably representing the larger follicles within the gland. L = lipid plaque, CCA = common carotid artery, U = ulcer, P = plaque, F = fascia (carotid sheath), N = vagus nerve.

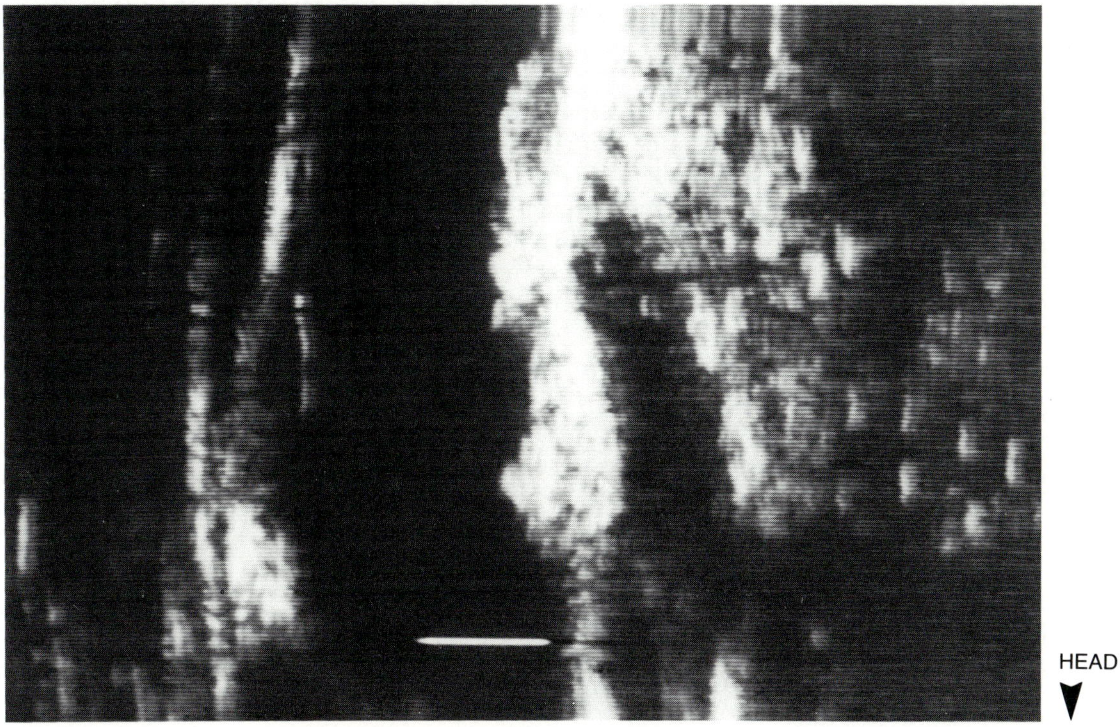
HEAD

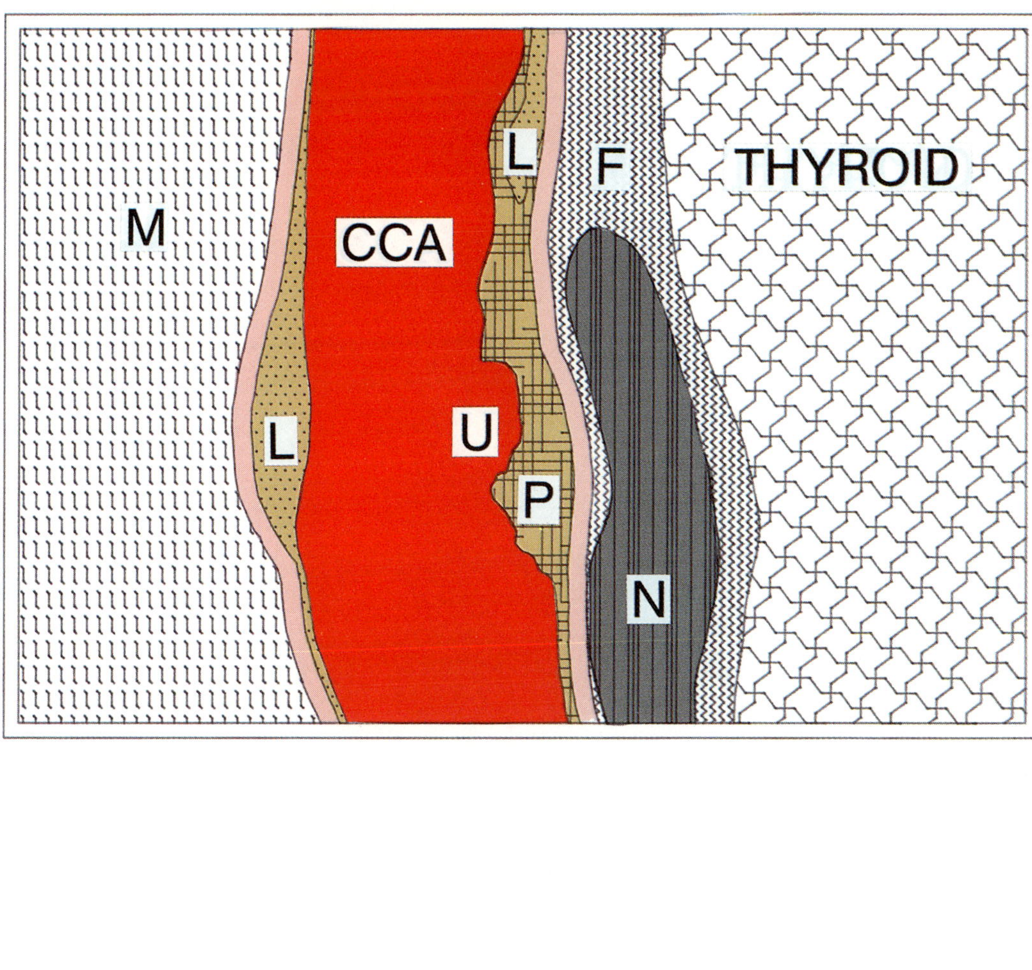
M
CCA
L
L
F
THYROID
U
P
N

Figure 78. ULCERATED COMPLEX PLAQUE—INTERNAL CAROTID ARTERY

This is a longitudinal view of the right carotid bifurcation with a large heterogeneous, highly echogenic, moderately irregular plaque causing approximately a 70% stenosis of the origin of the internal carotid artery (ICA). The residual lumen measures 1.2 mm in diameter. Note the punched-out appearance of this moderate sized ulcer (U), which is 1.8 mm in depth and 2.5 mm in width. The plaque (P) is of brighter echogenicity near the surface than near the arterial wall. Perhaps some intraplaque hemorrhage (H) has dissected along the base of the plaque. The particularly bright section of plaque below the ulcer is calcified with acoustic shadowing (not drawn) to the right. The external carotid artery (ECA) must originate directly superficial to the internal carotid artery without rotation in order to obtain this "tuning-fork" configuration. This particular view is often difficult to achieve because of variations in rotation of the vessels at the bifurcation. The sternocleidomastoid muscle (M) is to the left. SQ = subcutaneous tissue, CCA = common carotid artery.

HISTORY *This ulcer had been found on a screening carotid scan 20 months previously. The patient had symptomatic lower extremity vascular disease. He was without any cerebrovascular symptoms up until the time of this ultrasound scan, 20 months later.*

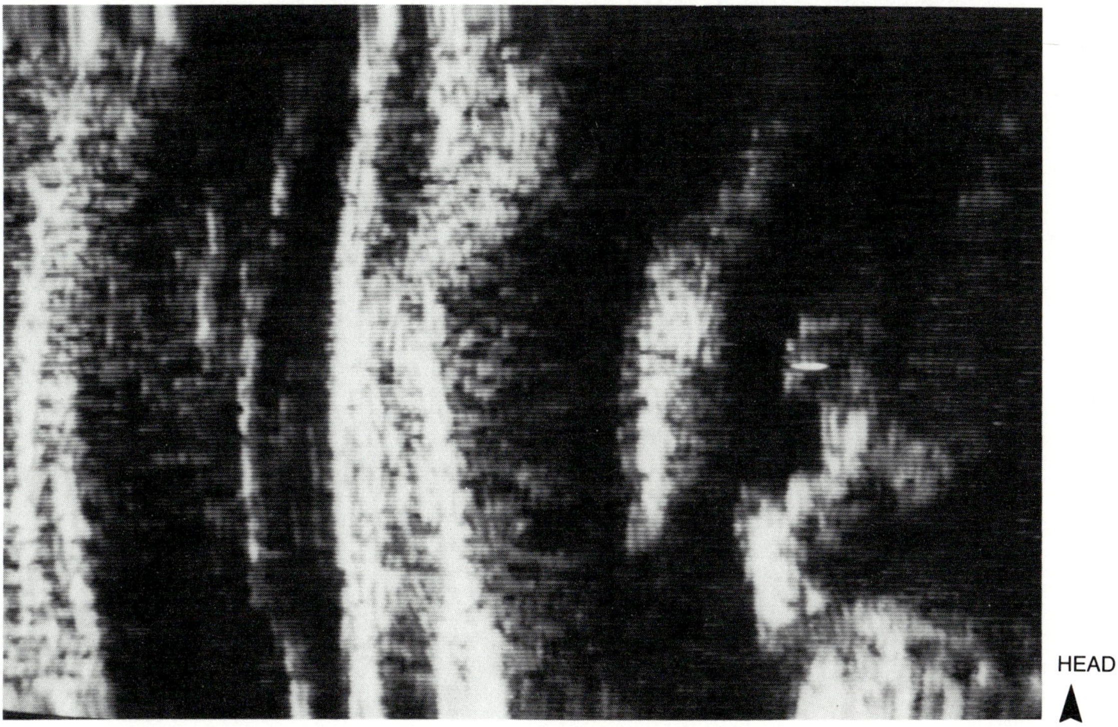
HEAD

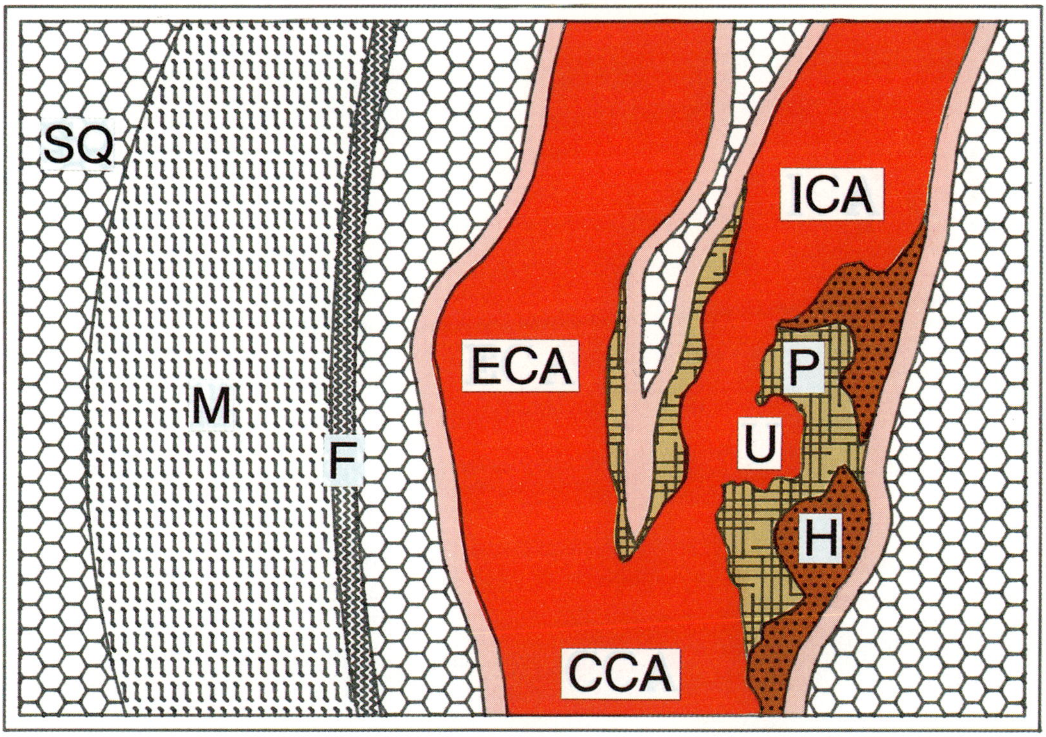
SQ
M
F
ECA
ICA
P
U
H
CCA

Figure 79. LARGE INTERNAL CAROTID ULCER

This is a longitudinal view of the left carotid bifurcation with the internal carotid artery (ICA) containing a large ulcer (U) with quite abrupt shelving edges above and below the crater. This ulcer crater measures 2.5 mm in depth by 6.5 mm in width. Distally, where the Doppler cursor is located, the ICA becomes severely stenotic with a residual lumen of 0.5 mm. This plaque is not only ulcerated, but also brightly echogenic and very heterogeneous with evidence of intraplaque hemorrhage (H). This is termed a complex plaque. P = plaque, CCA = common carotid artery, ECA = external carotid artery, SQ = subcutaneous tissue, M = sternocleidomastoid muscle, F = fascia.

HISTORY *Despite the very large size of the ulcer, this 72-year-old patient had been asymptomatic with complaints only of occasional episodes of dizziness.*

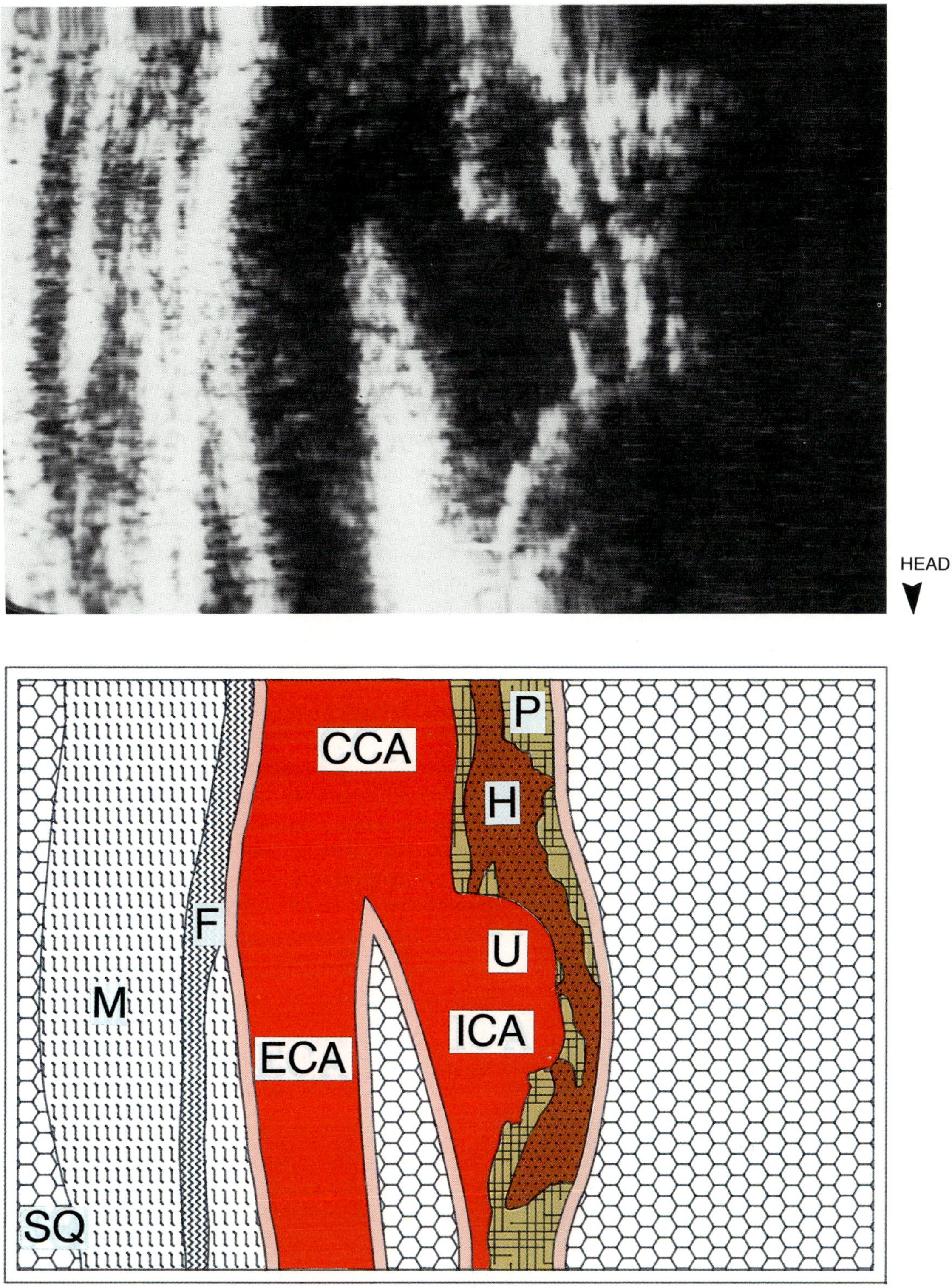
HEAD
CCA
P
H
F
U
M
ICA
ECA
SQ

Figure 80. SMALL CAROTID ULCER

This is one of the smallest ulcers (U) in our clinical experience in which a definite crater with overhanging edges can be seen. This ulcer crater measures 1.5 mm in depth and in width. The plaque (P) on the superficial wall is moderately heterogeneous with a bright "fibrous" type layer covered by more faintly echogenic material characteristic of lipid. Most of this plaque is so faintly visible that when the gains are low (as seen on the left) it is very difficult to see the outlines. When the overall brightness is increased (as seen on the right) the plaque becomes more clearly visible, although there is saturation of the gray scale echoes within the superficial tissues and carotid sheath. The brightening of the image in this case was done photographically. It can also be done by means of the gain controls on the machine and also by computerized post-processing of the image, a technique that is available from many manufacturers of ultrasound instruments. It has been our experience, however, that while post-processing of these images can serve to highlight details involving particular shades of gray, it will not, render visible any plaque or other feature that is totally invisible on the original image. Once one becomes accustomed to the particular shades of gray associated with plaque, one will find that these other techniques are superfluous and offer little advantage over the human eye. This is a learning process, however, and most interpreting physicians find that it takes about 3 months of reading ultrasound scans before they are comfortable in distinguishing plaque from artifact in poor quality ultrasound scans. S = skin, M = platysma muscle, SQ = subcutaneous tissue, SCM = sternocleidomastoid muscle, F = fascia (carotid sheath), CCA = common carotid artery, ICA = internal carotid artery, ? = tissue of uncertain composition.

HISTORY *This is a 71-year-old male who had presented 4 years prior to this ultrasound scan with a transient ischemic attack involving left upper extremity paresis. Following this ultrasound scan the patient underwent an arteriogram that also revealed a defect consistent with an ulcer. The patient was treated with aspirin and dipyridamole until a subsequent ultrasound scan showed progression of stenosis 1 year later. At that time he underwent endarterectomy.*

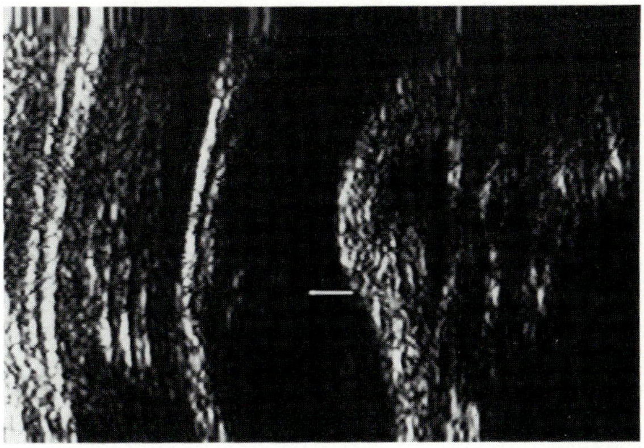
HEAD

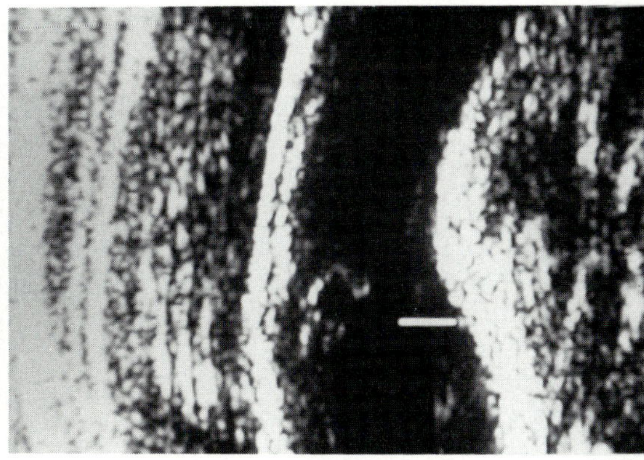
HEAD

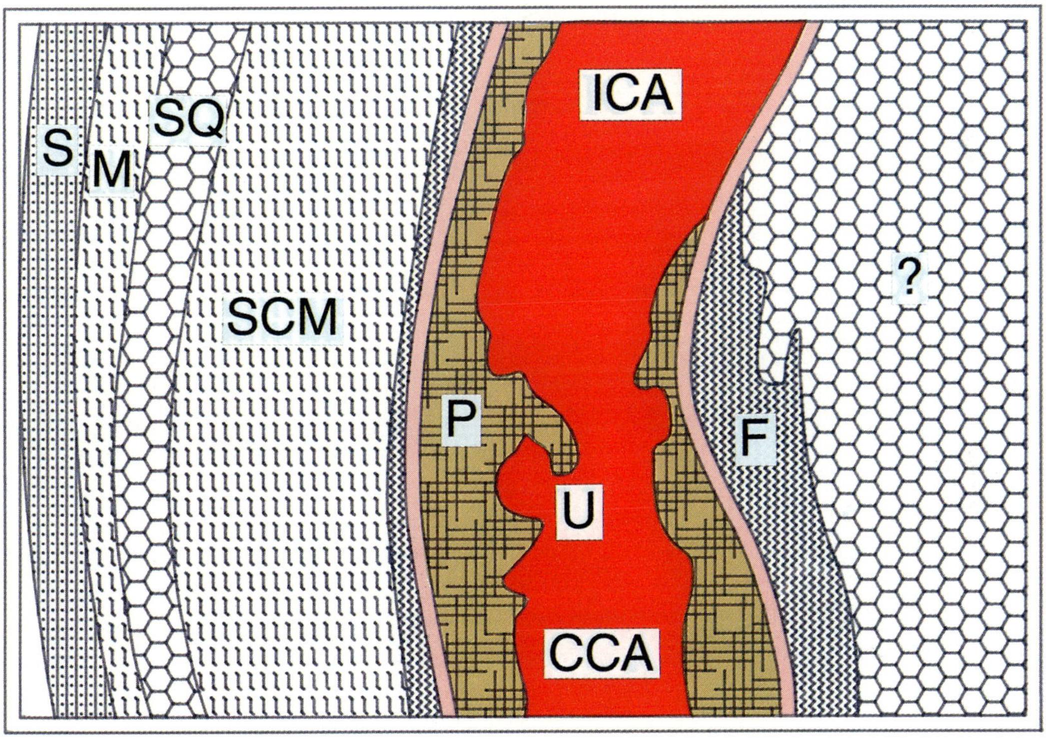
S
M
SQ
SCM
P
ICA
U
CCA
F
?

Figure 81. SMALL ULCERATED PLAQUE

This longitudinal view of the right internal carotid artery (ICA) above the bifurcation is notable for a quite small ulcer within moderately echogenic plaque on the posterior wall of the artery. The ulcer measures approximately 0.7 mm in depth and 1.5 mm in width. Note again the rounded crater formed by the ulcer. The internal jugular vein (IJV) is seen above and to the left with artifact within the superficial aspect of both vessels because of the high gain used to brighten this picture. SQ = subcutaneous tissue, M = muscle (platysma and sternocleidomastoid), F = fascia.

HISTORY *This 77-year-old female complained of diminished vision (scotoma) involving the contralateral eye. She had no symptoms referable to this ulcer.*

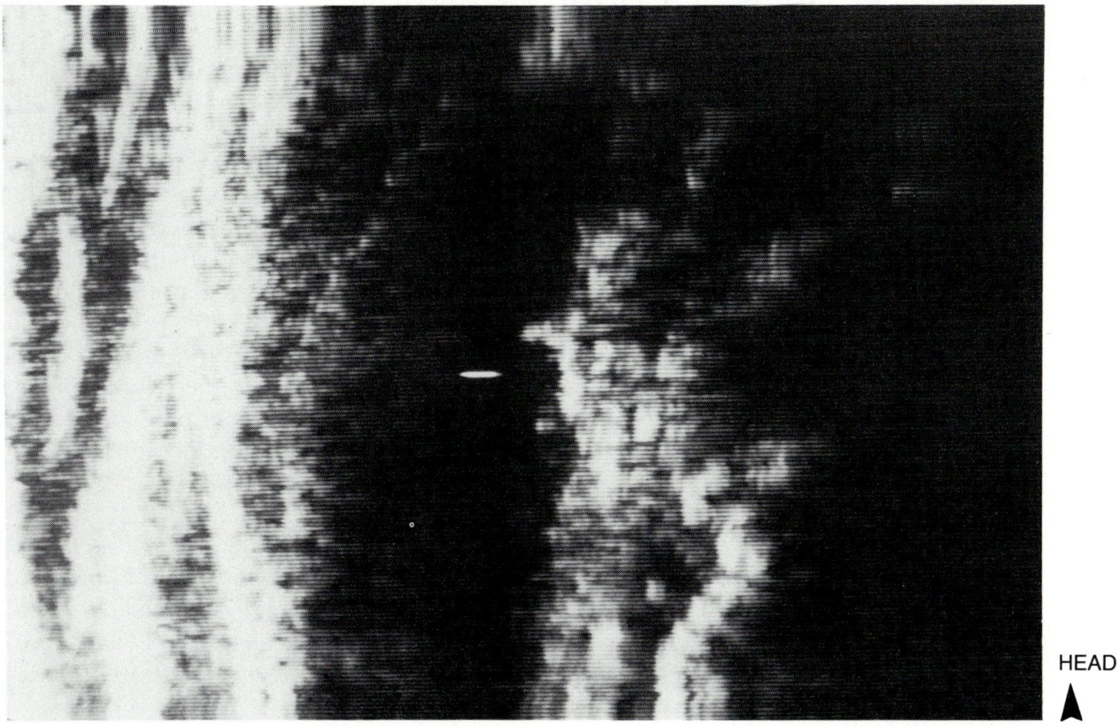
HEAD

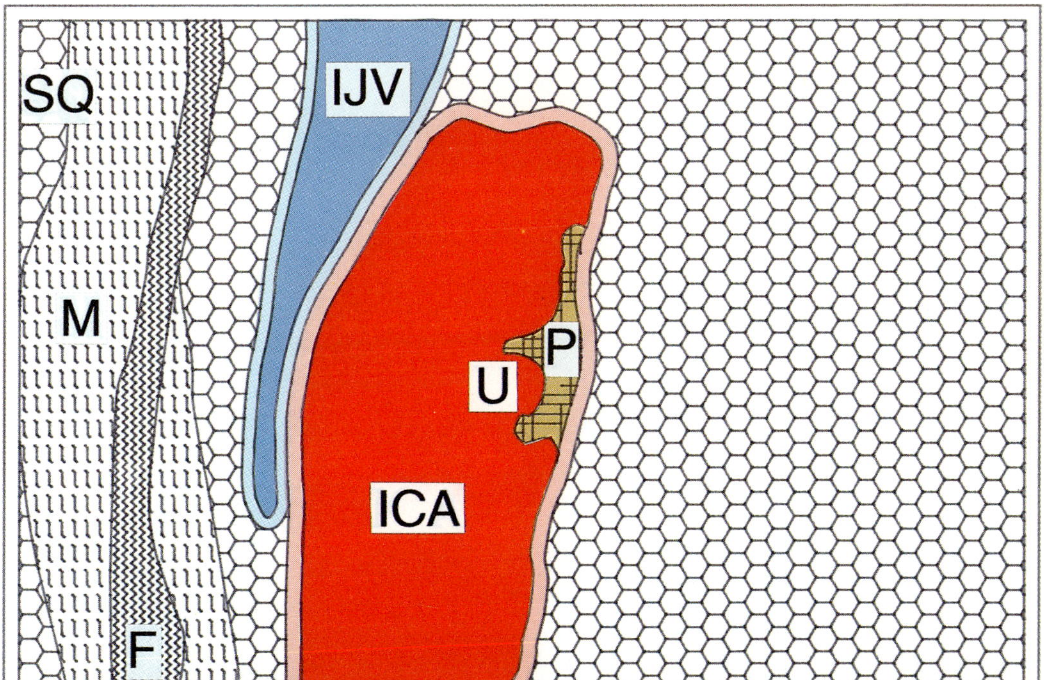
SQ
IJV
M
P
U
ICA
F

Figure 82. INTERNAL CAROTID ULCERATION

In this longitudinal view of a left internal carotid artery (ICA), brightly echogenic, somewhat heterogeneous plaque (P) is seen on the deep wall of the vessel with a pair of rather sharply punched-out defects in the plaque. The crater in the center of the ultrasound scan has the appearance of a definite ulcer (U). The defect in the deep wall plaque toward the bottom of the scan (higher in the artery) is possibly an ulcer (?U). However, it may also be a normal section of artery between the end of one plaque and the beginning of another. Whether this is a defect in a single plaque or a separation between two plaques cannot be determined. Both possibilities exist. Usually, ulcers do not present a difficult diagnostic problem. They tend not to penetrate all the way through to the arterial wall, exposing a significant length of it; rather they leave some residual plaque in the base, as in the upper of the two ulcers in the scan. SQ = subcutaneous tissue, M = sternocleidomastoid muscle, F = fascia, V = internal jugular vein.

HISTORY *This is an 81-year-old male who presented with slurring of speech and right lower extremity weakness, as a transient ischemic attack, 1 week prior to the ultrasound scan. An angiogram 13 days following the ultrasound scan failed to show any evidence of ulcerated plaque, but 1 day after the angiogram the patient underwent a left carotid endarterectomy, at which time ulcerated plaque was found.*

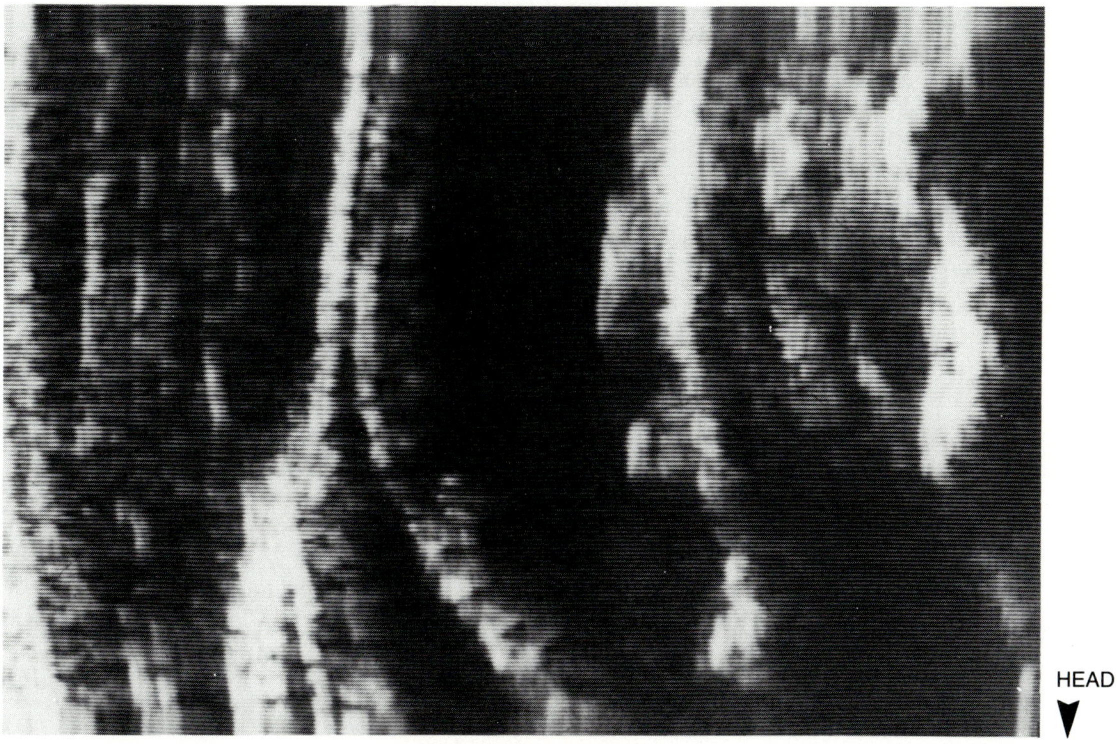
HEAD

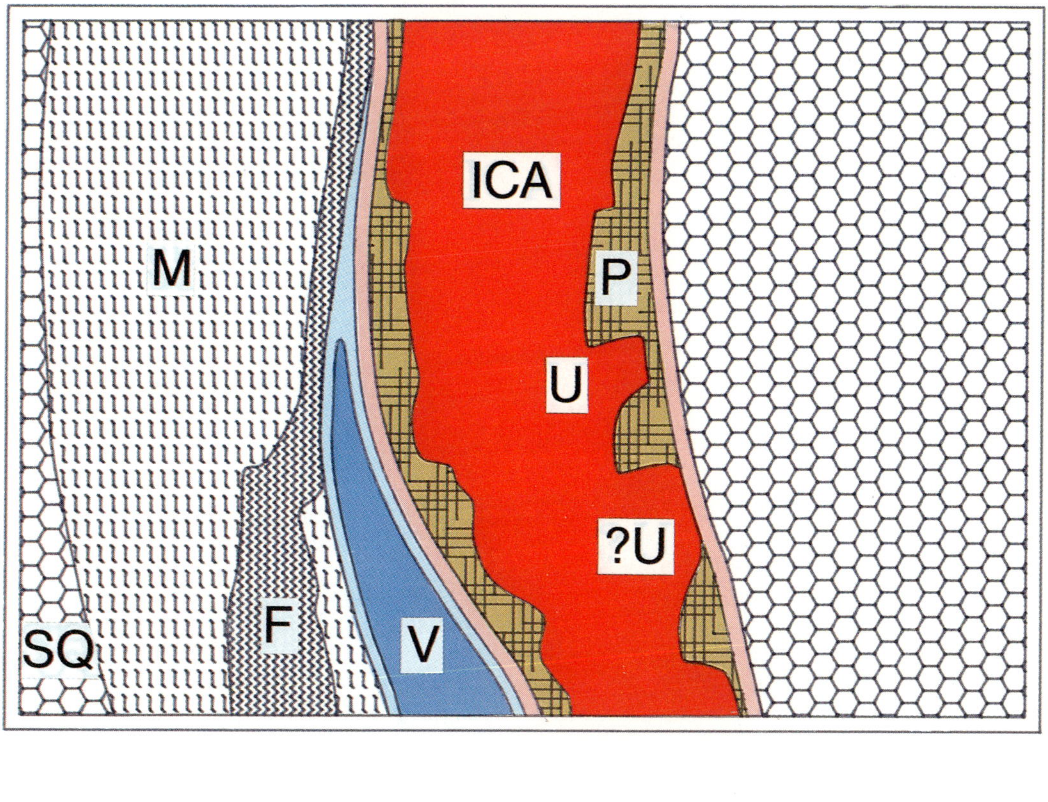
ICA
P
U
?U
M
F
V
SQ

Figure 83. CAROTID ULCER—OBLIQUE CUT

This view and the following two views demonstrate a rather large ulcer (U) within the left internal carotid bulb (ICA). The common carotid artery (CCA) is seen at the top of the scan, and the bifurcation of the external carotid artery is not seen but is located at the level where the plaque (P) begins. The probe is held in longitudinal orientation relative to the neck and arteries. The obliquity of the beam path relative to the ulcer crater does not permit visualization of the open channel that communicates with the residual lumen. This is shown, however, in the following view (Figure 84). The residual lumen is narrower than the overlying Doppler cursor (not drawn). The ulcer cavity is seen just immediately to the right. This mostly deep wall plaque has been separated by hemorrhage with intraplaque thrombus (T) surrounding the ulcer crater. The 4 MHz probe is occasionally useful for giving good overall views of long plaques for purposes of evaluating the contour. G = gel, S = skin, SQ = subcutaneous tissue, IJV = internal jugular vein.

HISTORY *This 70-year-old female had complaints of multiple episodes of right upper extremity numbness over the 6 months prior to this ultrasound scan.*

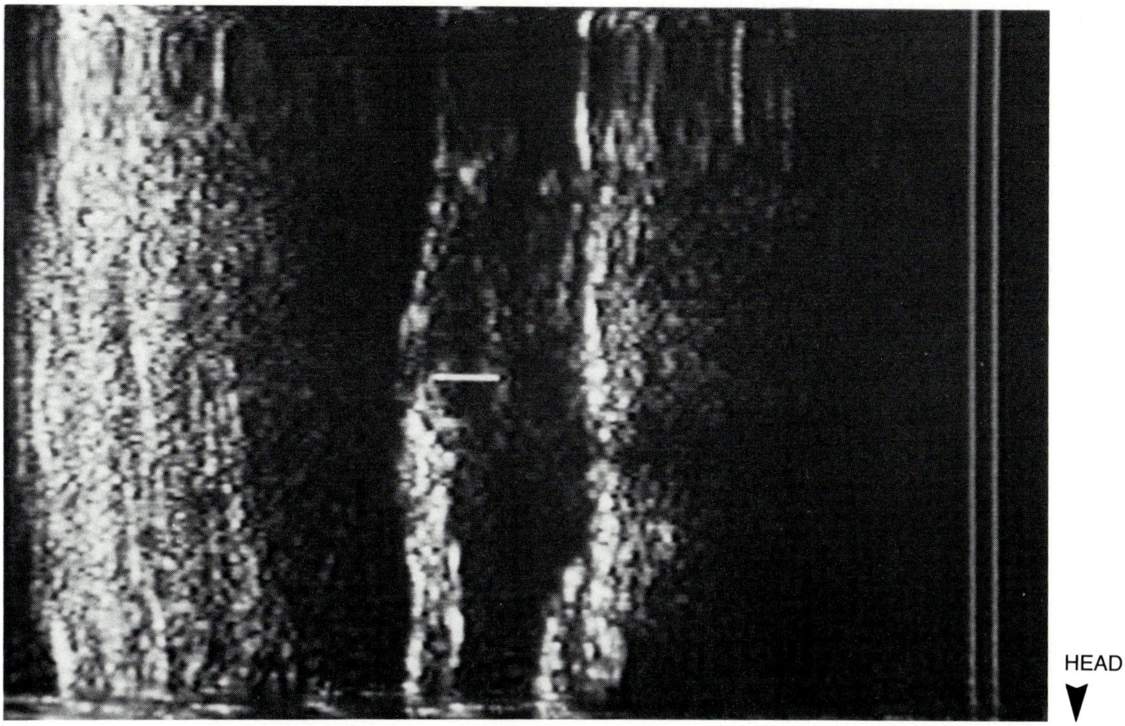
HEAD

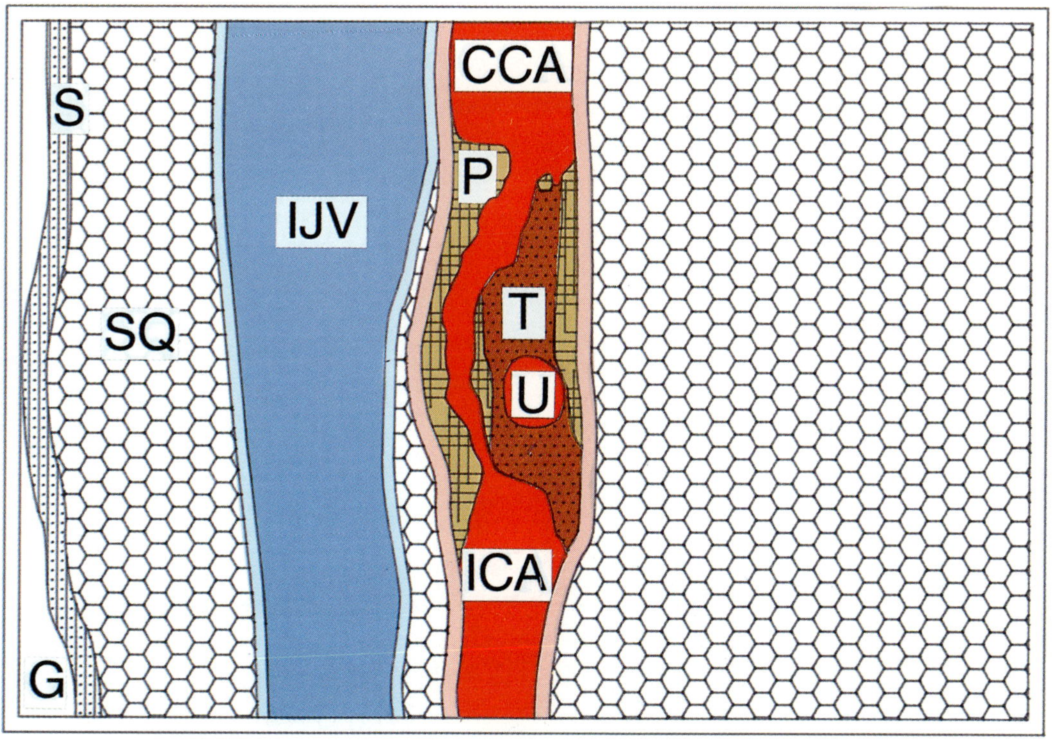
S
CCA
P
IJV
T
SQ
U
ICA
G

Figure 84. CAROTID ULCER—TRANSVERSE VIEW

In this transverse view at the level of the ulcer (U), faintly echogenic plaque (P) and thrombus (T) are seen outlining a dumbbell-shaped cavity, the neck of which corresponds to the communication between the larger ulcer crater and the true residual lumen. Doppler signals were obtainable at both ends, but the right half of this dumbbell-shaped cavity disappears at planes above and below this level, thus corresponding to the ulcer cavity. The internal jugular vein (IJV) is seen above and to the left of the internal carotid artery (ICA). A small lymph node (LN) is observed below the ICA and slightly to the left. The external carotid artery (ECA) is seen below and to the right of the ICA. Line #1 corresponds to the plane of the 4 MHz view, which passes through the internal jugular vein (Figure 83), and line #2 corresponds to the plane of the 8 MHz view that misses the vein and passes through the ulcer crater but not through the true residual lumen (Figure 85). M = sternocleidomastoid muscle, SQ = subcutaneous tissue, AS = acoustic shadowing.

HISTORY *This small residual lumen was judged to be hemodynamically significant by duplex scanning, and in fact a 70% stenosis was identified by arteriography.*

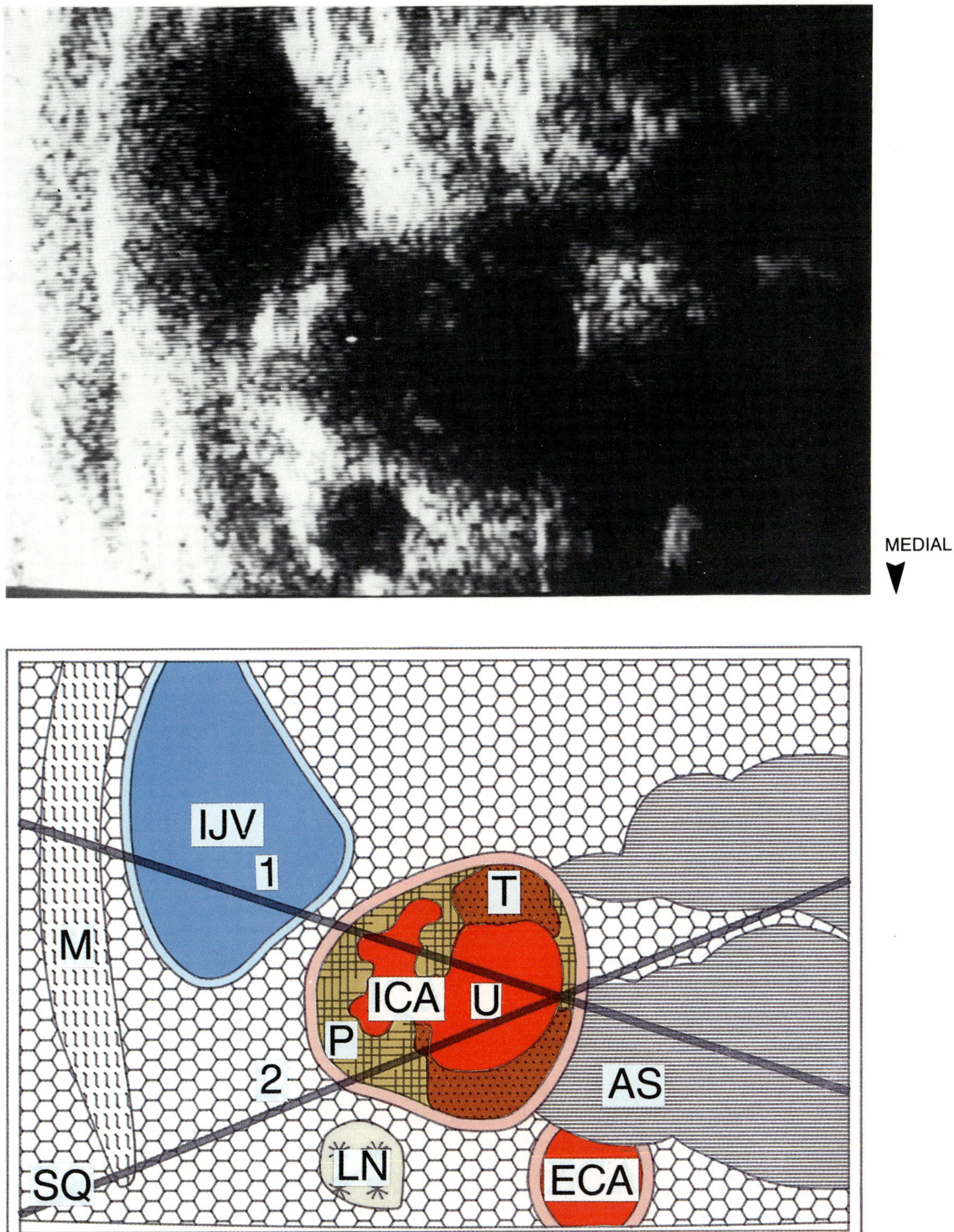
MEDIAL
IJV
1
T
M
ICA
U
P
2
AS
LN
SQ
ECA

Figure 85. CAROTID ULCER EN FACE

In this close-up view with the 8 MHz probe the open face of the ulcer (U) is surrounded by faintly echogenic material that is part lipid plaque (P) and part thrombus (T) at the base of the internal carotid artery (ICA). The common carotid artery (CCA) is seen at the top of the scan. The ulcer is situated just above the Doppler cursor (not drawn). This ulcer had easily detectable Doppler signals within it and could be seen to visibly pulsate in size in real time. Much of the artery appears to be totally occluded because of the plane of the beam through the vessel, which does not cut through the open residual channel. It is unusual to be able to see a cross section of the ulcer cavity as shown here. Usually, if the ulcer is large enough, it tends to be located on the deep wall of the artery. It is also difficult to position the probe far enough around the neck to see the ulcer en face. G = gel, S = skin, SQ = subcutaneous tissue, M = muscle (platysma and sternocleidomastoid).

HISTORY *The presence of this ulcer and the surrounding intraplaque hemorrhage was confirmed by arteriography, subsequent operation, and pathological examination 1 week later.*

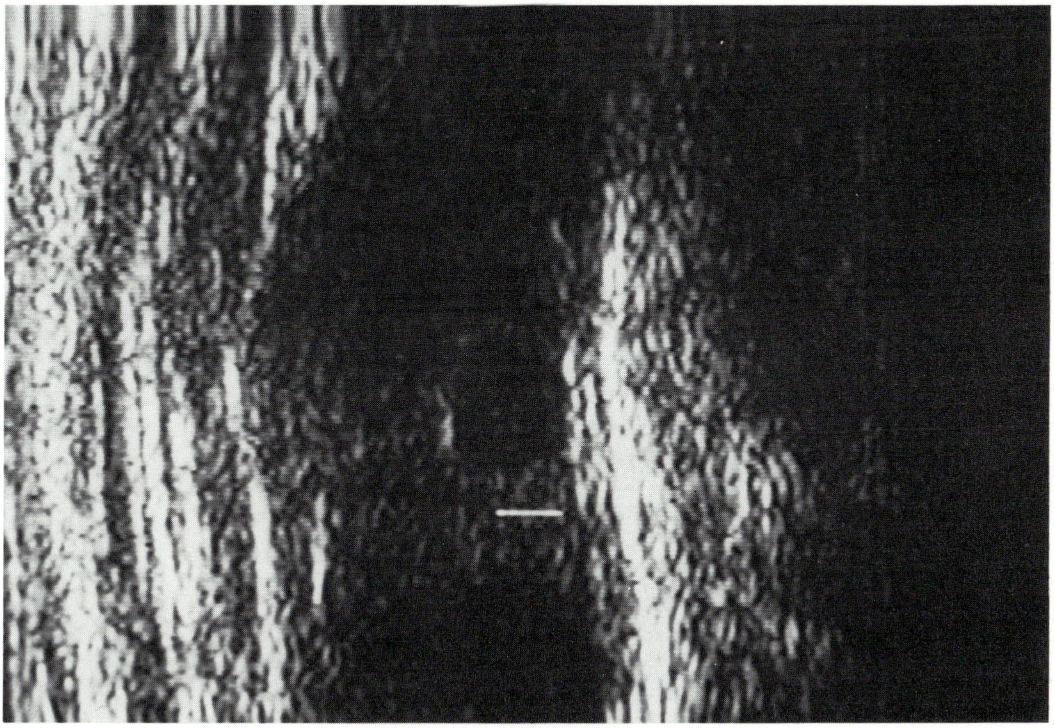

HEAD

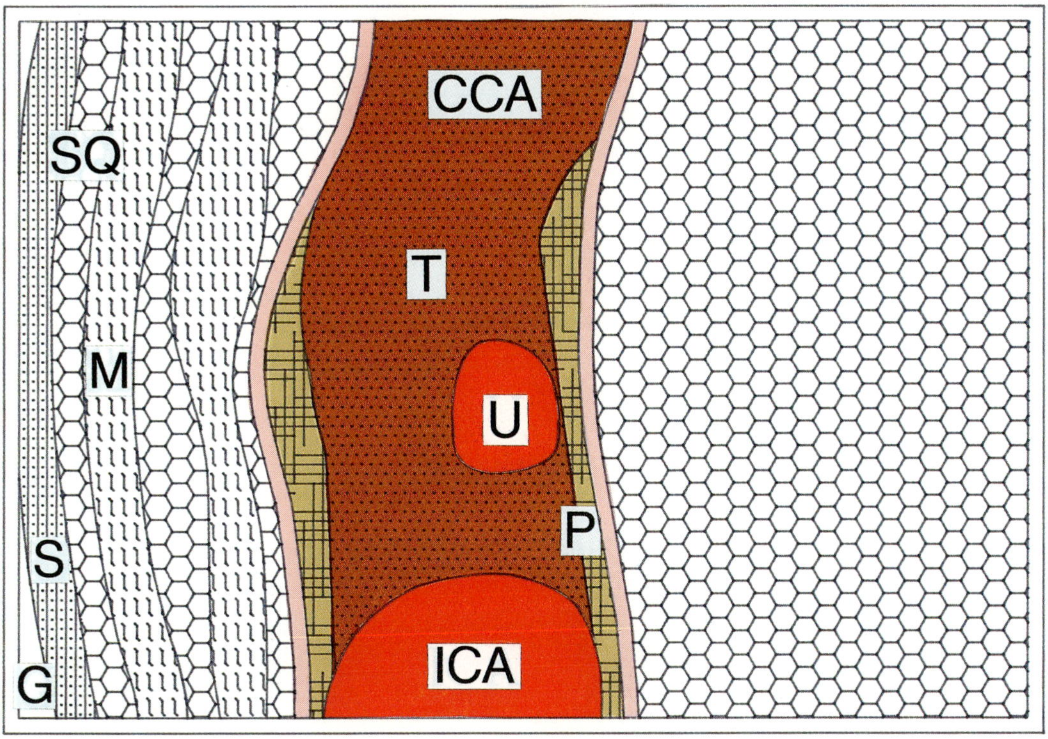

Figure 86. ULCER-CONTAINING THROMBUS

This is an interesting longitudinal view of a small ulcer (U) on the posterior wall of the internal carotid bulb. There is very faintly visible thrombus (T) within the ulcer crater itself. One might be inclined to think that this is artifact or that the faintly echogenic material in this crater is actually the back wall of the ulcer crater. However, compare the following Figure 87. The plaque (P) is characterized as moderately echogenic and homogeneous on the superficial wall to the left and mildly heterogeneous on the deep wall to the right. Except for the presence of this ulcer the plaque would be classified as moderately but not highly irregular. This photograph is somewhat underexposed throughout. Note the rather dark appearance of the skin and subcutaneous tissue. G = gel, S = skin, SQ = subcutaneous tissue, M = sternocleidomastoid muscle, F = fascia (carotid sheath), CCA = common carotid artery, ICA = internal carotid artery, DIST = distal internal carotid, ? = tissue of uncertain composition.

HISTORY *This 92-year-old female presented with bilateral lower extremity paresis as well as left facial paresis.*

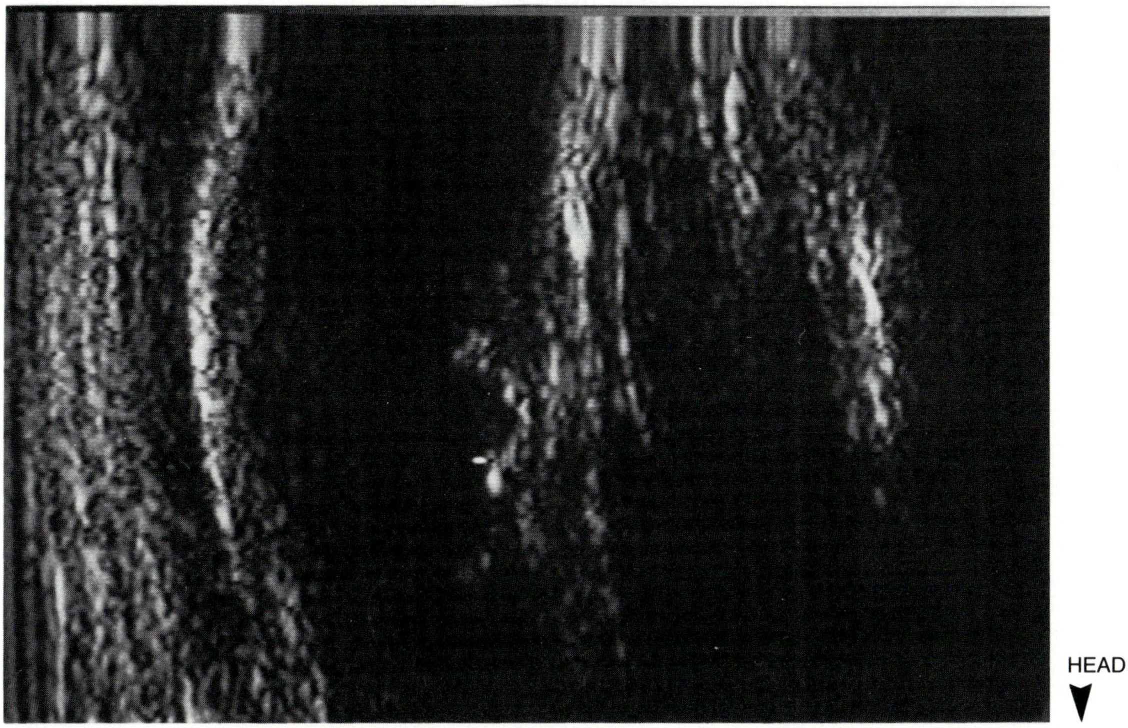
HEAD

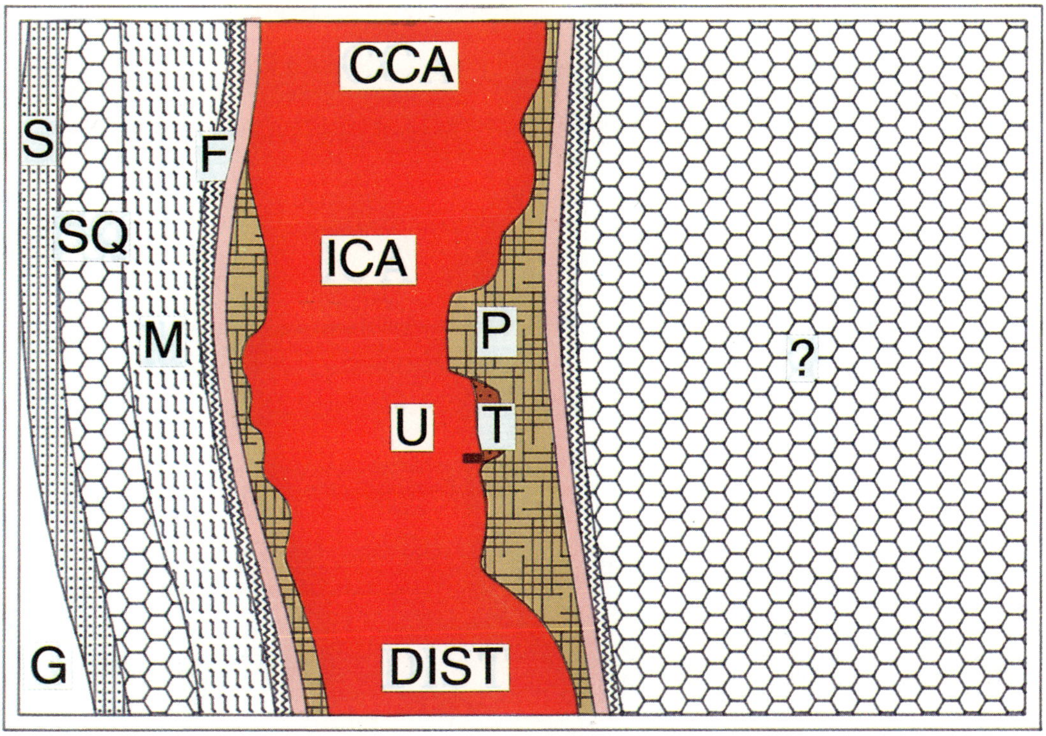
CCA
S
F
SQ
ICA
M
P
?
U
T
G
DIST

Figure 87. ULCER-CONTAINING THROMBUS

This is a second view of the same ulcer as seen by rocking the probe slightly to obtain a different cut through the common carotid artery (CCA) and internal carotid artery (ICA). The margins of the ulcer crater (U) are somewhat more prominent. Note the persistence of faintly echogenic thrombus (T) filling in the cavity within the ulcer. The plaque (P) is not as well seen on the deep wall because of shadowing but is somewhat more distinct on the superficial wall. G = gel, S = skin, SQ = subcutaneous tissue, M = sternocleidomastoid muscle, F = fascia (carotid sheath), ? = tissue of uncertain composition.

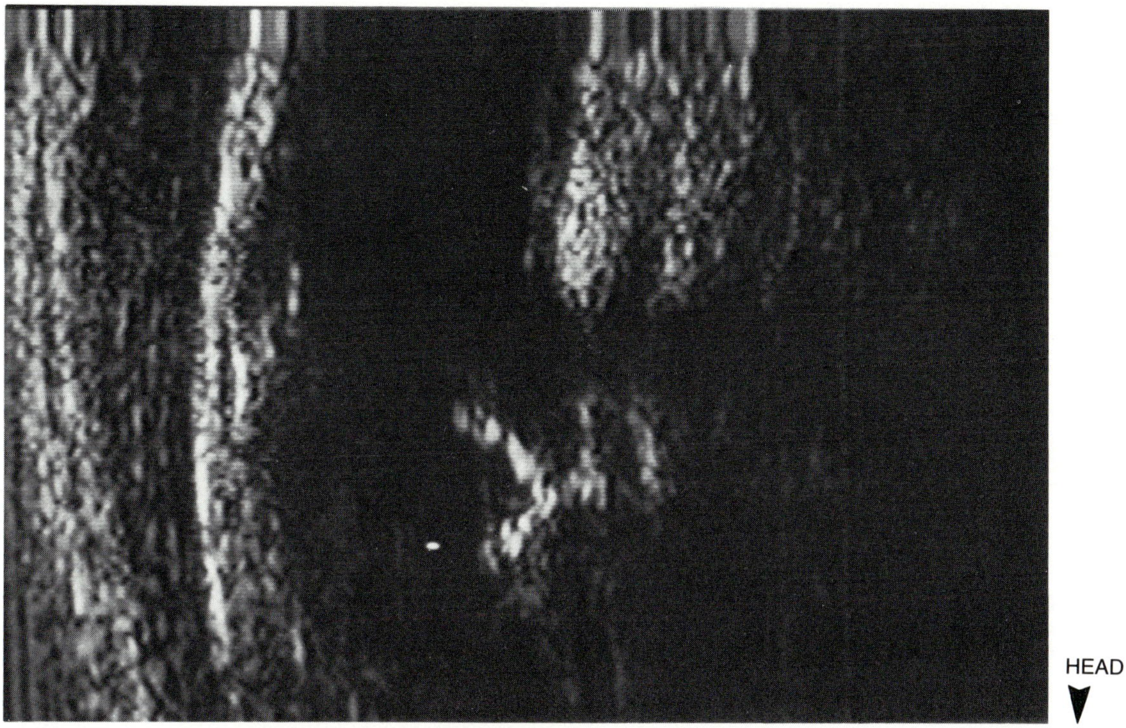
HEAD

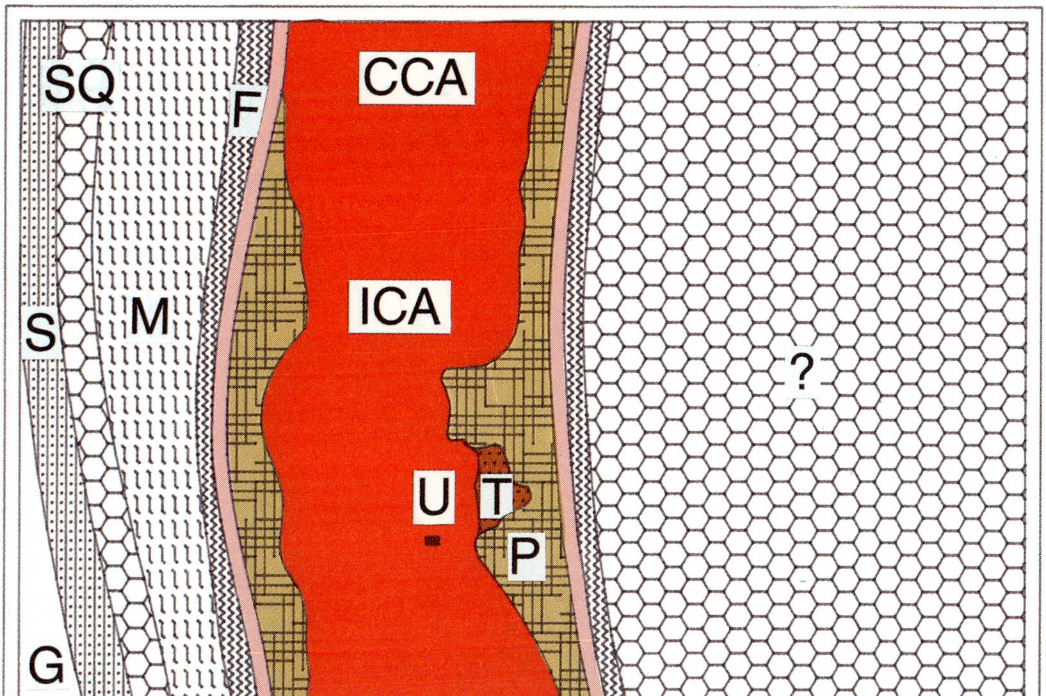
SQ
CCA
F
ICA
S
M
?
U
T
P
G

Figure 88. INTERNAL CAROTID WEB

This is a rather bizarre example of through-and-through ulceration of a faintly echogenic, homogeneous plaque (P) within the internal carotid artery (ICA), leaving behind a thin web (W) from the original plaque surface with the true lumen being located to the right of the web. The false lumen that had developed through the plaque, located to the left of the web, was shown to be patent with a pulsatile Doppler signal on both sides of the web. The internal and external carotid arteries are very superficial in this patient who had previously undergone a radical neck dissection with removal of the sternocleidomastoid muscle as well as post-operative radiation for squamous carcinoma of the larynx several years earlier. The presence of this web with a double lumen was confirmed at the time of endarterectomy. The web had been present for some time with endothelialized surfaces on both sides. This bifurcation is "reversed" with the ICA located superficial and medial to (below) the external carotid artery (ECA). S = skin, SQ = subcutaneous tissue.

HISTORY *This 58-year-old male presented with transient ischemic attacks involving his right hand 2 months prior to the ultrasound scan. He underwent left carotid endarterectomy 3 days after the ultrasound scan and has been asymptomatic over the following 18 months.*

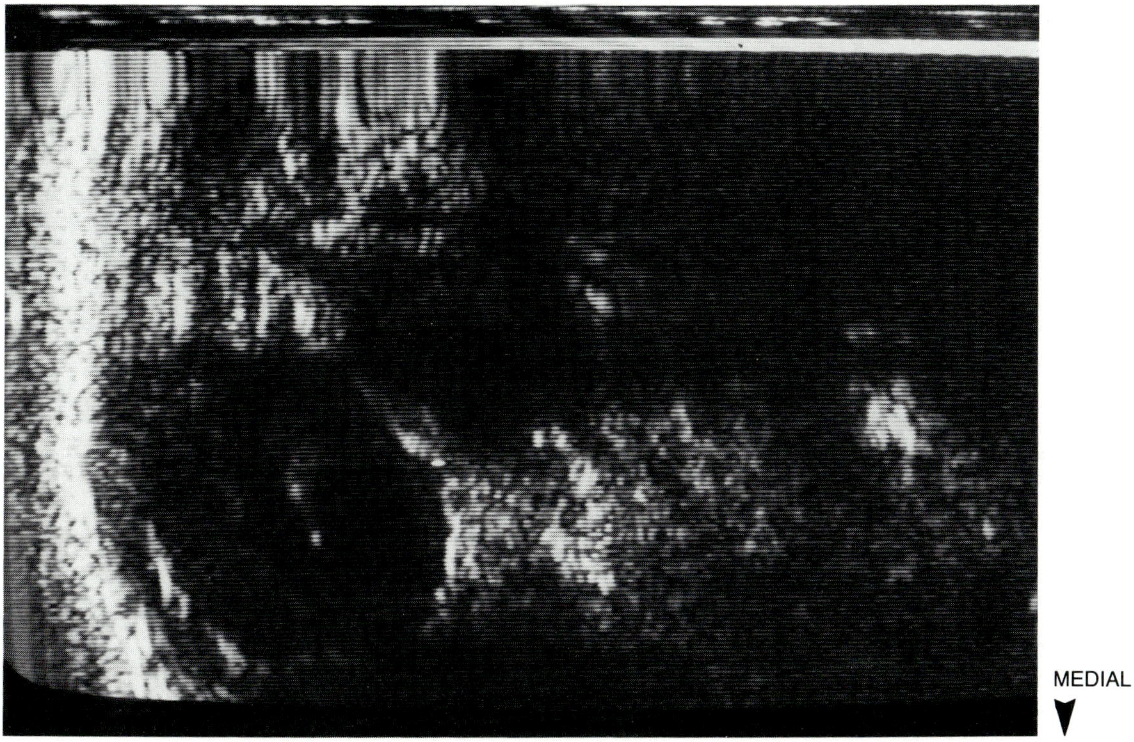
MEDIAL

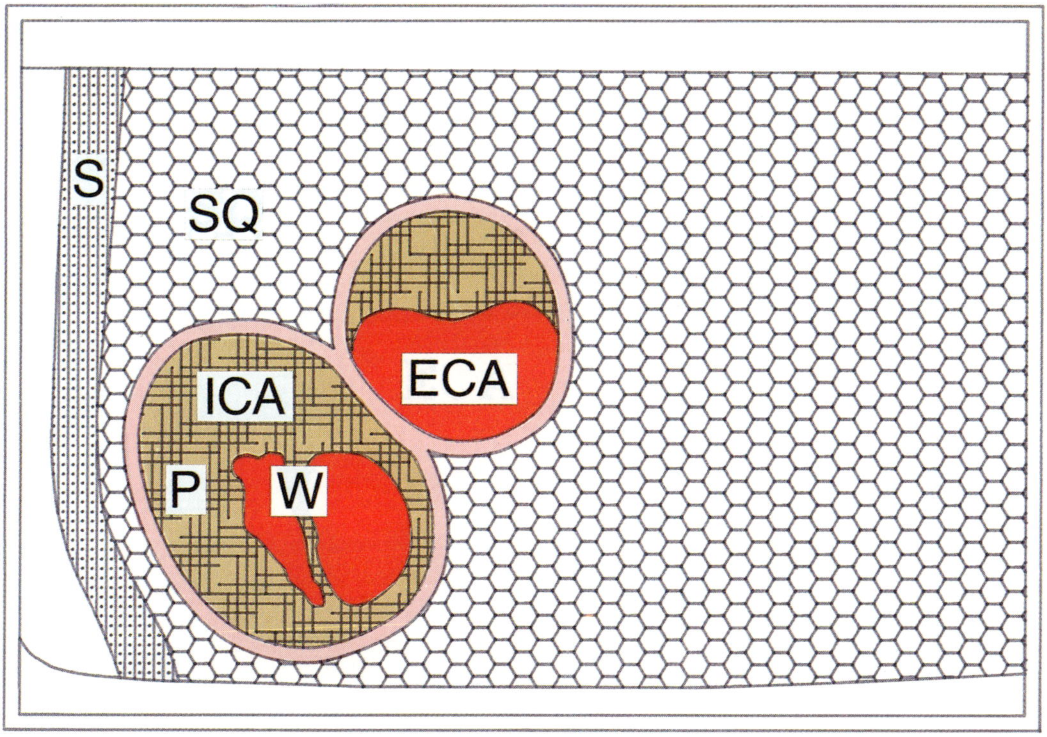
S
SQ
ECA
ICA
P
W

CHAPTER 5

TOTAL OCCLUSIONS

Figure 89. CHRONIC THROMBOSIS—INTERNAL CAROTID ARTERY

This photograph demonstrates a total occlusion of the left internal carotid artery (ICA) at its origin. Total arterial occlusions are distinguished by two characteristics as follows: (1) the lack of a visible lumen within the affected segment and (2) the lack of a Doppler flow signal within the segment. A helpful, but not absolute, criterion is the presence of a drumbeat type of Doppler signal just proximal to the point of occlusion. Another criterion is lack of visible expansion of the distal artery, but this is sometimes difficult to assess.

Acute thrombosis of a vessel can be distinguished from chronic occlusion by six additional criteria. First, an acute thrombosis tends to have a rounded or cup-shaped meniscus at the proximal extent. The second criterion is that the material within the occluded segment has the typical faint but speckled, only slightly heterogeneous appearance of clotted blood. In contrast, chronic occlusions tend to be more strikingly heterogeneous. The third characteristic, which is appreciated only in real time, is an up/down pulsatility that one can detect by watching the meniscus bounce longitudinally, as the systolic pressure beats against the freshly congealed and rather soft thrombus. This is perhaps the most important of all the criteria. The fourth characteristic is that acute occlusions tend to be associated with preservation of the normal diameter of the clotted arterial segment. In chronic thrombosis, this segment of the artery appears to shrink with time. The fifth characteristic is that because acute thrombus is faintly echogenic, the clotted arterial segment tends to have clearly visible walls. With time, the artery appears to fade into the background, as the plaque and thrombus acquire an echogenicity similar to the surrounding tissue. Often a chronically occluded arterial segment cannot be seen, since it blends in so well with the surrounding tissue. A sixth criterion is that the location of the meniscus in some but not all acute occlusions may be found more distally within the unbranched segment of artery beyond an arterial bifurcation. In chronic occlusions, this clot tends to propagate back to the point of bifurcation and is thus more consistently found to be an occlusion of the artery at its origin. This particular ultrasound scan demonstrates the following criteria for chronic occlusion: (1) the meniscus is not pulsatile; (2) the meniscus is also located at the origin of the artery, although admittedly it is cup shaped; (3) the artery beyond is relatively small in diameter, and especially distally the arterial walls are not well seen (see Figure 90); and (4) the material within the occluded segment, while less heterogeneous than sometimes found, is more heterogeneous than freshly clotted blood. ICA = internal carotid artery, CCA = common carotid artery, T = thrombus, V = internal jugular vein (partially compressed).

HISTORY *This patient had nonhemispheric symptoms 103 days prior to the duplex scan. Seven days after the scan a surgeon attempted an endarterectomy of the occluded carotid artery and confirmed a chronic occlusion with a fibrous cord distally within the artery.*

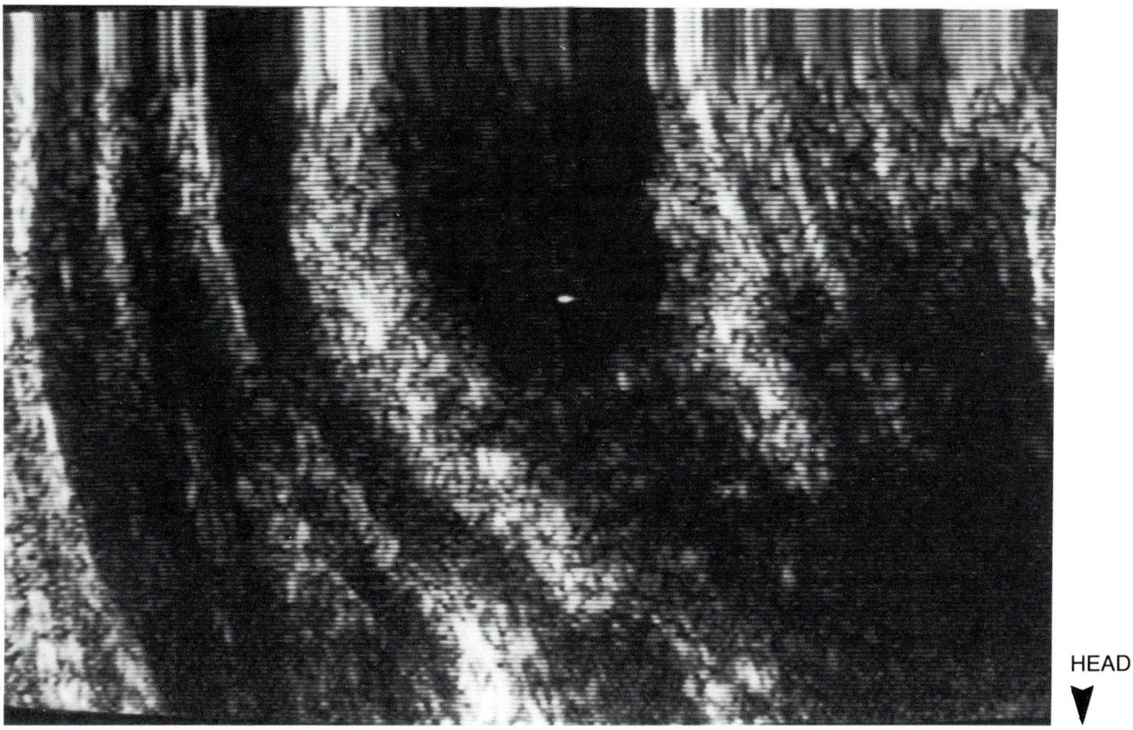
HEAD

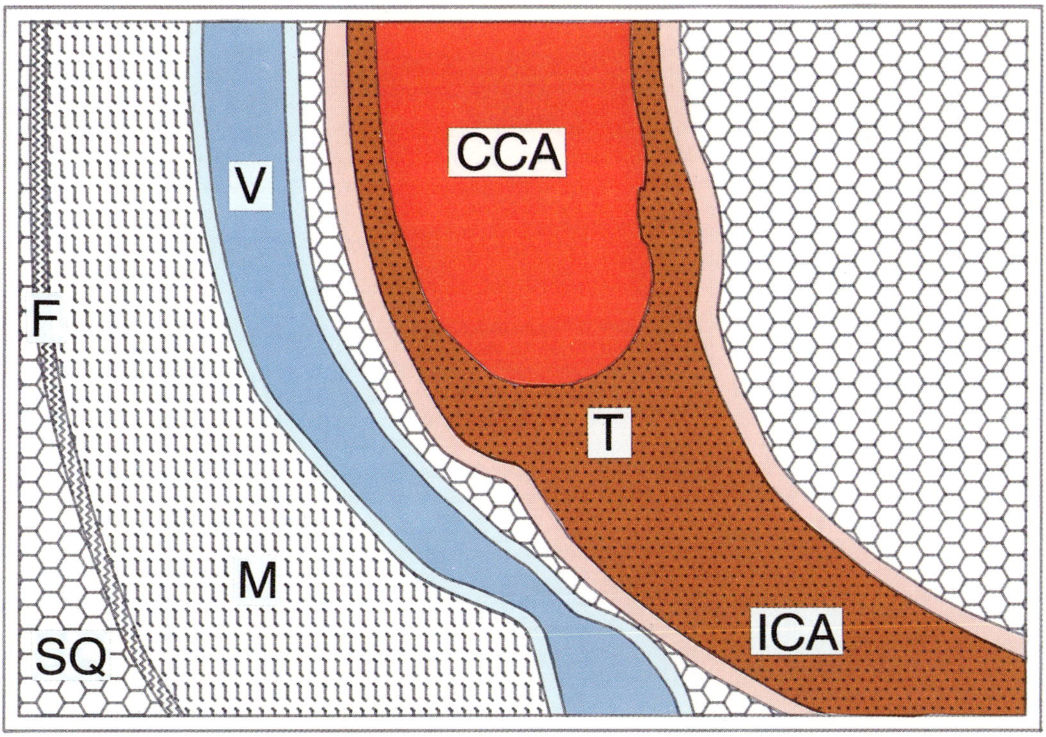
CCA
V
F
T
M
ICA
SQ

Figure 90. CHRONIC INTERNAL CAROTID OCCLUSION

In the transverse view of the same patient at a level slightly above the bifurcation, the entire left internal carotid artery (ICA) is seen to be filled in with moderately heterogeneous material. This heterogeneous obliteration of an artery, rendering it difficult to see, is typical of a chronic occlusion. There is also a thin rim of plaque (P) within the external carotid artery (ECA). The diameters of the internal and external carotid arteries are 4.5 mm and 4.0 mm, respectively, at this level. Just above the Doppler cursor (not drawn) is seen a dark area corresponding to the vagus nerve (VN). The internal jugular vein (V) lies below and to the left of the arteries. SQ = subcutaneous tissue, SCM = sternocleidomastoid muscle.

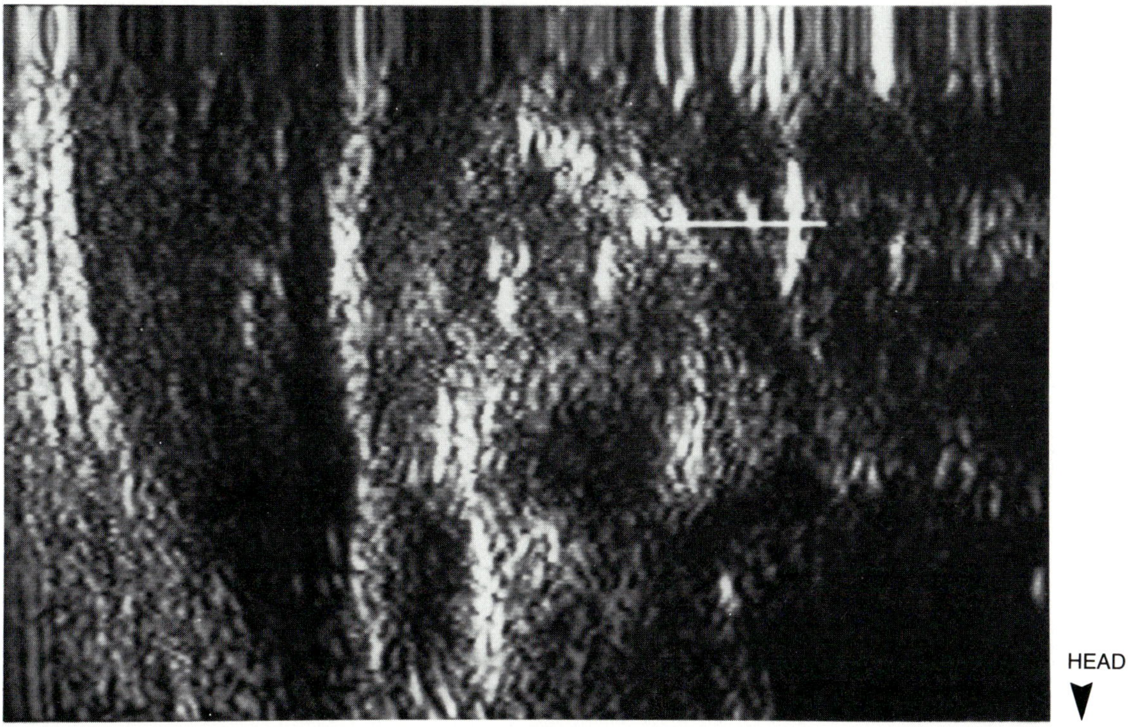
HEAD

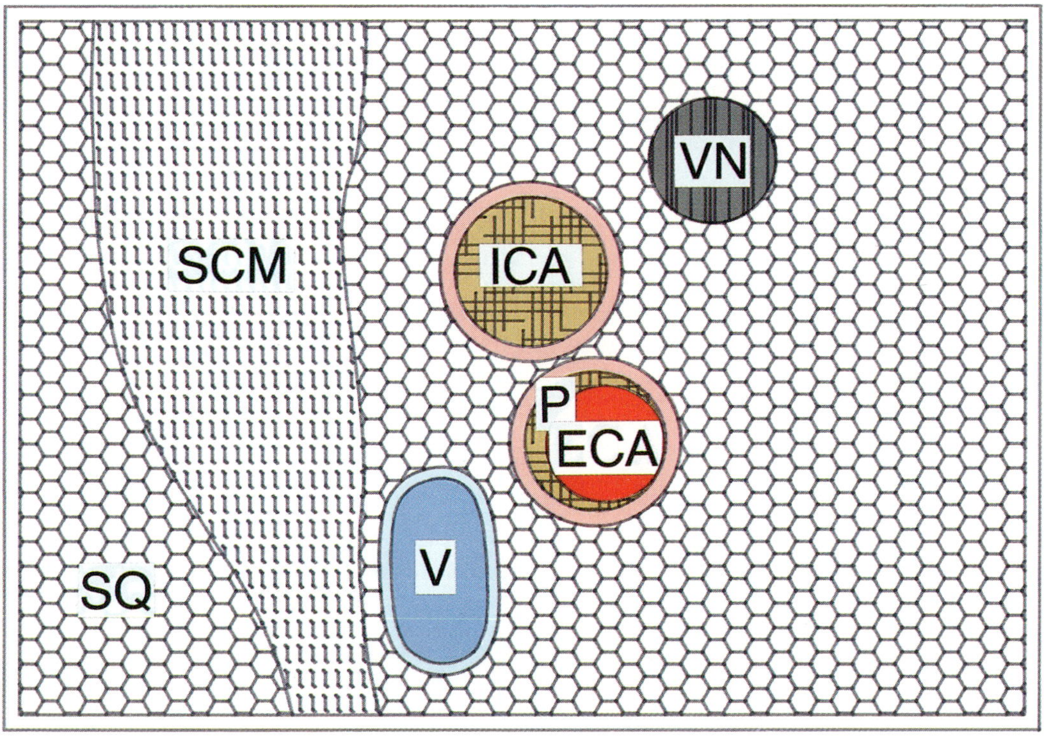
VN
ICA
SCM
P
ECA
V
SQ

Figure 91. ACUTE CAROTID THROMBOSIS

This is a longitudinal view of an acute occlusion of a right internal carotid artery (ICA) by extremely faintly echogenic thrombus (T). The plaque (P) that surrounds the thrombus is also faintly echogenic but somewhat brighter than the clot itself. The clot extends down to the internal carotid bulb with a smooth meniscus (M) at the level of the Doppler cursor (C). This meniscus manifested up/down pulsatility in real time. The junction of the internal carotid artery (ICA) and common carotid artery (CCA) is at the level of the CCA lettering. Note the extremely faint echogenicity of this acute thrombus. G = gel, S = skin, SQ = subcutaneous tissues (including platysma muscle), SCM = sternocleidomastoid muscle, IJV = internal jugular vein, BULB = internal carotid bulb.

HISTORY *This is of a 50-year-old male who presented with transient ischemic attack of $\frac{1}{2}$-hour duration, consisting of left upper and lower extremity paresis. The findings of a total occlusion were confirmed by arteriogram 5 days following the scan. A computed tomographic scan with enhancement on the same day as the arteriogram suggested patency of the intracranial carotid arteries. The occlusion was believed to be acute.*

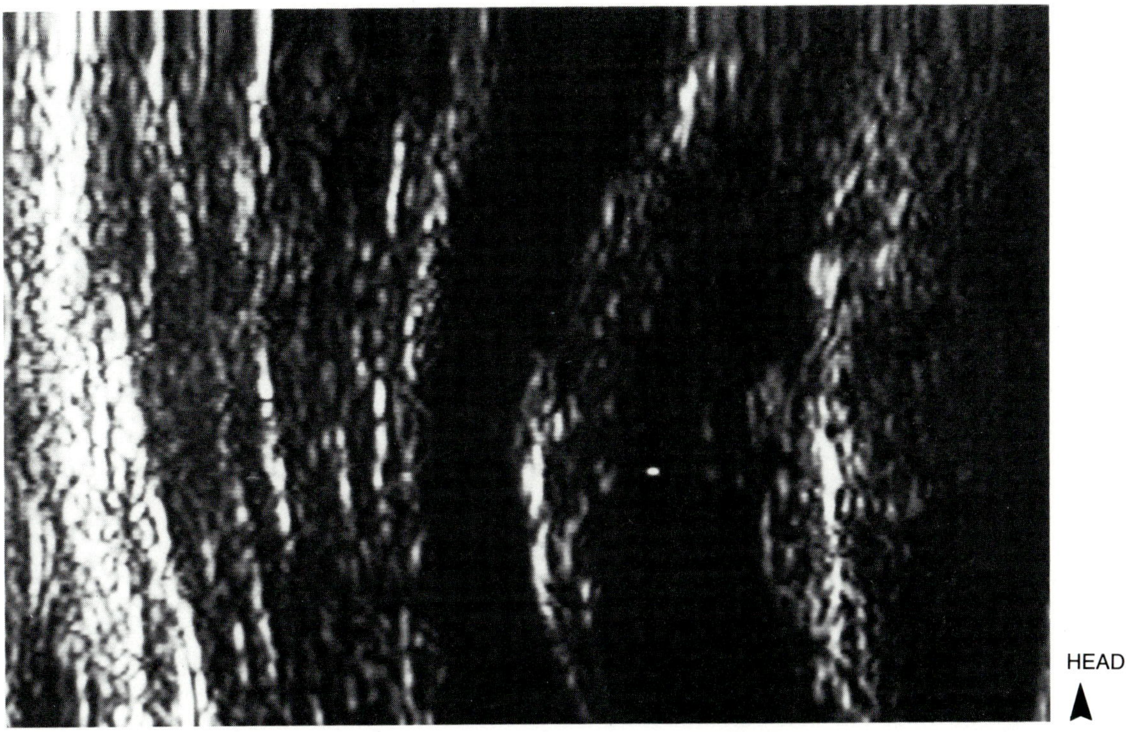
HEAD

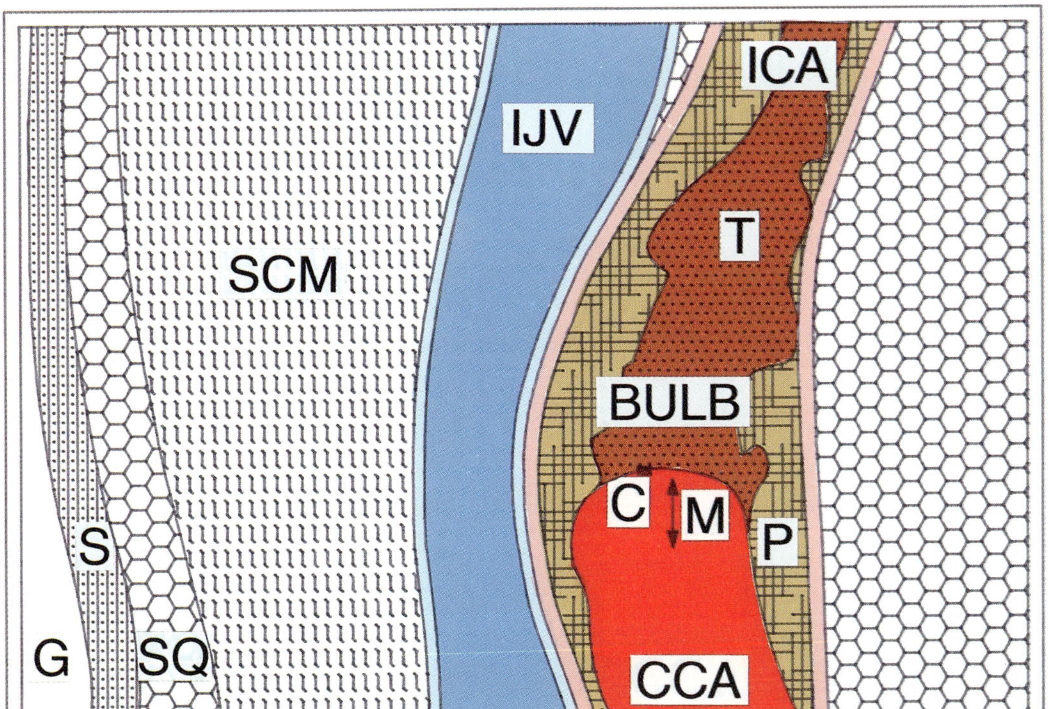
ICA
IJV
T
SCM
BULB
C
M
P
S
G
SQ
CCA

Figure 92. ONE WEEK LATER

The same right internal carotid artery (ICA) is seen 1 week later. The thrombus (T) within the internal carotid artery (ICA) has become slightly more echogenic, although it remains darker than the plaque (P) on the superficial and deep walls. This view is slightly more distal along the artery than in Figure 91, and the presence of a pre-existing stenosis above the internal carotid bulb is more apparent. There is a particularly dark area within the clot at the Doppler cursor (not drawn), but the fact that this is clot and not flowing blood was confirmed by the absence of a Doppler signal at this point. The actual meniscus to the occlusion is almost off the field of view to the bottom of the ultrasound scan where the common carotid artery (CCA) is located. At the time of this scan, 1 week following Figure 91, there was no longer any up/down pulsatility to the meniscus. There has also been a slight degree of shrinkage of the distal arterial lumen. The internal jugular vein (IJV) is located to the left. SQ = subcutaneous tissue, M = sternocleidomastoid muscle (note the typical vertical striations of muscle).

HISTORY *This scan was obtained 1 week later than that in Figure 91 and immediately prior to an attempted endarterectomy. The ICA could not be reopened more than 10 cm above the bifurcation because of carotid syphon disease. However, currant jelly–like clot was removed from the ICA, confirming the acute nature of the thrombus at this level.*

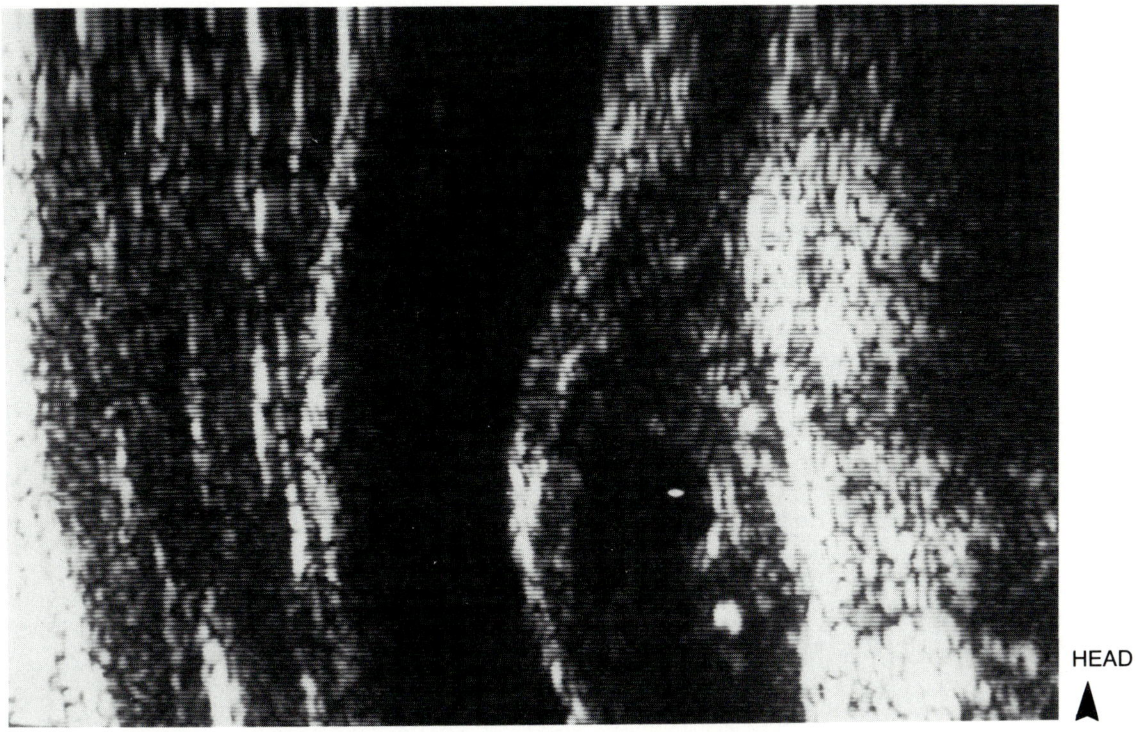
HEAD

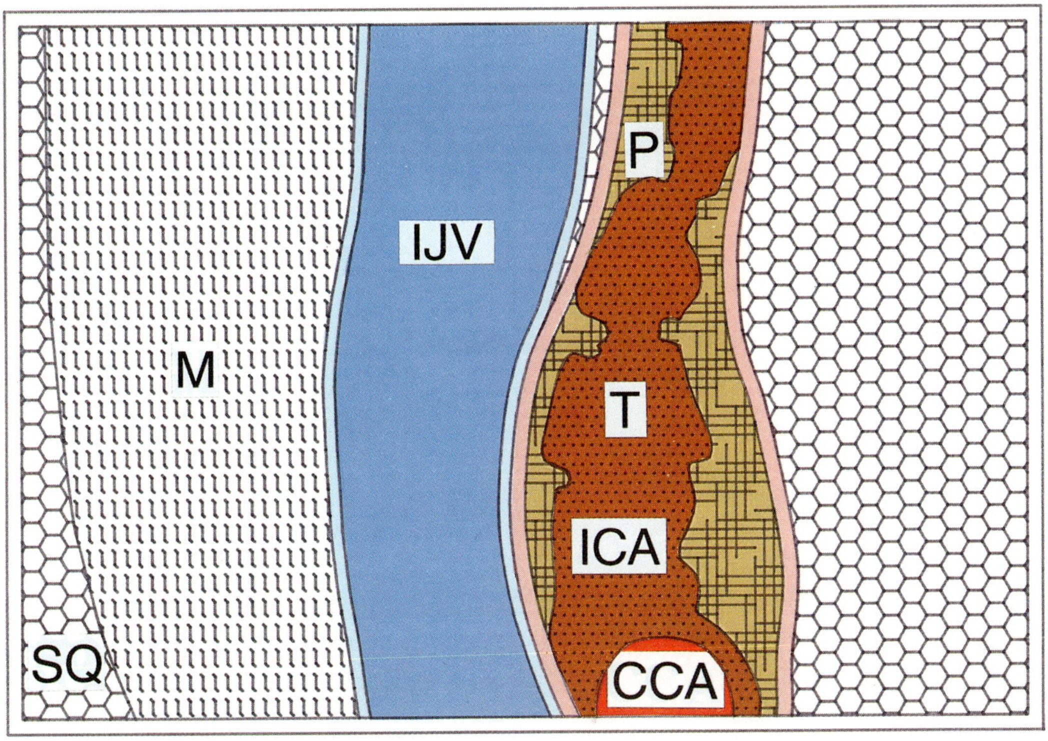
P
IJV
M
T
ICA
SQ
CCA

Figure 93. ICA OCCLUSION—CHRONIC THROMBOSIS

This is a longitudinal view of the left carotid bifurcation showing a total occlusion of the internal carotid artery (ICA), which is chronic. This occlusion is at least 1 year old (see subsequent History). The material (P) within the ICA has the finely speckled heterogeneity of thrombus rather than of atherosclerotic plaque. This thrombus propagated back from a distal occlusion of the ICA. The clot was quite firm without up/down pulsatility and with an oblique meniscus rather than the concavity found with most acute occlusions. The origin of the external carotid artery (ECA) is seen to the right, but the vessel travels obliquely out of the plane of view. S = skin, SQ = subcutaneous tissue (including platysma muscle), M = sternocleidomastoid muscle, F = fascia, CCA = common carotid artery, IJV = internal jugular vein.

HISTORY *This 66-year-old male had a total occlusion of the left ICA by duplex scan 1 year earlier and a cerebrovascular accident (CVA) several years earlier.*

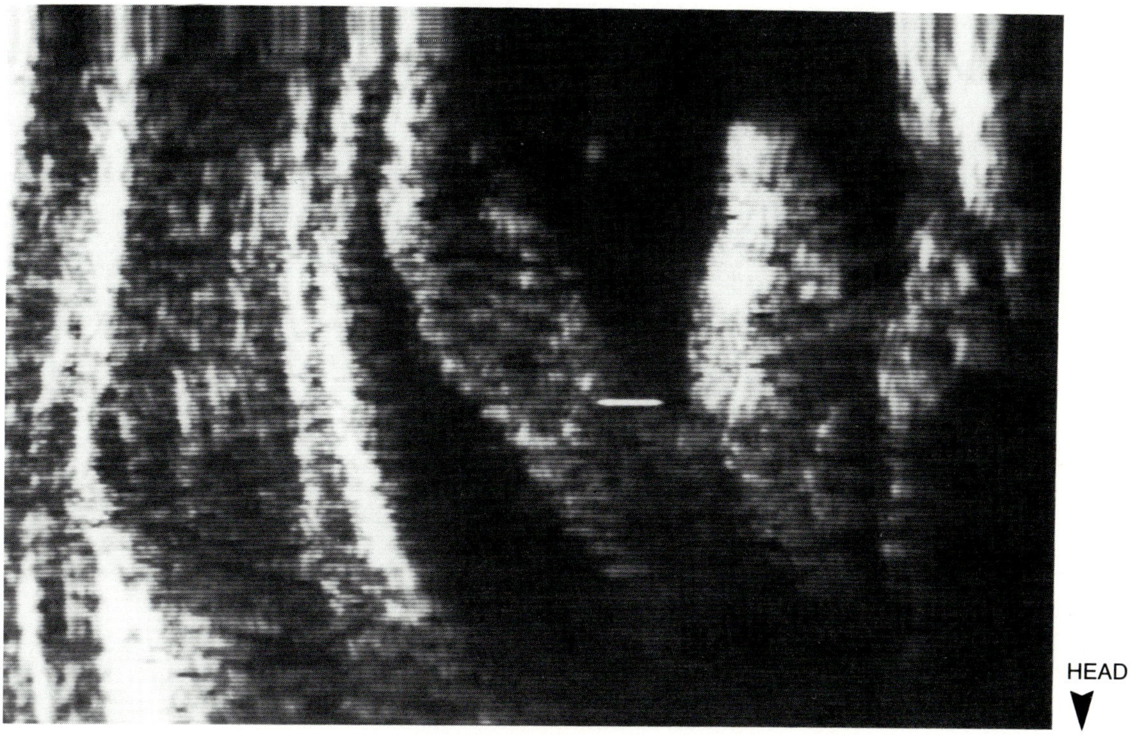
HEAD

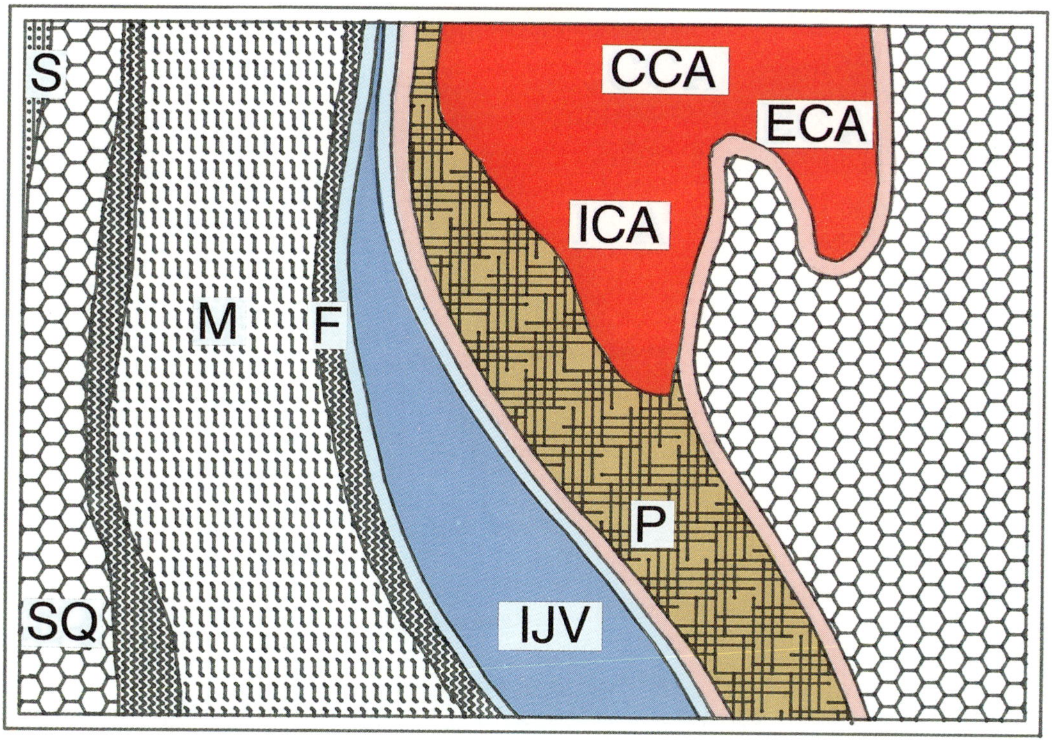
S
CCA
ECA
ICA
M
F
P
SQ
IJV

Figure 94. CHRONIC OCCLUSION—ICA

This is an example of a chronic arterial occlusion. Note the very heterogeneous, brightly echogenic material filling the internal carotid artery (ICA). The plaque extends out of the origin of the ICA into the common carotid (CCA), where it has an irregular contour rather than the smooth concavity present with most acute menisci. The occluded segment of artery is also quite small in diameter. Some fascial partitions are seen within the sternocleidomastoid muscle (M) to the left but are not drawn. ECA = external carotid artery.

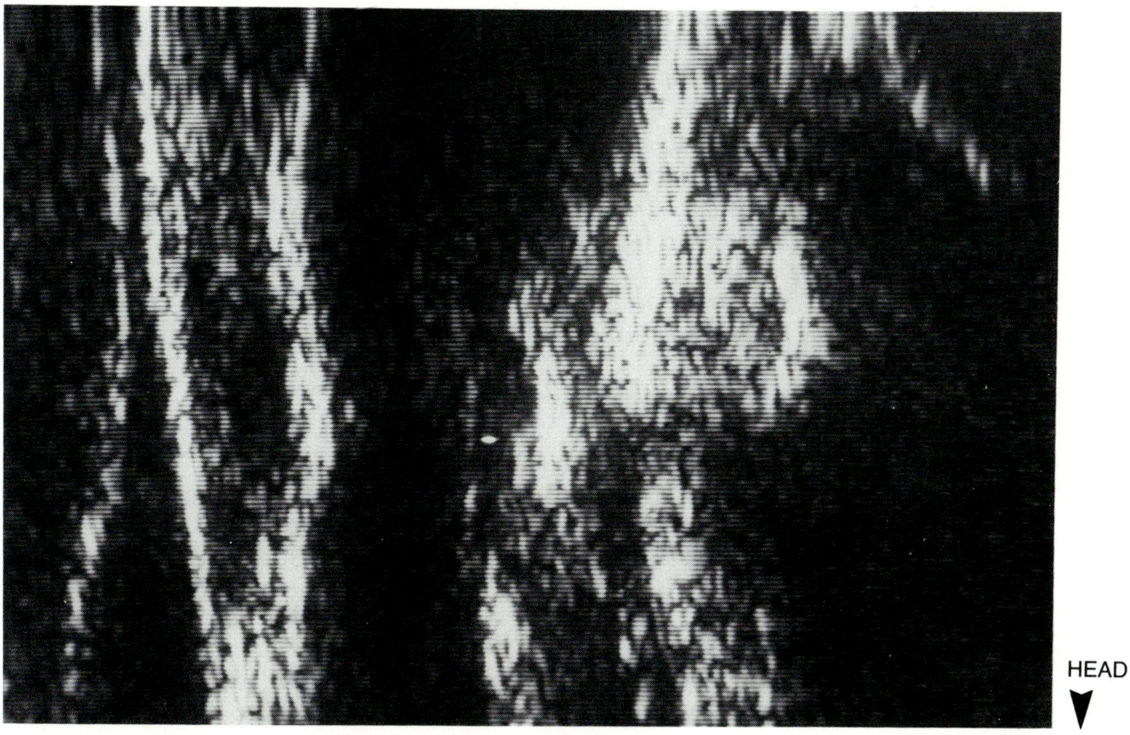
HEAD

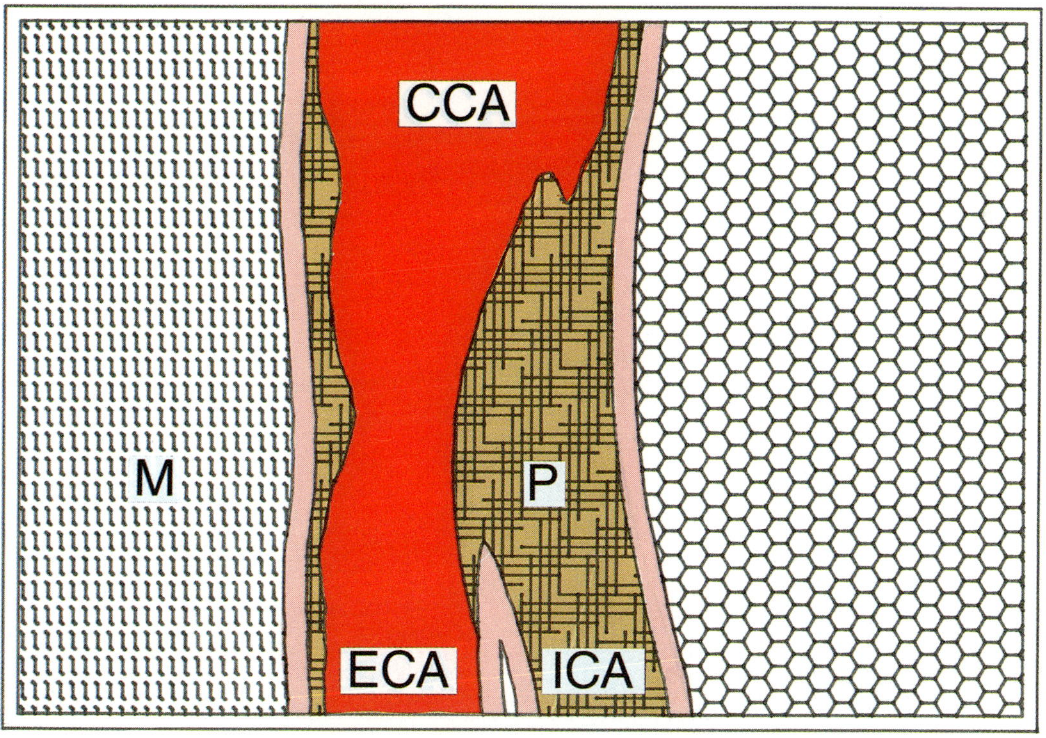
CCA
M
P
ECA
ICA

Figure 95. ACUTE INTERNAL CAROTID OCCLUSION

This is another example of acute thrombosis of the right internal carotid artery (ICA) with a well-defined meniscus across the center of the vessel. This meniscus has the typical concavity of an acute thrombosis. Note the thrombus (T) at the level of the Doppler cursor, which is faintly echogenic and fairly homogeneous in appearance. This thrombus shows two additional characteristics of acute occlusion as follows: the presence of up/down pulsatility in real time and the location of the meniscus at the level of the mid bulb of the ICA rather than at the origin of the vessel. The sternocleidomastoid muscle (M) to the left in this ultrasound scan demonstrates particularly well the fine longitudinal striations of the muscle seen in good quality scans. SQ = subcutaneous tissue, IJV = internal jugular vein (seen in an oblique cut).

HISTORY *This is of a 35-year-old diabetic who presented with right amaurosis fugax.*

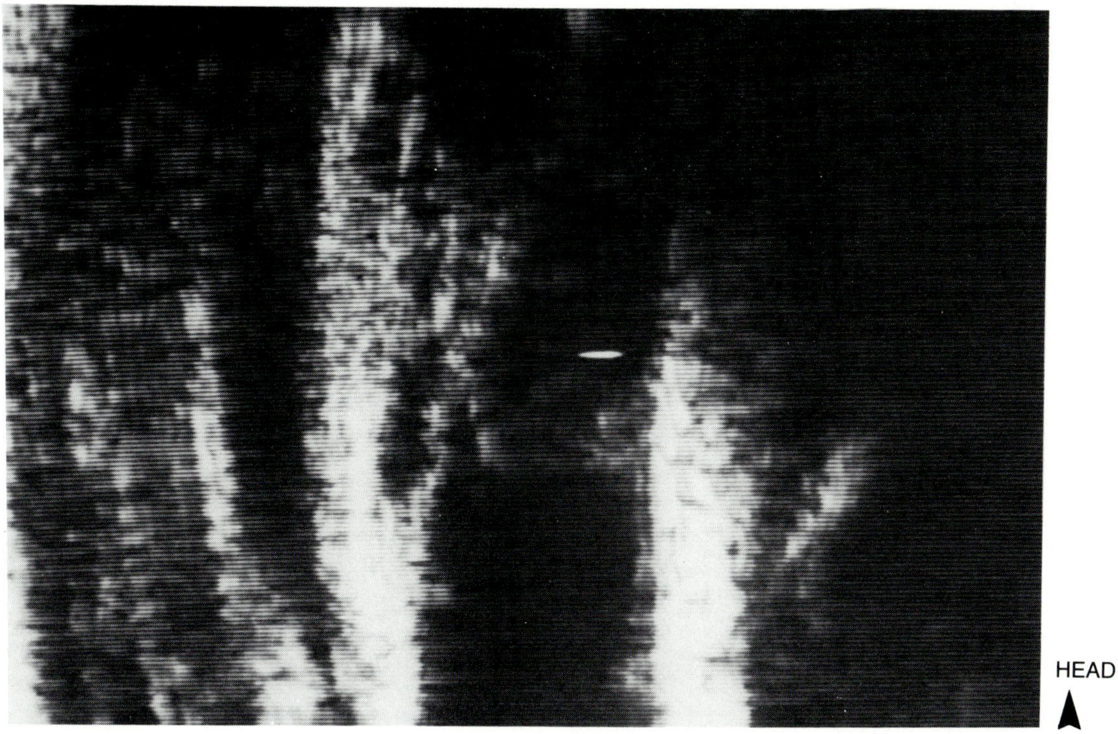
HEAD

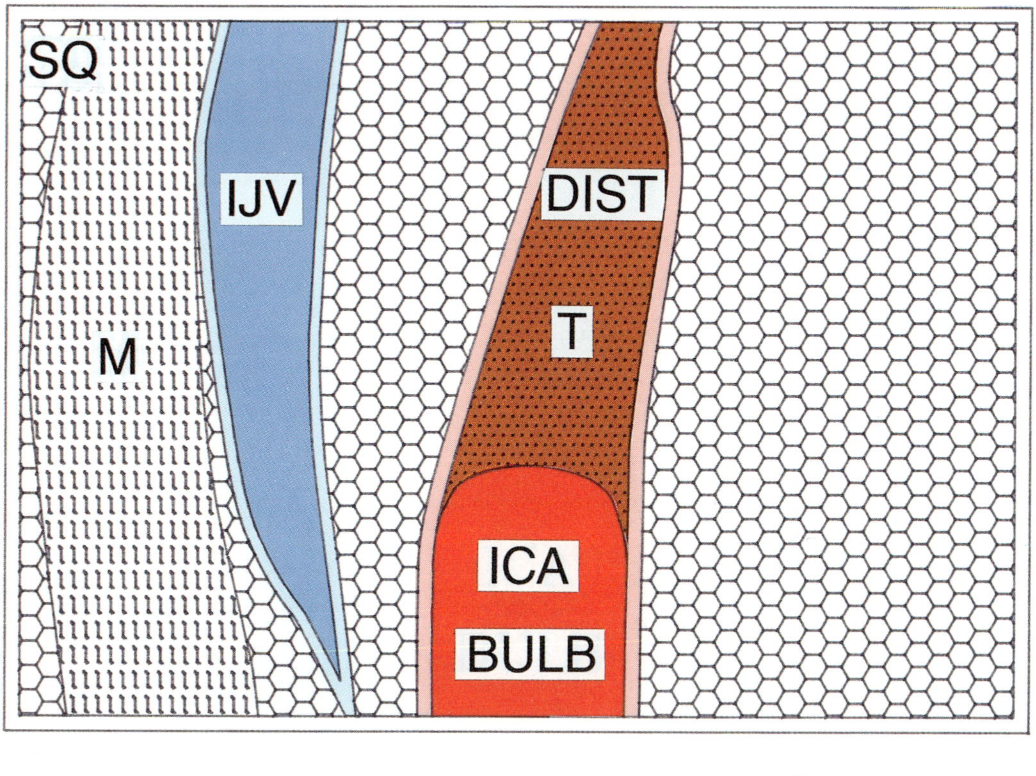
SQ
IJV
M
DIST
T
ICA
BULB

Figure 96. TOTAL OCCLUSION—CHRONIC

This is another example of a chronic total occlusion of the right internal carotid artery (ICA) down to the bifurcation where an irregular surface can be seen projecting into the common carotid artery's (CCA) lumen itself. In this case the total occlusion resulted from progression of the plaque rather than thrombosis extending down from above. The plaque (P) is very heterogeneous and of moderate echogenicity. Note how indistinct the arterial borders become, as one follows the ICA above the bifurcation, because of the nature of echoes produced by the intraluminal plaque. To re-emphasize, the surface of this plaque is moderately irregular at the origin of the ICA and does not demonstrate up/down pulsatility in real time. The origin of the superior thyroid artery (ST) is seen arising from the base of the external carotid artery (ECA). SQ = subcutaneous tissue, M = muscle (sternocleidomastoid), F = fascia (carotid sheath).

HISTORY *This 62-year-old male was asymptomatic with respect to the chronic occlusion confirmed by angiography 4 years previously. He had an infarct in the left parietal lobe with hemiparesis 5 weeks prior to the scan that revealed a 60% left internal carotid stenosis. These findings were again confirmed by a repeat angiogram. He has been asymptomatic at 1 year follow-up.*

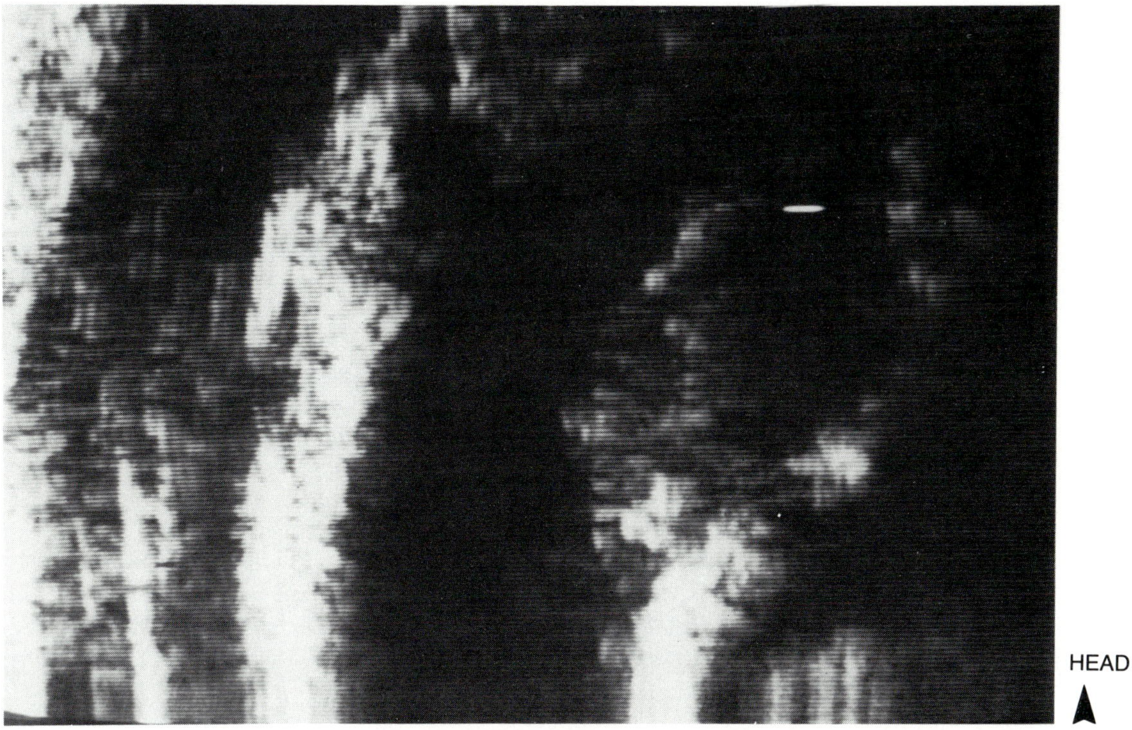
HEAD

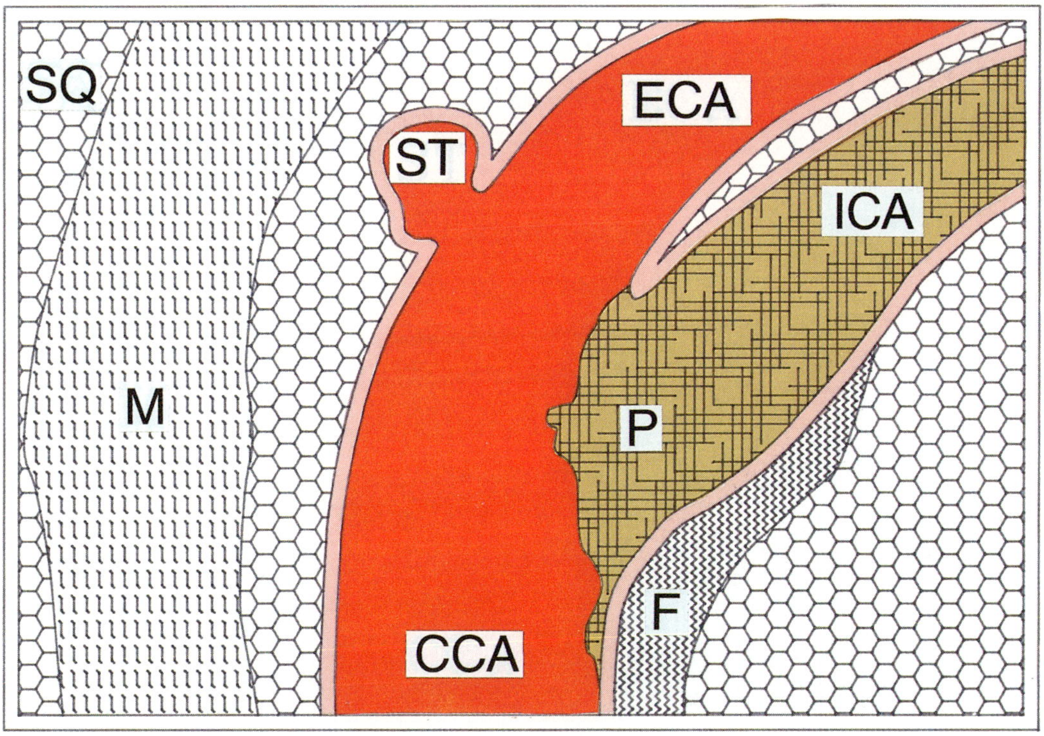
SQ
ECA
ST
ICA
M
P
F
CCA

Figure 97. ACUTE INTERNAL CAROTID THROMBOSIS

This is another example of an acute thrombosis of a left internal carotid artery (ICA). There is some plaque (P) of brighter echogenicity along the deep wall of the junction between the common carotid artery (CCA) and the ICA. There is also a lesser amount of plaque along the superficial wall of the CCA. In addition, there is more faintly echogenic material consistent with thrombus (T) filling the residual lumen with a meniscus (M) visible at the level of the Doppler cursor (not drawn). There was no Doppler signal obtainable within the distal ICA. SCM = sternocleidomastoid muscle, SQ = subcutaneous tissue, ? = tissue of uncertain composition.

HISTORY *This is a 60-year-old female who developed confusion and garbled speech on the second day following a left carotid endarterectomy. This ultrasound scan was obtained 7 days later. The endarterectomy had been performed because of a large ulcer seen on angiography that was coexistent with a 40% stenosis of the internal carotid bulb. She had been symptomatic with a left hemispheric cerebrovascular accident (CVA) 5 months prior; she also had a 90% stenosis of the cavernous portion of the left ICA, which may have been responsible for the postoperative occlusion. A computed tomography scan confirmed left cerebral infarction.*

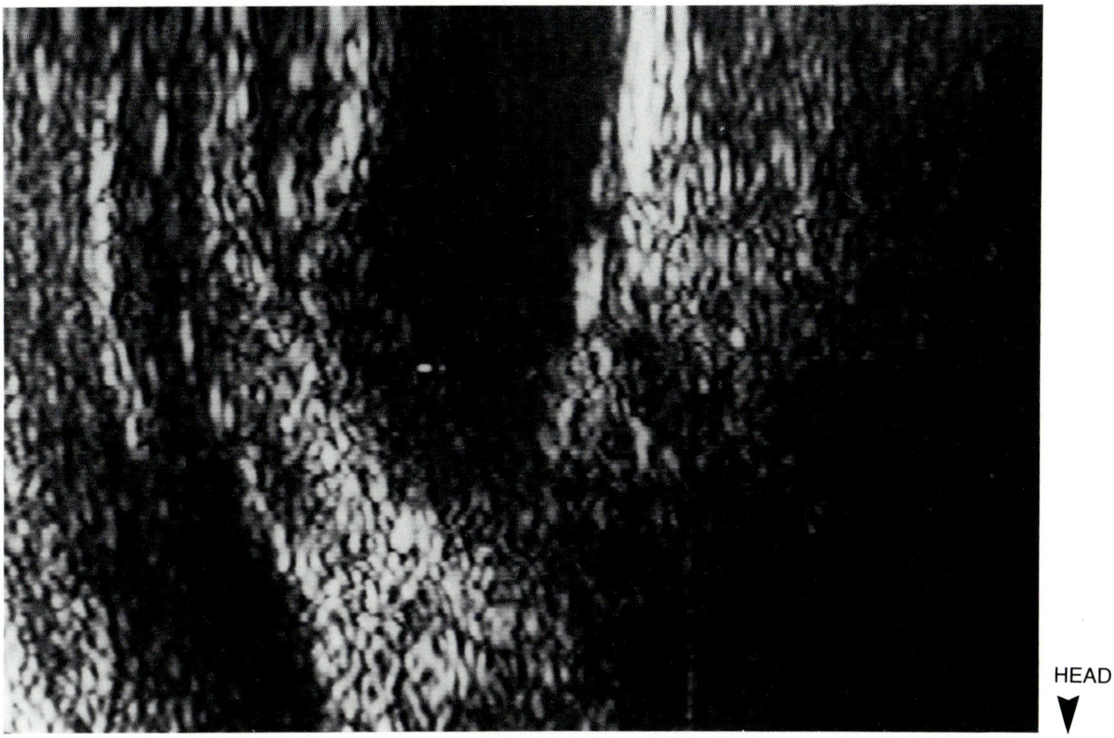
HEAD

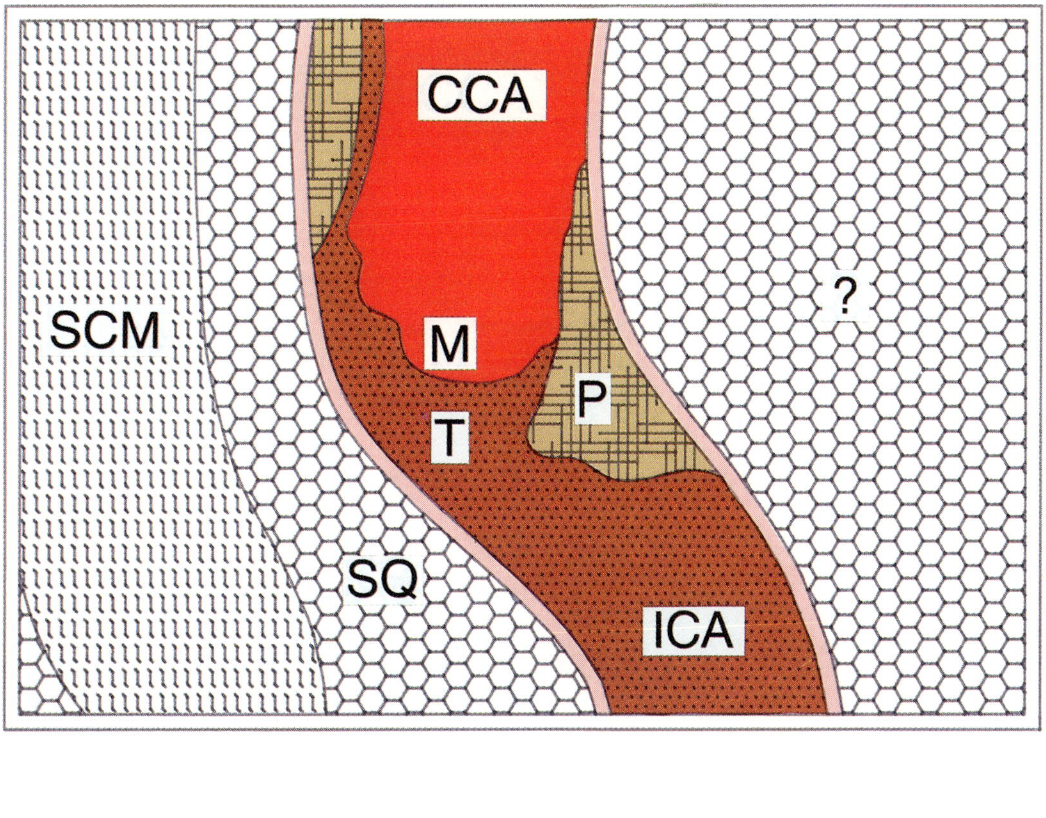
CCA
SCM
M
?
P
T
SQ
ICA

Figure 98. HIGHLY HETEROGENEOUS CHRONIC OCCLUSION

In this 4 MHz longitudinal view of a chronically occluded left internal carotid artery (I), there is very heterogeneous plaque (P) filling the rather small internal carotid bulb. The outline of a meniscus (M) can be seen crossing the mouth of the internal carotid artery. The external carotid artery (E) is almost out of the plane. The 5.5-mm diameter common carotid artery (CCA) contains some artifact (AF) before the bifurcation, which can be distinguished from plaque only in real time. This is the typical appearance of a chronic occlusion. G = gel, S = skin, PL = platysma muscle, F = fascia, SCM = sternocleidomastoid muscle, V = internal jugular vein, ? = tissue of uncertain composition, SQ = subcutaneous tissue.

HISTORY *This 62-year-old male developed some loss of vision in the nasal half of his left eye. An ophthalmic examination confirmed cholesterol emboli. Immediately following this scan an arteriogram was performed, which suggested a patent internal carotid artery with a "string sign." Because of the arteriographic findings, the patient was explored with the intention of doing an endarterectomy. At operation, the duplex scan findings of a chronic occlusion were confirmed. The internal carotid artery was therefore closed at its origin, following endarterectomy of the external carotid artery.*

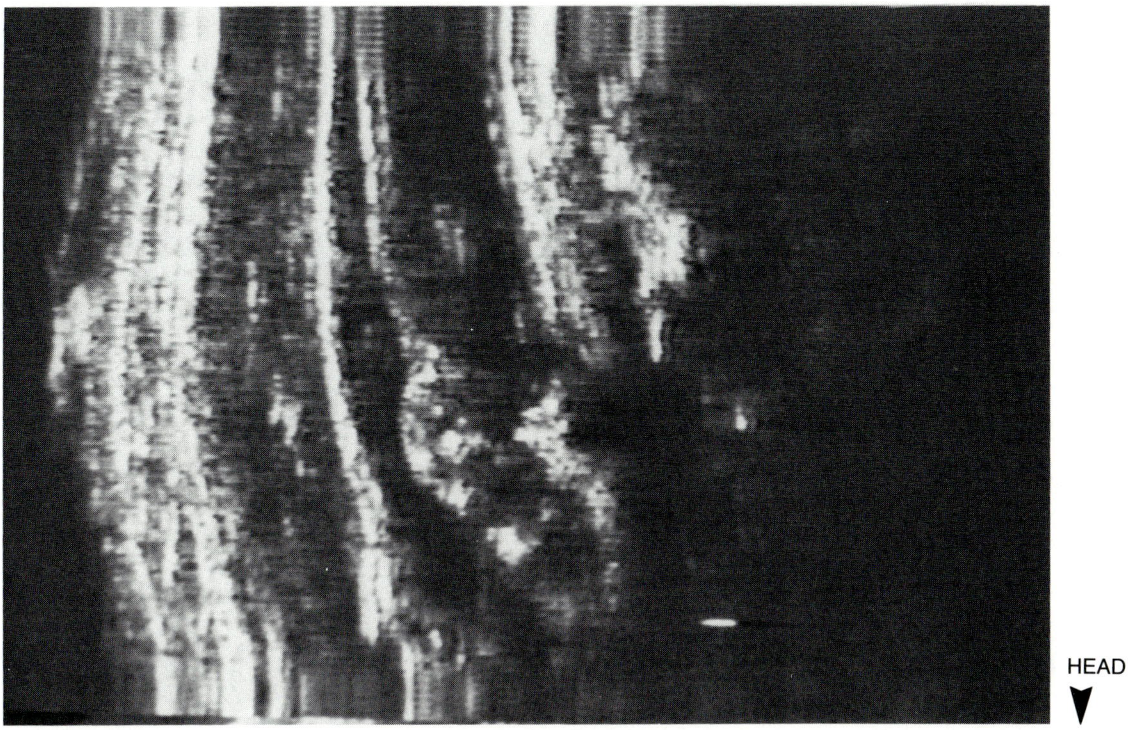
HEAD

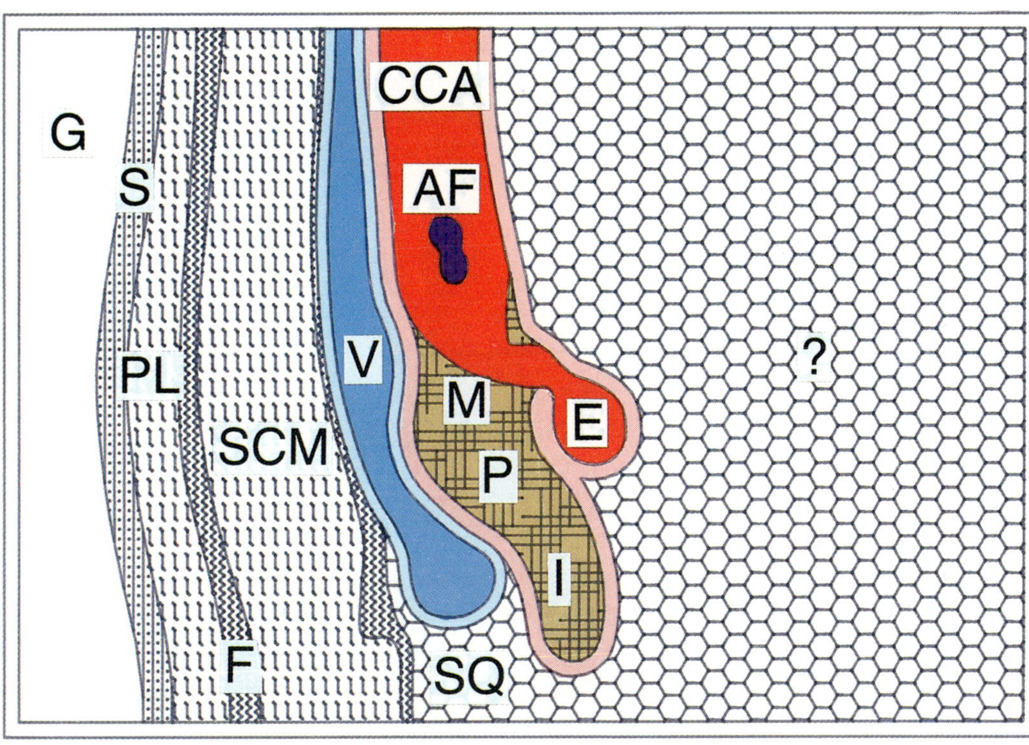
CCA
G
S
AF
PL
V
?
M
E
SCM
P
I
F
SQ

Figure 99. APPARENT TOTAL OCCLUSION

When visualized in longitudinal orientation, it is possible to make this very heterogeneous calcified plaque (P) appear as a total occlusion within the internal carotid artery (ICA). This view is obtained by an extremely posterior position of the probe on the neck so as to direct the beam from side-to-side through the plaque rather than through the open lumen from front-to-back. If the probe had been rocked more anteriorly, the open lumen would have become apparent. (See also Figures 54 and 55 for comparative views.) Note the acoustic shadowing (AS) extending behind the calcified plaque. The origin of the external carotid artery (ECA) is seen before the artery travels out of plane. A small patch of "back wall" plaque is seen within the common carotid artery (CCA) just below the bifurcation. Isolated "islands" of plaque can give this appearance when the beam makes contact with the highest projections of the plaque from the "back walls." In many cases, this phenomenon occurs because the beam is directed off center, within the artery. If the projection is particularly high, however, it may be present even within a well-centered view. SCM = sternocleidomastoid muscle, F = fascia, SQ = subcutaneous tissue.

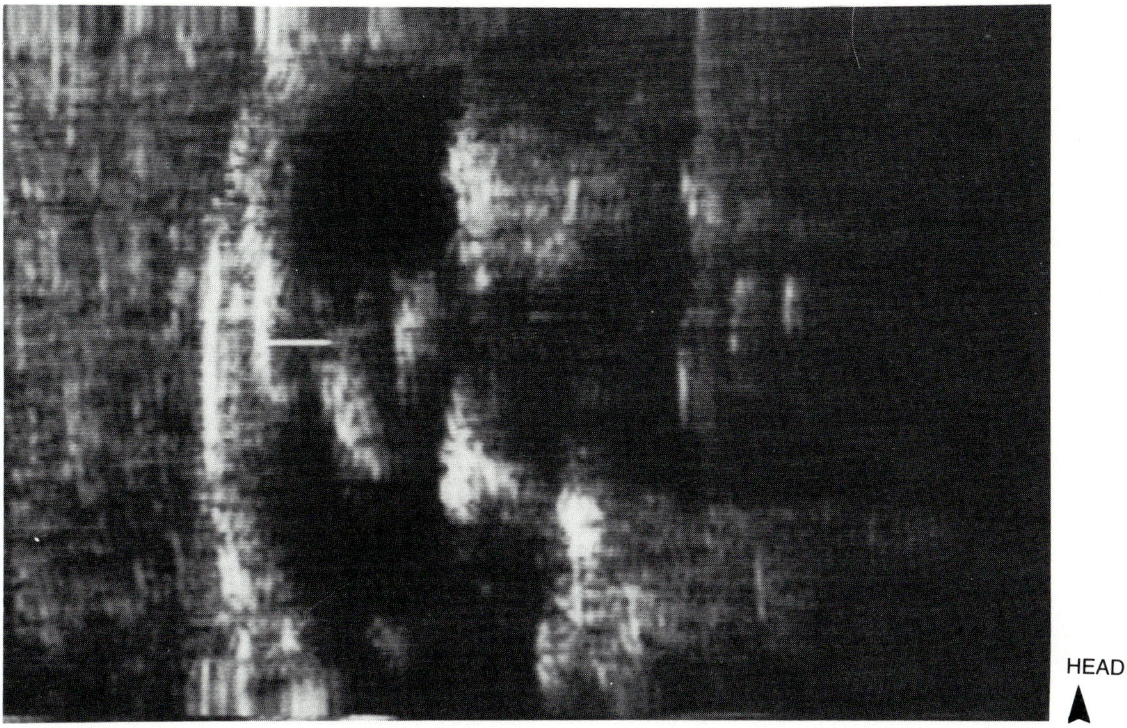
HEAD

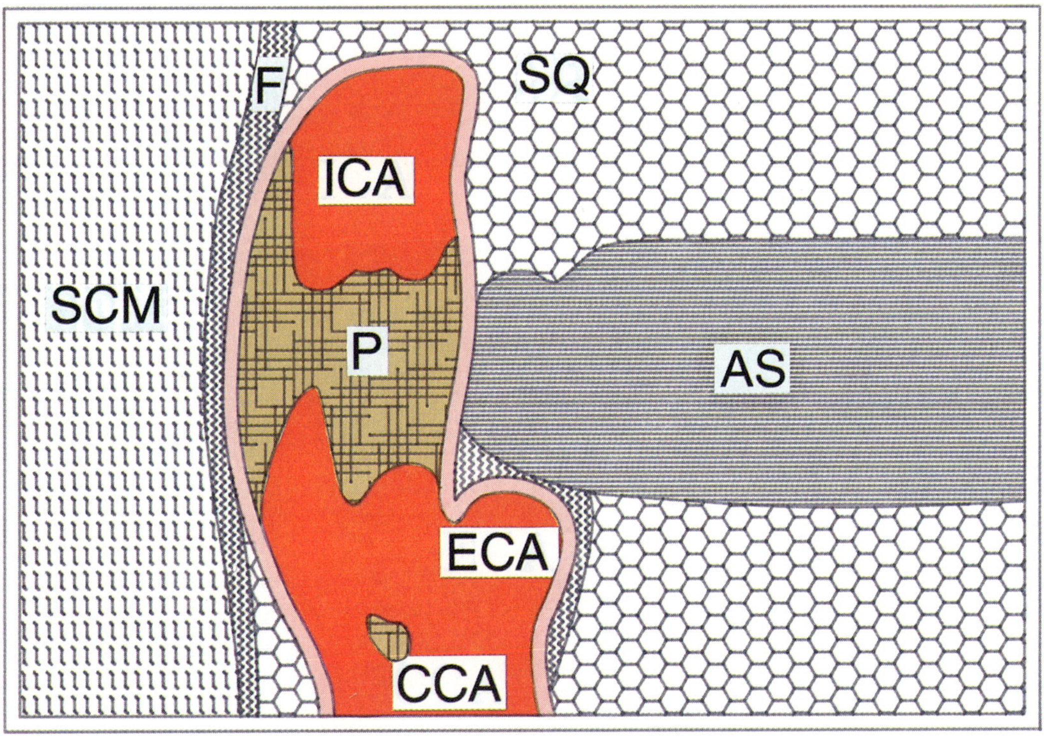
F
SQ
ICA
SCM
P
AS
ECA
CCA

CHAPTER 6

POST-OPERATIVE FINDINGS

Figure 100. POST-ENDARTERECTOMY SUTURE LINE

In this longitudinal view of the left carotid bifurcation, one can see the suture line (SL) on the anterior wall of the common carotid artery (CCA) and internal carotid artery (ICA). These sutures typically appear as bright, white, elliptical dots spaced in a somewhat regular fashion along the arterial wall. By ultrasound, this portion of the arterial wall often appears to be somewhat thickened, but it is assumed that anything within and outside the suture line is arterial wall and not plaque. In this example, there is only a small amount of plaque (P) high in the ICA at the bottom of the ultrasound scan. SQ = subcutaneous tissue (skin obscured), M = sternocleidomastoid muscle, IJV = internal jugular vein.

HISTORY *This 60-year-old diabetic male had had an endarterectomy 4 years prior for retinal artery emboli. He had remained asymptomatic for the subsequent 4 years until the time of this scan and also for 3 years following. The lack of significant stenosis was confirmed by arteriogram 6 months prior to this ultrasound scan.*

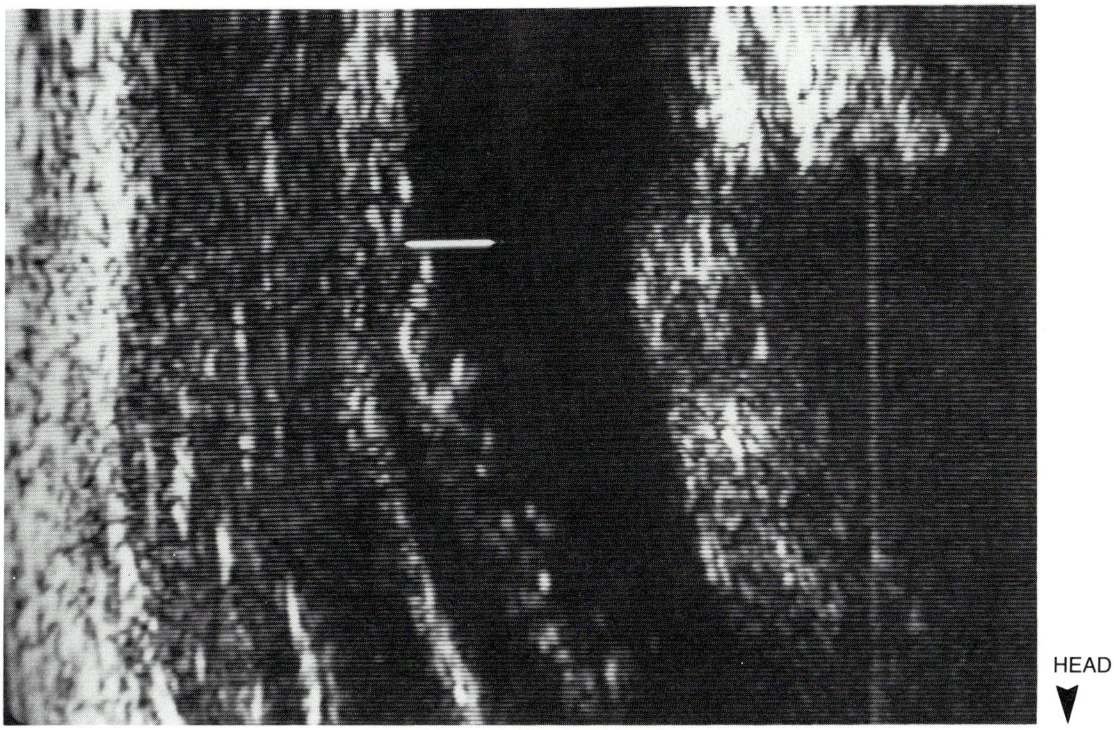
HEAD

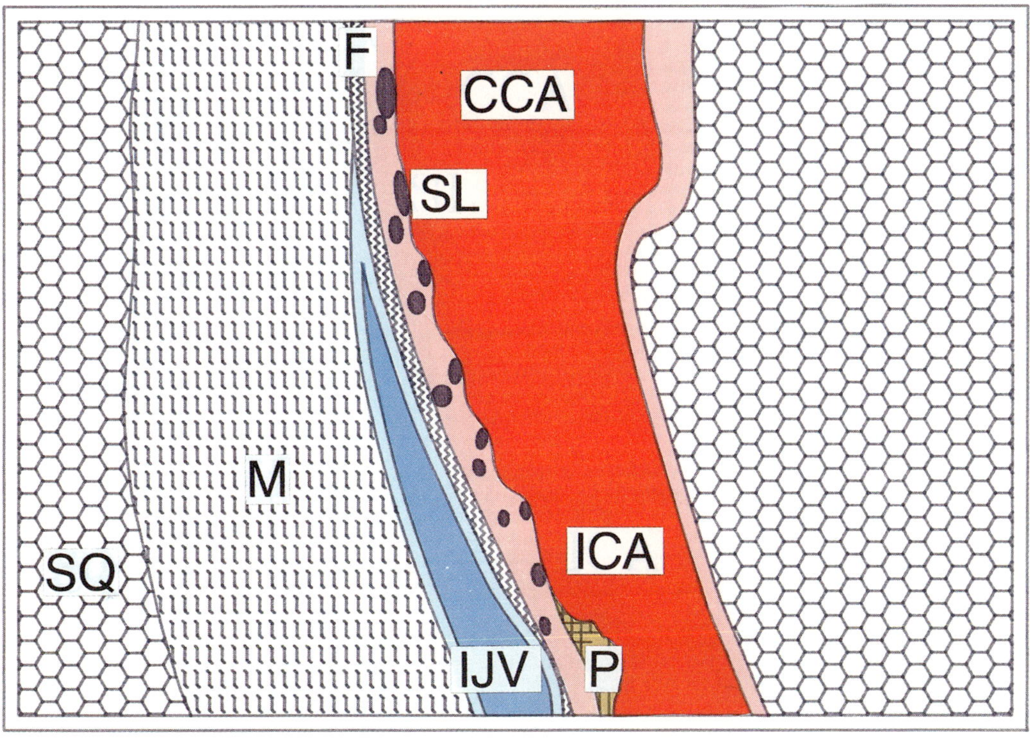
F
CCA
SL
M
ICA
SQ
IJV
P

Figure 101. BIFURCATION AFTER ENDARTERECTOMY

This scan was performed 10 months after endarterectomy and is a longitudinal view of the right internal carotid artery (ICA) in which there is no recurrent plaque. There is no stenosis of the distal ICA (at the top of the scan) due to closure of the arteriotomy. The upper portion of the suture line (SL) is seen. It follows the normal tapering of the vessel without any impingement of the lumen. SQ = subcutaneous tissue (platysma obliterated), M = sternocleidomastoid muscle, F = fascia (part carotid sheath, part scar, and part investing fascia of the sternocleidomastoid).

HISTORY *This 65-year-old male underwent endarterectomy 2 years prior for crescendo transient ischemic attacks (TIAs) while on heparin. The TIAs consisted of paresis of the left arm. He has remained asymptomatic for the past 3 years since the endarterectomy.*

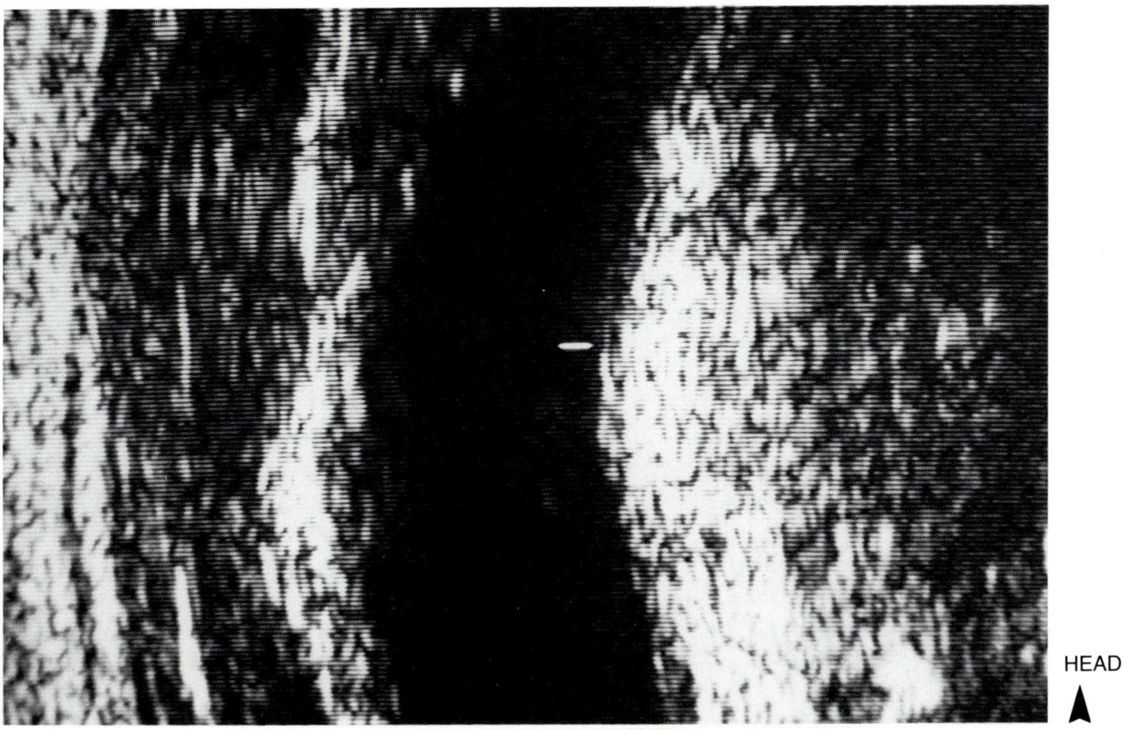
HEAD

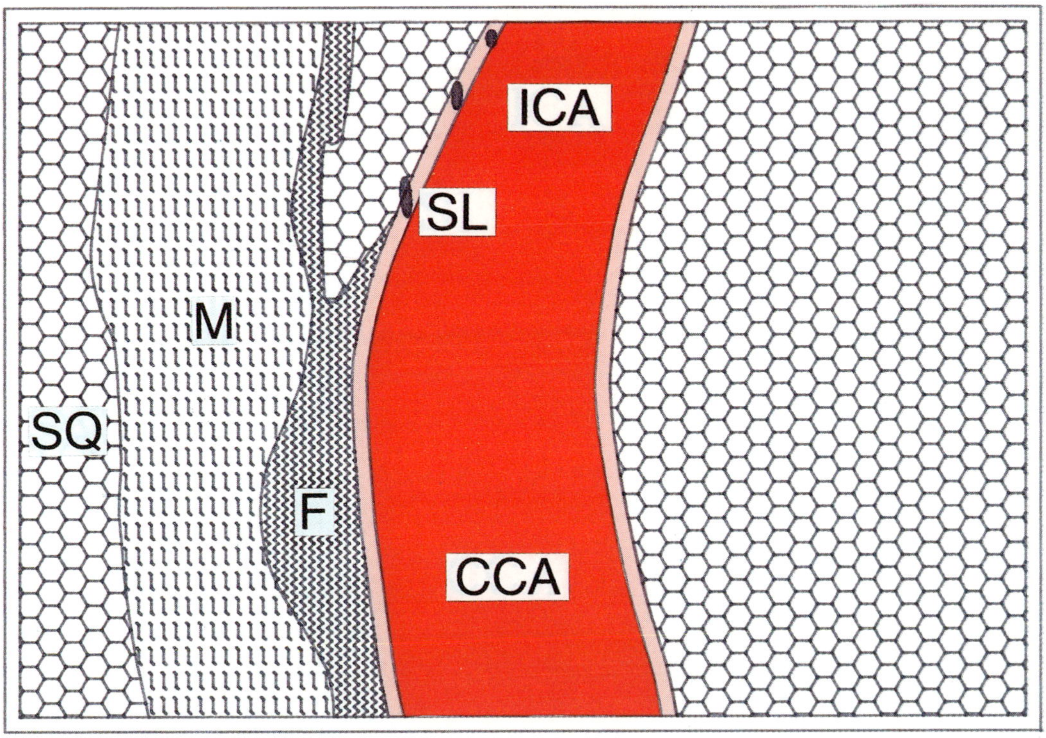
ICA
SL
M
SQ
F
CCA

Figure 102. ENDARTERECTOMY SUTURE LINE

In this longitudinal view of the right carotid bifurcation, the suture line (SL) from an endarterectomy performed 6 weeks prior is well visualized and causes approximately a 15% diameter stenosis of the internal carotid artery (ICA). Although there is some thickening (T) of the superficial wall of the ICA, this thickening is not due to recurrent or residual plaque but rather to the gathering effect of the sutures themselves. If one assumes a complete endarterectomy, any thickening of the arterial wall outside the sutures cannot be plaque. This is otherwise a very good result at this point in time. SQ = subcutaneous tissue, M = muscle (sternocleidomastoid), CCA = common carotid artery, ICA = internal carotid artery.

HISTORY *This 65-year-old male had undergone a right carotid endarterectomy owing to the presence of a 90% stenosis with the appearance of clot, extending into the ICA. This occurrence was associated with cross perfusion of the right cerebral circulation via the left ICA, which also had a 60% stenosis. He presented with a single episode of transient right hemiparesis referable to the left carotid lesion but was asymptomatic with regard to the right side. He has remained asymptomatic over the subsequent 2 years.*

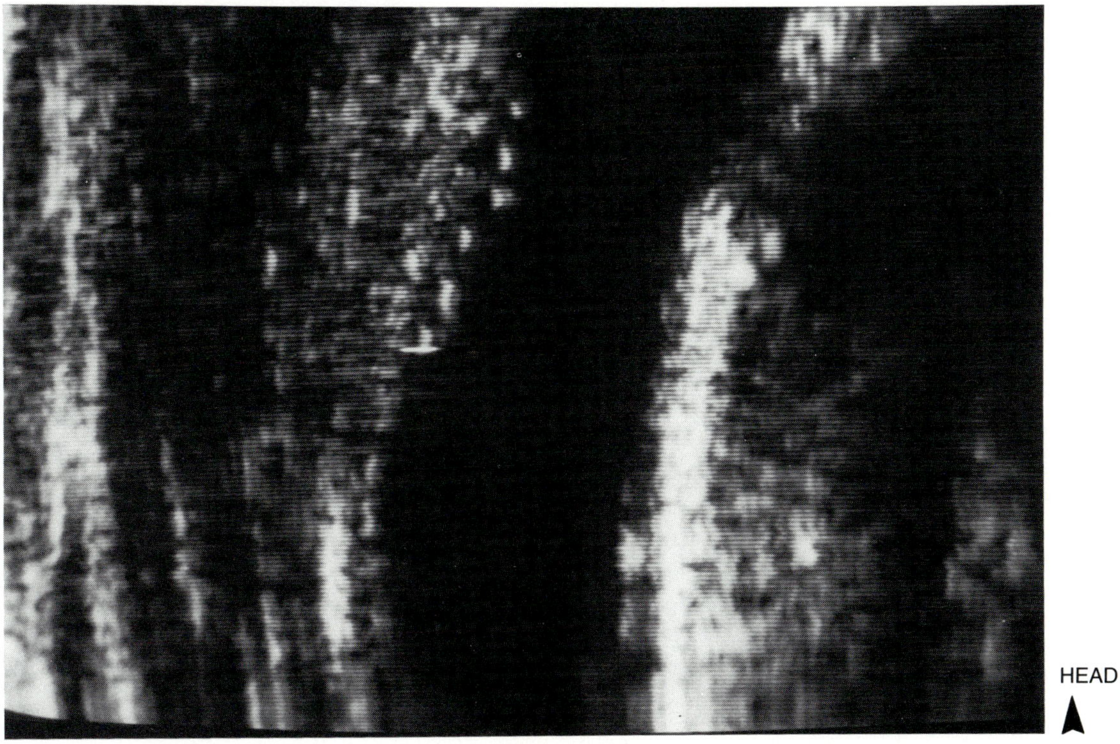
HEAD

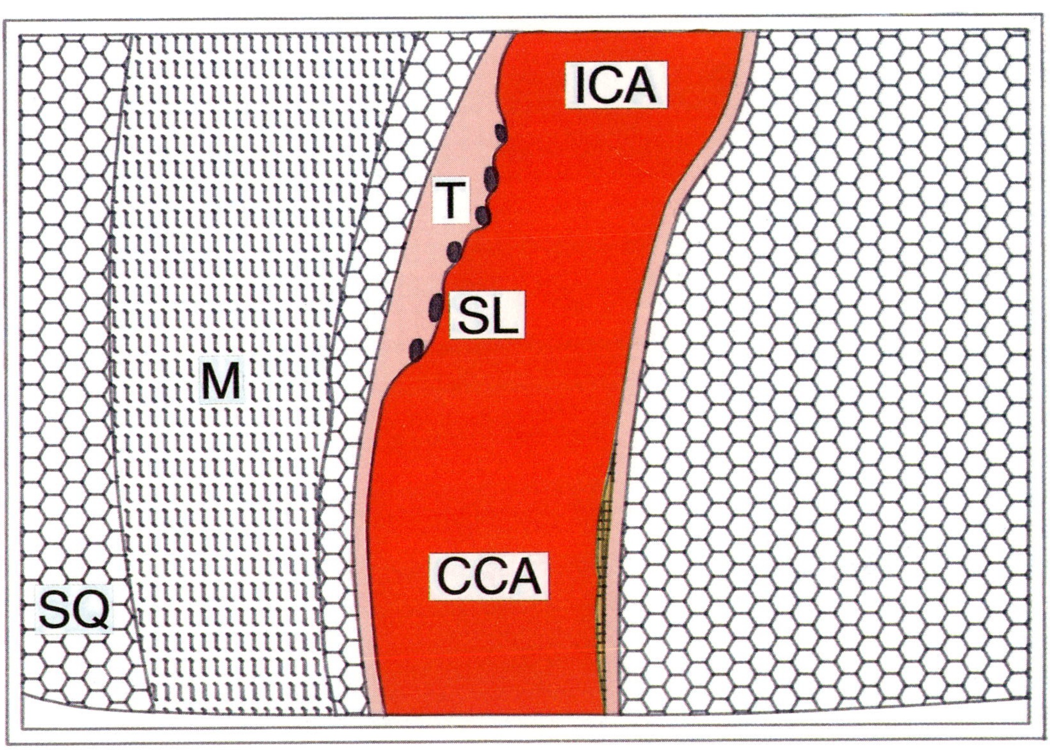
ICA
T
SL
M
CCA
SQ

Figure 103. POST-ENDARTERECTOMY SUTURE LINE

Note again the presence of the easily visualized suture line (SL) on the superficial walls of the common carotid artery (CCA) and internal carotid artery (ICA). The superficial wall has been thickened by bunching of the artery caused by the sutures, but this thickening is not due to plaque. To restate, recurrent plaque must appear medial to the sutures within the vessel not lateral to them. Note also the absence of a clearly defined "intimal stripe" in this endarterectomized bifurcation along either the superficial or deep arterial wall. The longitudinal striations of the sternocleidomastoid muscle (M) are also nicely seen. S = skin, SQ = subcutaneous tissue, F = fascia (superficial portion of the carotid sheath).

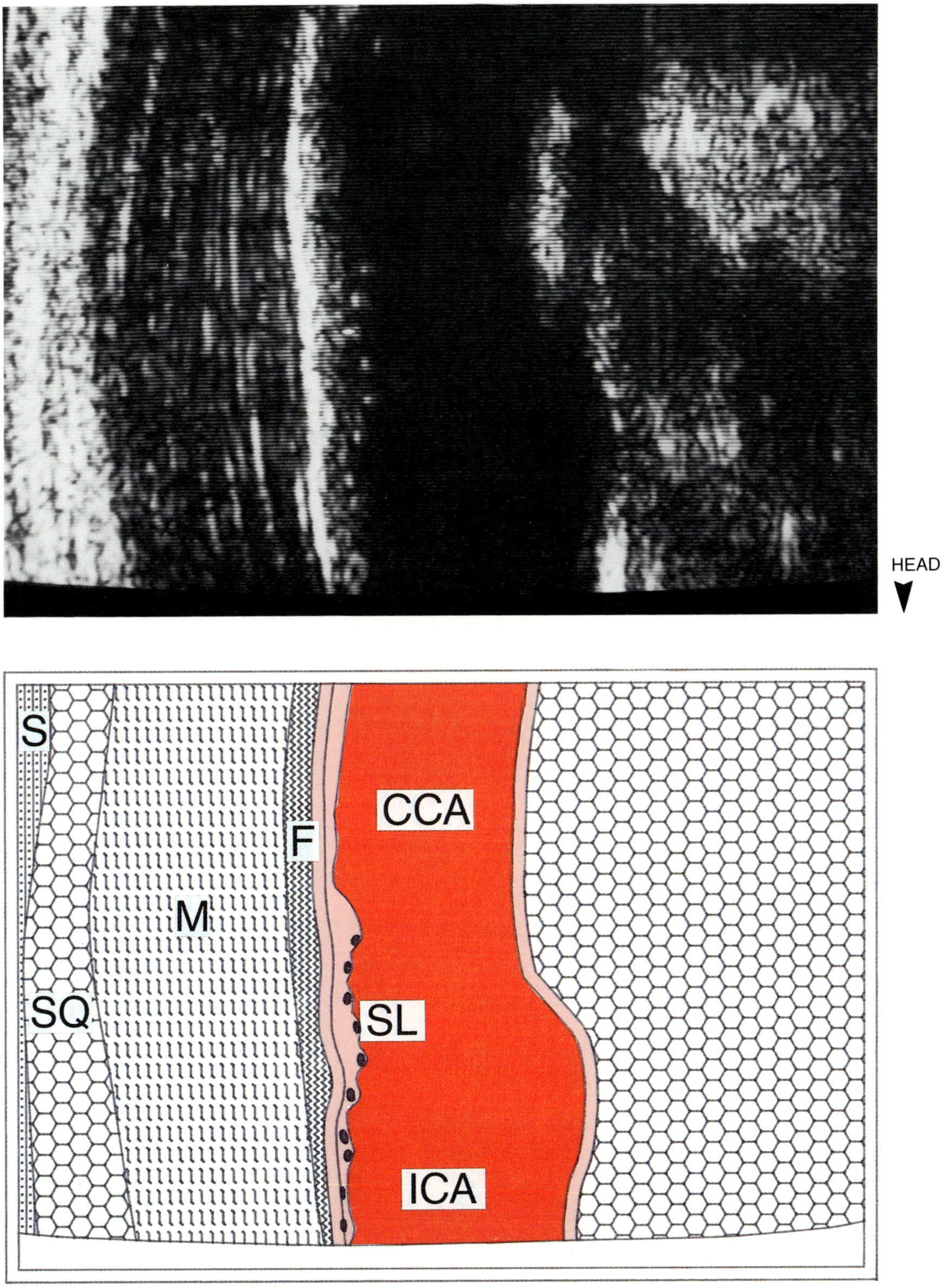
HEAD
S
CCA
F
M
SQ
SL
ICA

Figure 104. ENDARTERECTOMY TRANSITION POINT

This longitudinal view of an endarterectomized right internal carotid artery (ICA) is shown to demonstrate the ability of ultrasound to reveal the distal transition point (TP) between the endarterectomized portion of the artery, consisting mostly of media, and some pseudo-intima (PI) near the bottom of the scan. Note the contrast between this fuzzy border below and the quite sharp, smooth and bright surface of the "intimal stripe" (I) above. Any plaque present below the transition point would be classified as recurrent stenosis, and it would have to have developed after the time of the endarterectomy. By contrast any plaque present in the portion of the artery in the top half of the scan, especially if the scan was performed soon after the endarterectomy, would be classified as residual stenosis. It would be presumed that plaque at this level had been left behind at the time of the endarterectomy. At later points in time, it would not be possible to say either how much plaque was present at the time of the endarterectomy or how much of the plaque was a progression of atherosclerosis since the endarterectomy. SQ = subcutaneous tissue, M = sternocleidomastoid muscle, F = fascia (carotid sheath), A = adventitial portion of the artery.

HISTORY *This scan of this 78-year-old male was obtained 12 years following a right carotid endarterectomy. The lack of any recurrent or residual stenosis was also noted by arteriogram 8 years following the endarterectomy and 4 years prior to this ultrasound scan.*

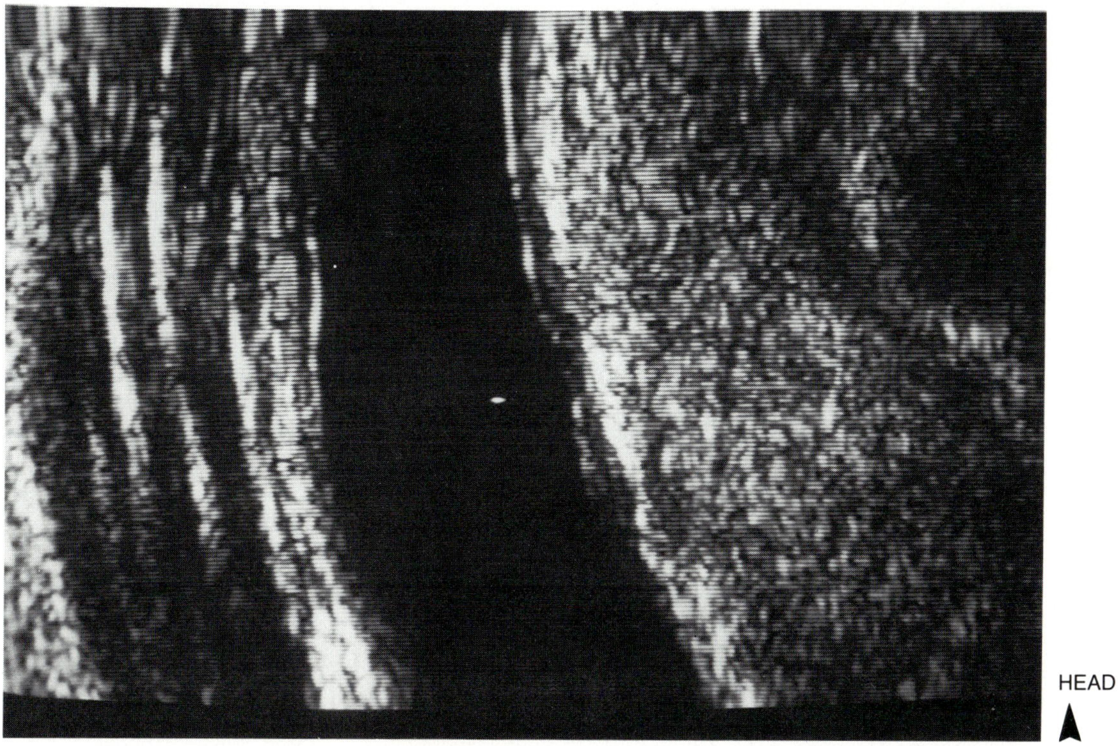
HEAD

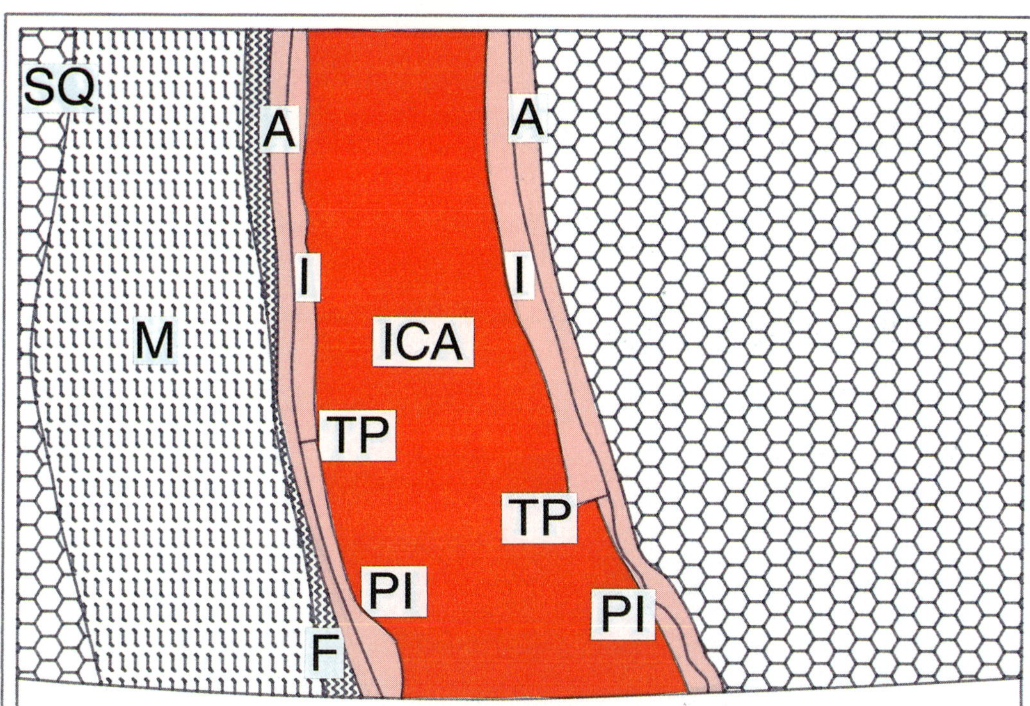
SQ
A
A
I
I
M
ICA
TP
TP
PI
PI
F

Figure 105. RECURRENT IRREGULAR PLAQUE

This is a longitudinal view of the left internal carotid artery (ICA) showing recurrent moderately irregular, moderately echogenic, homogeneous plaque (P) within the artery following an endarterectomy. This plaque is recurrent in the sense that it is now present in the endarterectomized portion of the artery. The distal ICA at the bottom of the screen, above the level of the endarterectomy, shows the transition points (TP) to the smooth intimal stripes of the untouched artery beyond. There is a questionable ulcer (?U) in the deep wall plaque in the mid internal carotid bulb. The common carotid artery (CCA) is barely visualized at the top of the scan, and the back wall (BW) of the external carotid artery is seen tangentially near the external carotid artery (ECA) origin. Near the bottom of the scan the ECA travels into the plane of view and is seen in a slightly oblique orientation. Fascial layers (F) are seen on both sides of the sternocleidomastoid muscle (M). (The skin and platysmal muscle are not seen.) SQ = subcutaneous tissue.

HISTORY *This 78-year-old male had a cerebrovascular accident (CVA) 14 years prior to this scan followed by bilateral carotid endarterectomies 12 years prior to this scan. He presented with transient ischemic attacks, consisting of dizziness and ataxia, 4 years prior to the scan and on arteriography was found to have a vertebral artery occlusion on the left and a 50% vertebral stenosis on the right as well as a 50% left ICA stenosis. This ultrasound scan (4 years after the arteriogram) shows no further progression of ICA stenosis, again estimated at 50% by ultrasound. Contrast these findings with the scan of this patient's opposite bifurcation seen in Figure 104.*

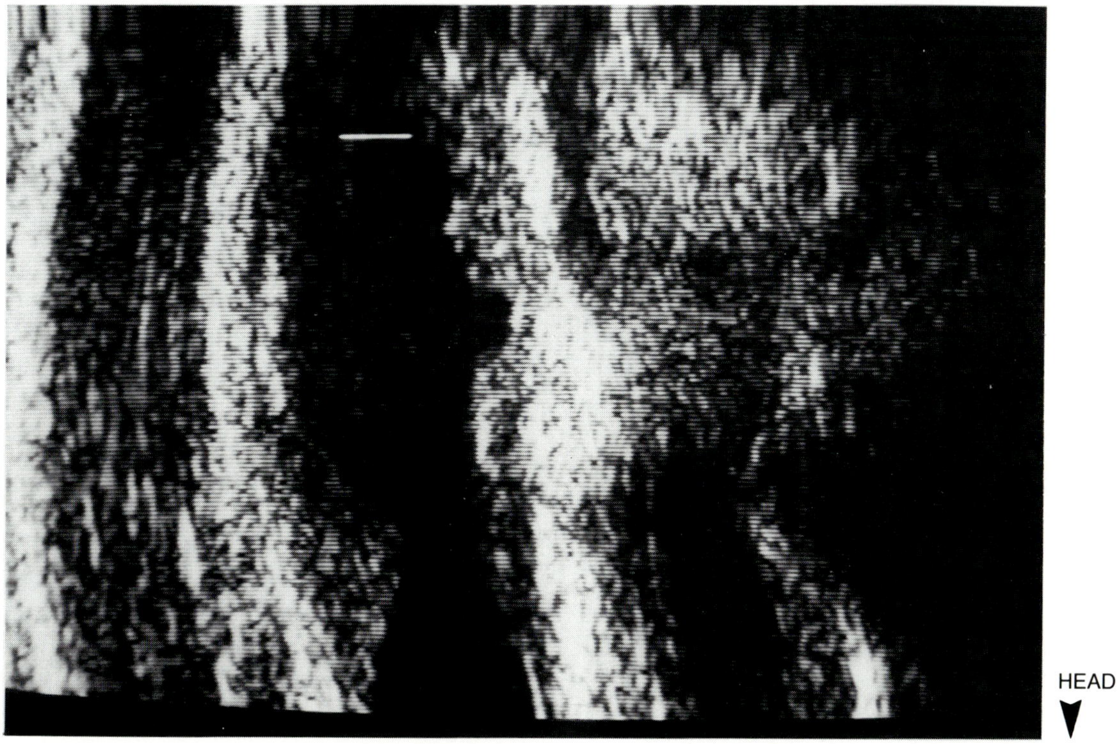
HEAD

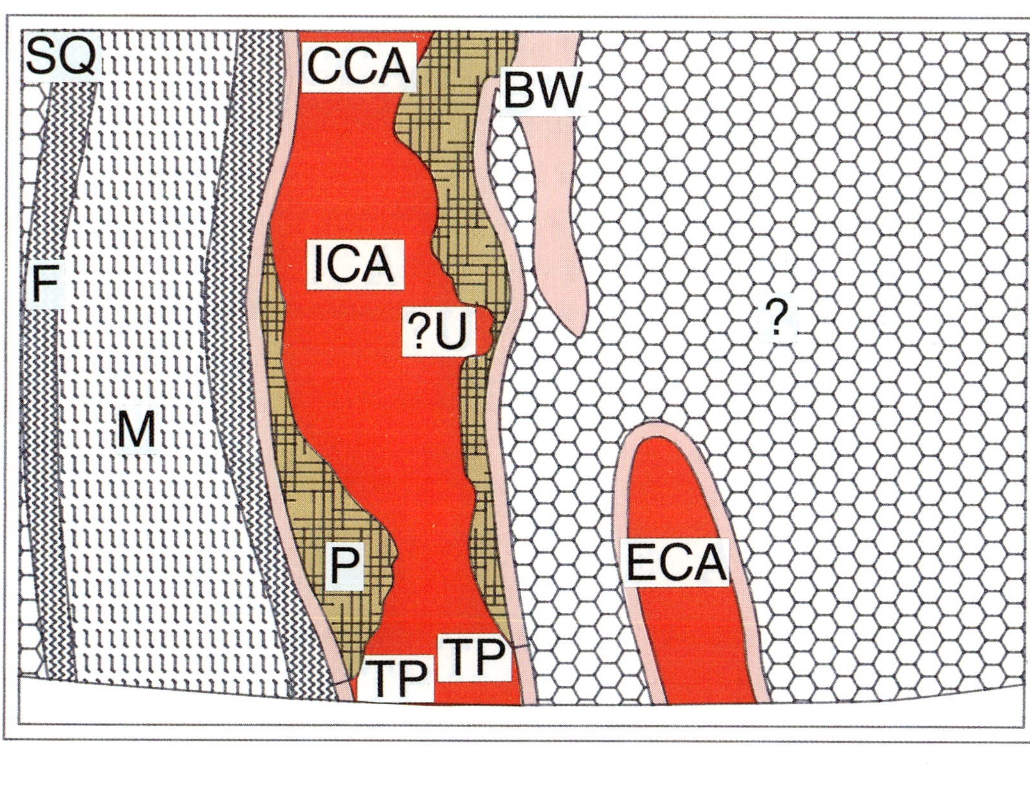
SQ
CCA
BW
F
ICA
?U
?
M
P
ECA
TP
TP

Figure 106. CAROTID STENOSIS POST-ENDARTERECTOMY

This is another longitudinal view of the same left internal carotid artery (ICA) as in Figure 105 from a more posterior approach on the neck. The recurrent carotid plaque (P), seen in the previous view as a large mound on the superficial wall of the distal ICA, is now seen as a quite faintly echogenic triangular projection from the deep wall of the artery just above the Doppler cursor (not drawn). In this particular view the normal "intimal stripes" of the distal internal carotid artery (DIST) are not seen, partly because of the angle the vessel makes as it dives into the deeper tissue and partly because the plane of view is slightly off center within the artery. SQ = subcutaneous tissue, M = muscle, F = fascia, PROX = proximal internal carotid artery.

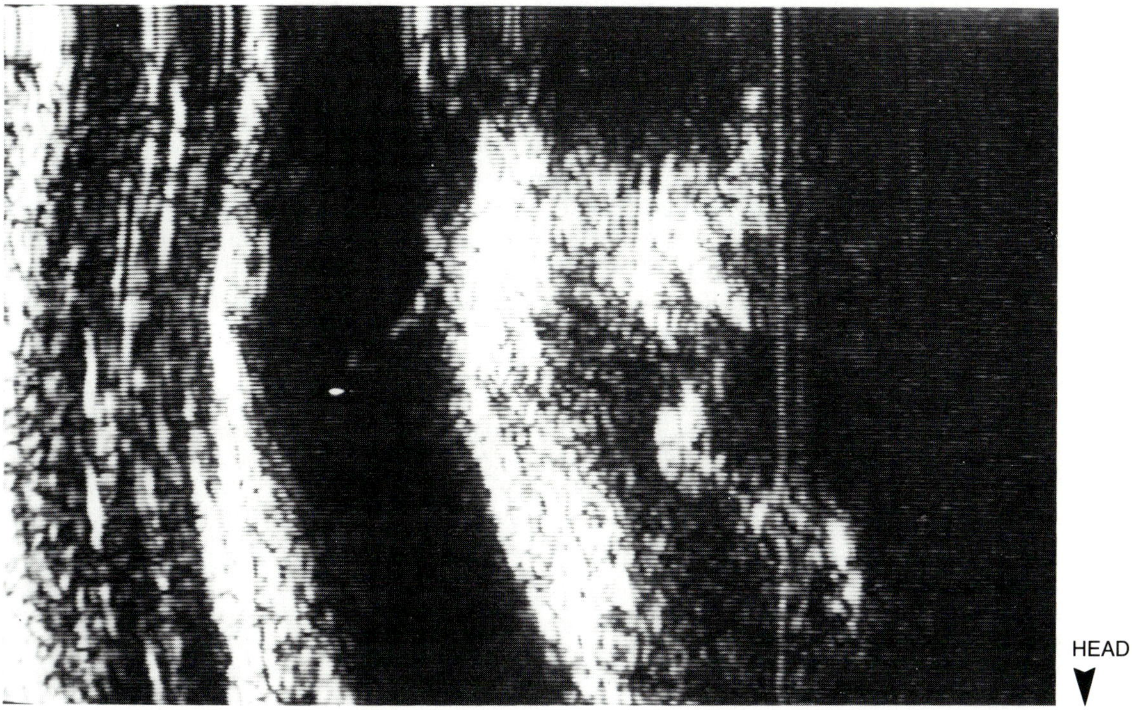
HEAD

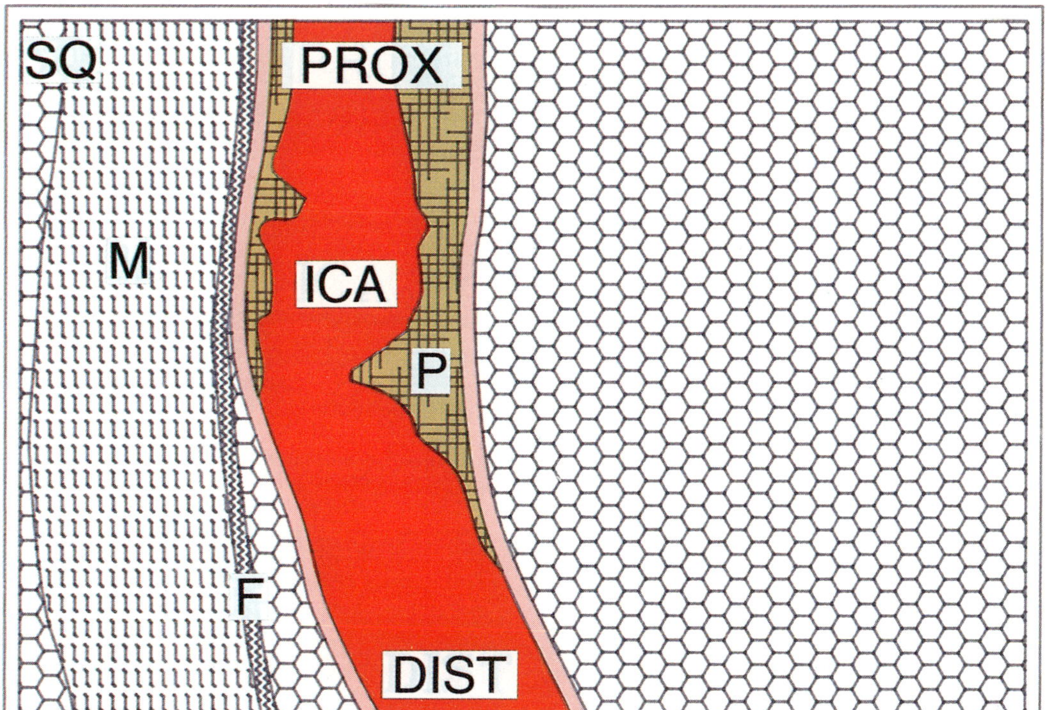
SQ
PROX
M
ICA
P
F
DIST

Figure 107. CAROTID STENOSIS POST-ENDARTERECTOMY

In this patient there is moderately echogenic, very homogeneous lipid-type plaque (P) within the right mid common carotid artery (CCA). This is residual plaque, located below the level of the endarterectomy and accompanied by a fairly well-defined smooth surface. Compare the plaque in this scan with that in Figure 105, which is a more irregular and recurrent, not residual, type plaque. It is the location of the plaque relative to the endarterectomy more than its ultrasonic characteristics that defines a plaque as being either recurrent or residual. SQ = subcutaneous tissue (including platysmal muscle), F = fascia, M = sternocleidomastoid muscle, IJV = internal jugular vein.

HISTORY *This 55-year-old female presented with waxing and waning neurological symptoms associated with a thrombosed right internal carotid artery for which she underwent an emergent carotid endarterectomy. She had some post-operative seizures but otherwise had a complete recovery. This scan was obtained 2 years following the endarterectomy.*

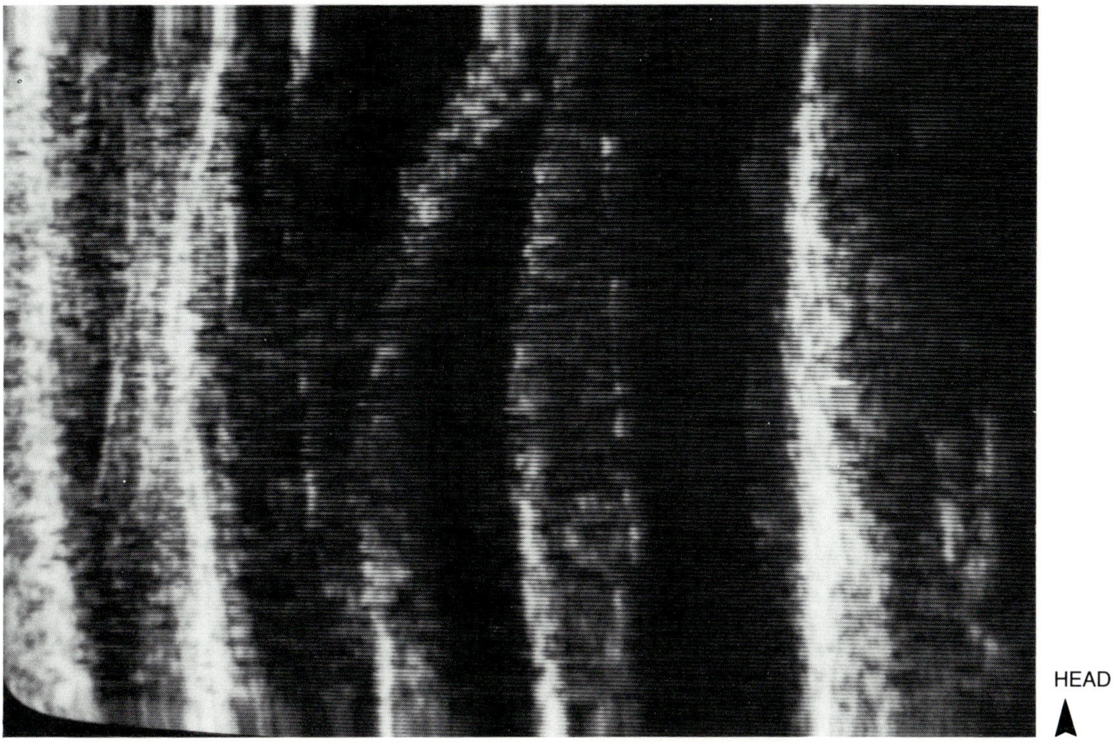
HEAD

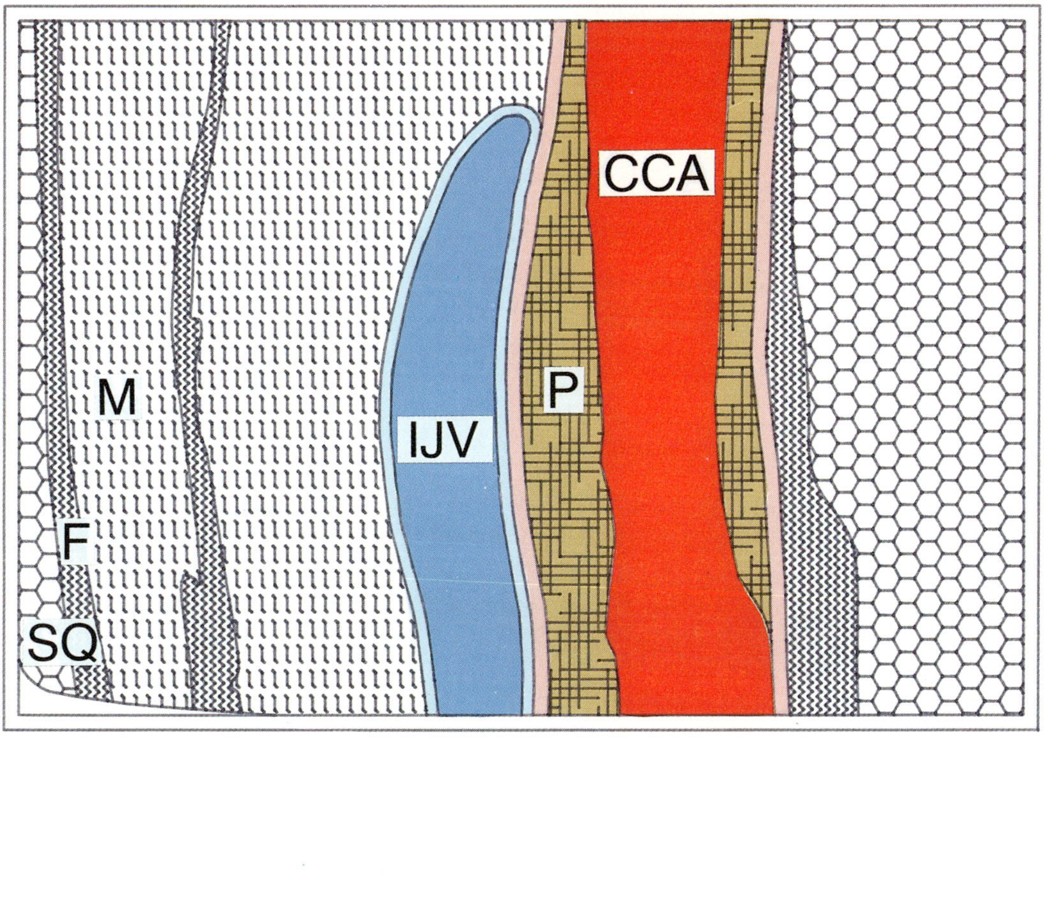
CCA
P
IJV
M
F
SQ

Figure 108. RECURRENT CAROTID STENOSIS

In this longitudinal view of the left internal carotid artery (ICA) recurrent, fairly smooth, homogeneous, moderately echogenic plaque is seen to cause a 75% stenosis of the artery with a residual lumen of 1.3 mm diameter and a distal ICA (at the bottom of the scan) of 5.5 mm diameter. Recurrent stenosis that develops from months to years after endarterectomy typically has the ultrasound characteristics of the plaque seen in this view, that is, the appearance of a stable, organized fibrous type lesion which is moderately echogenic and highly homogeneous. SQ = subcutaneous tissue, M = muscle, IJV = internal jugular vein, F = fascia (carotid sheath).

HISTORY *This is a 60-year-old male who had undergone a left carotid endarterectomy $6\frac{1}{2}$ years before and was asymptomatic at the time of this scan.*

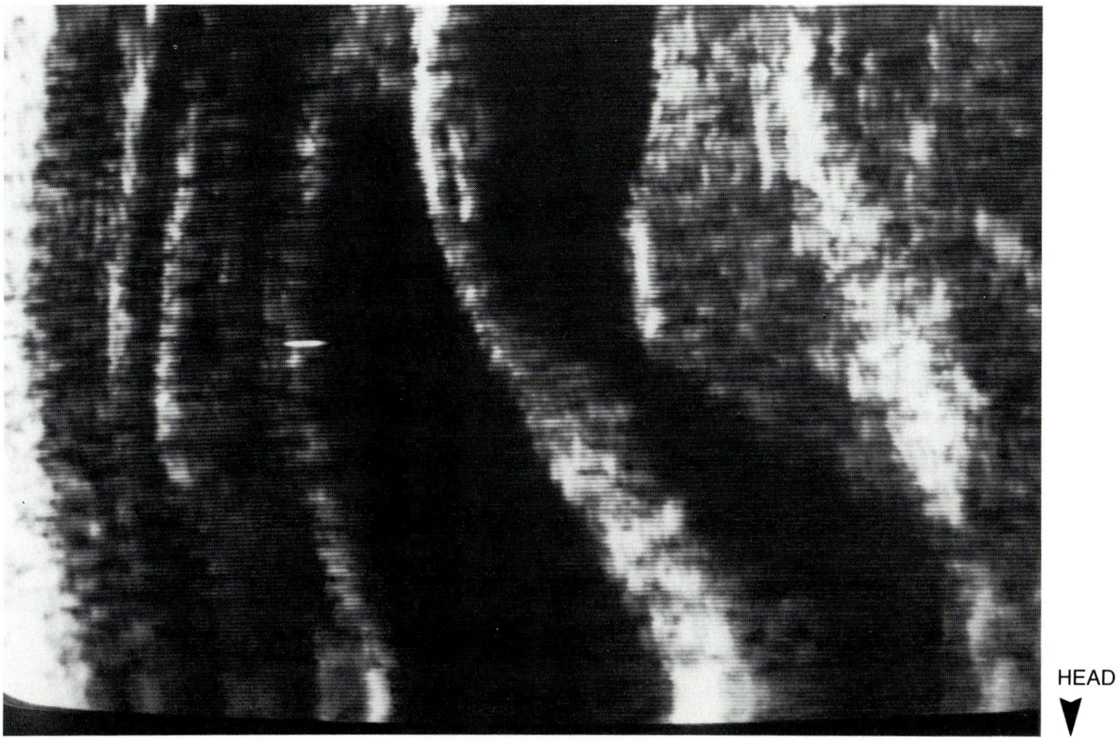
HEAD

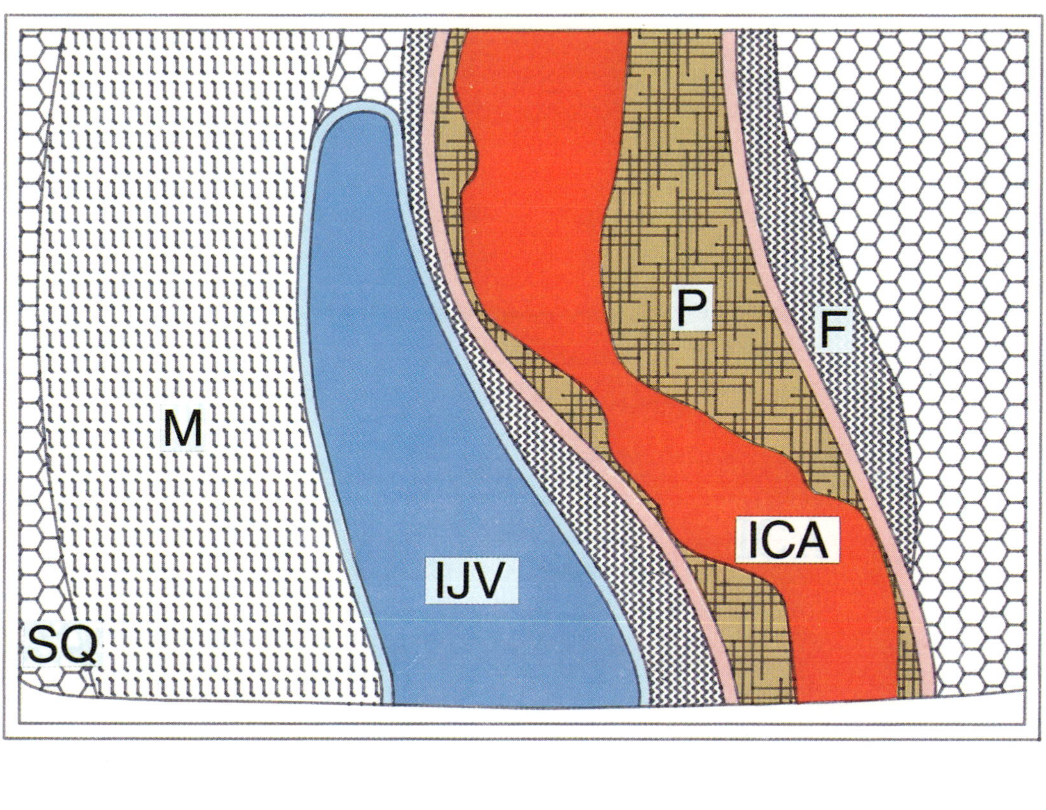
M
IJV
P
F
ICA
SQ

Figure 109. STENOSIS AT ENDARTERECTOMY

In this transverse view of the right common carotid artery (CCA), following a carotid endarterectomy 10 months prior, residual plaque (P) is seen at the level of the proximal endpoint of the endarterectomy. There is still a fairly large residual lumen within the artery, and the degree of plaque present at this level is not of great concern. M = sternocleidomastoid muscle, F = fascia, IJV = internal jugular vein, SQ = subcutaneous tissue.

HISTORY *This 67-year-old male had undergone an endarterectomy 10 months prior to the scan. He remained asymptomatic for the following 22 months despite the presence of this stenosis.*

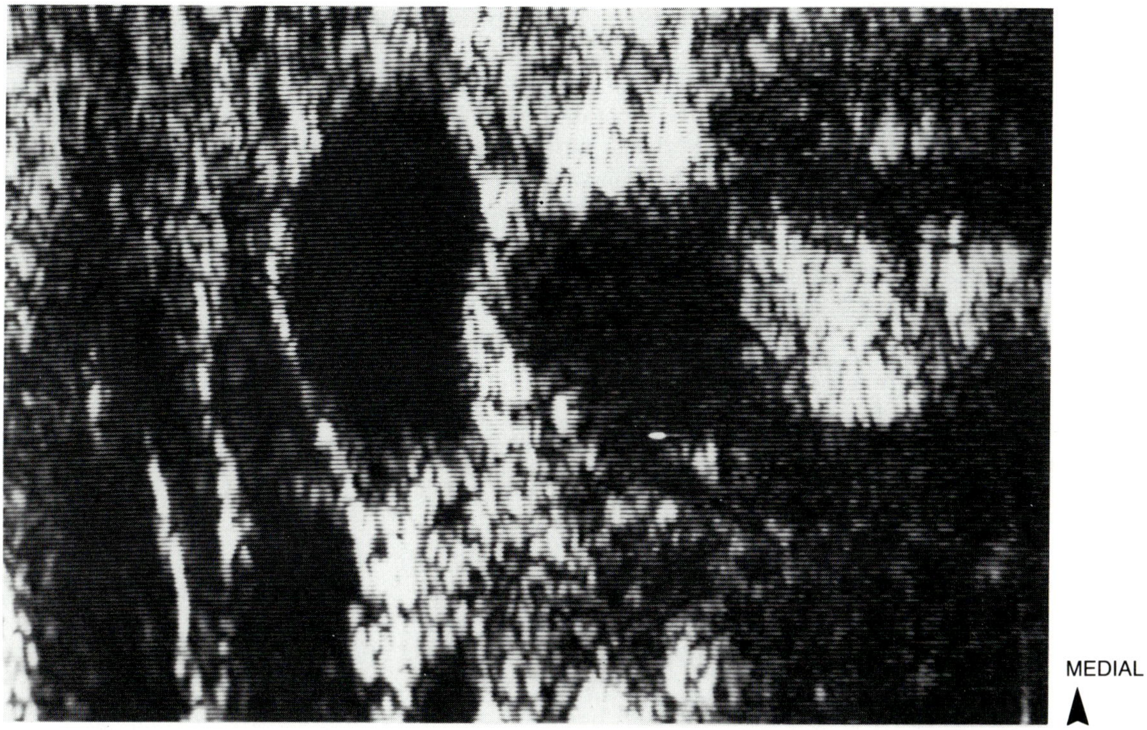
MEDIAL

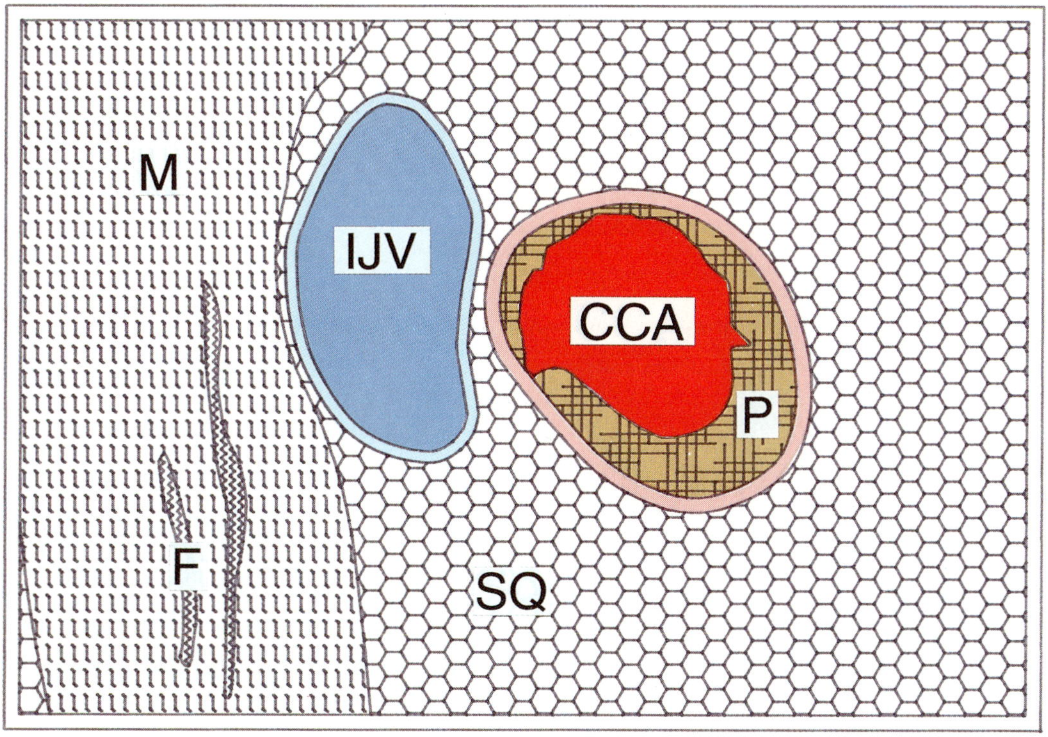
M
IJV
CCA
P
F
SQ

Figure 110. RESIDUAL STENOSIS BELOW ENDARTERECTOMY

This is a transverse view of the same common carotid artery (CCA) as in Figure 109 at mid neck below the level of the endarterectomy, showing residual plaque (P) that is moderately echogenic and heterogeneous. The residual lumen is quite a bit smaller. Carotid endarterectomies performed at the bifurcation occasionally miss significant disease present at a lower level. The residual lumen measures 2.3 mm in average diameter compared with an average arterial diameter of 7.5 mm. This corresponds to a 70% diameter stenosis. M = sternocleidomastoid muscle, F = fascia, IJV = internal jugular vein.

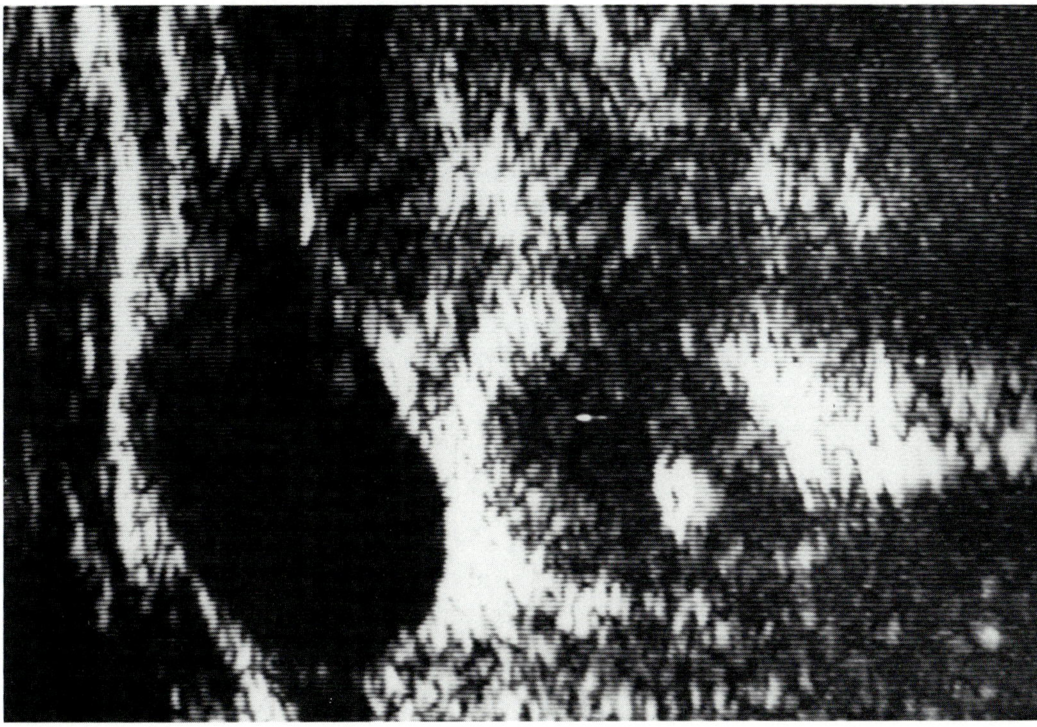

MEDIAL

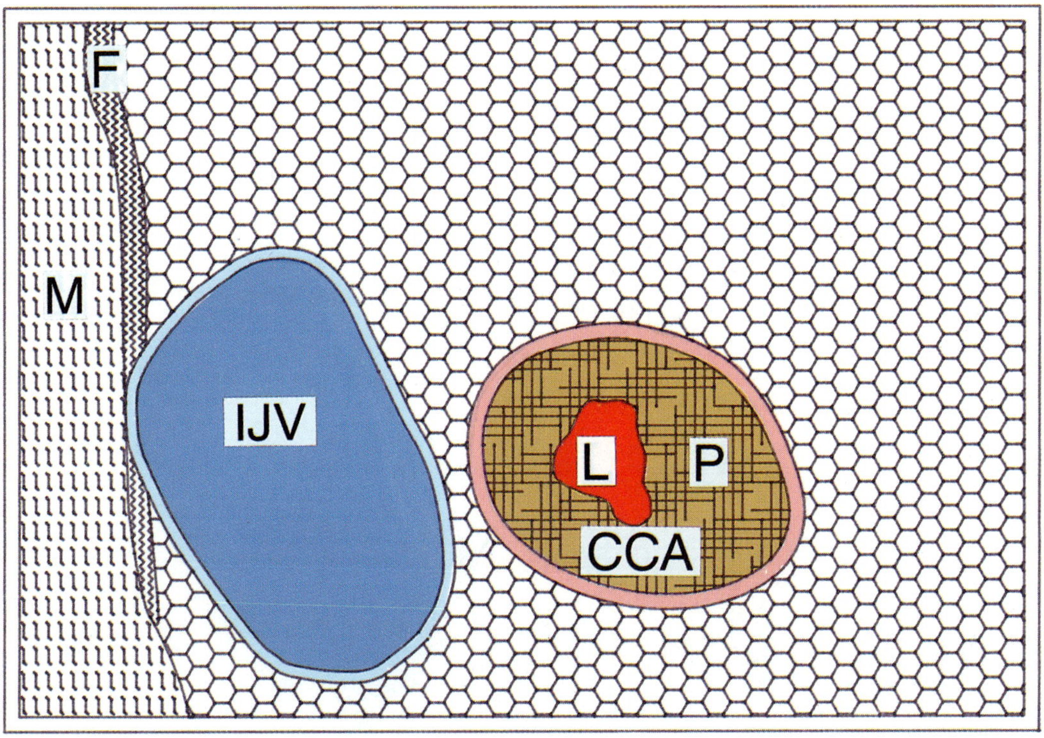

Figure 111. BIFURCATION POST-ENDARTERECTOMY

This is a longitudinal view of the left carotid bifurcation following a carotid endarterectomy. There is a considerable amount of residual plaque (P) within the common carotid artery (CCA), causing approximately a 50% diameter stenosis just proximal to the endarterectomized portion of the bifurcation. The proximal extent of the endarterectomy (EA) is seen as a rather abrupt, shelf-like ending of the plaque on the deep wall. These abrupt shelves are frequently seen after a carotid endarterectomy but are not as pronounced as in this case. Although the internal carotid artery (ICA) contained minimal residual plaque, there was a total occlusion of the external carotid artery (ECA). SQ = subcutaneous tissue, M = muscle (sternocleidomastoid), F = fascia (carotid sheath).

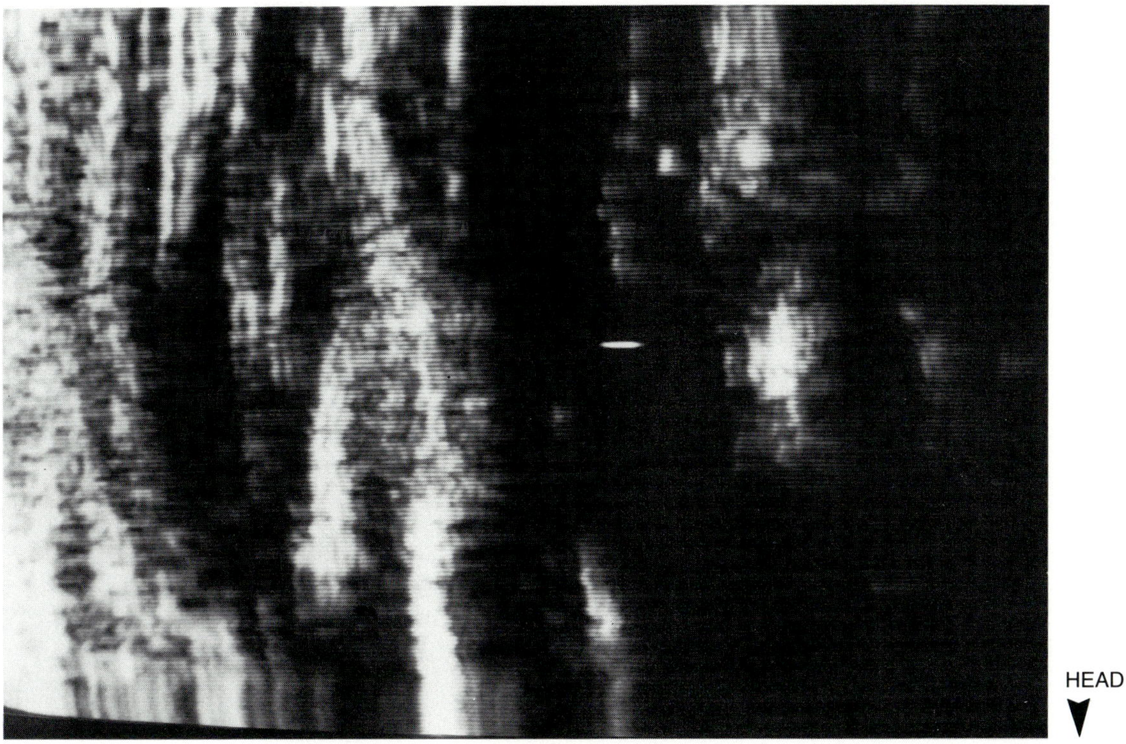
HEAD

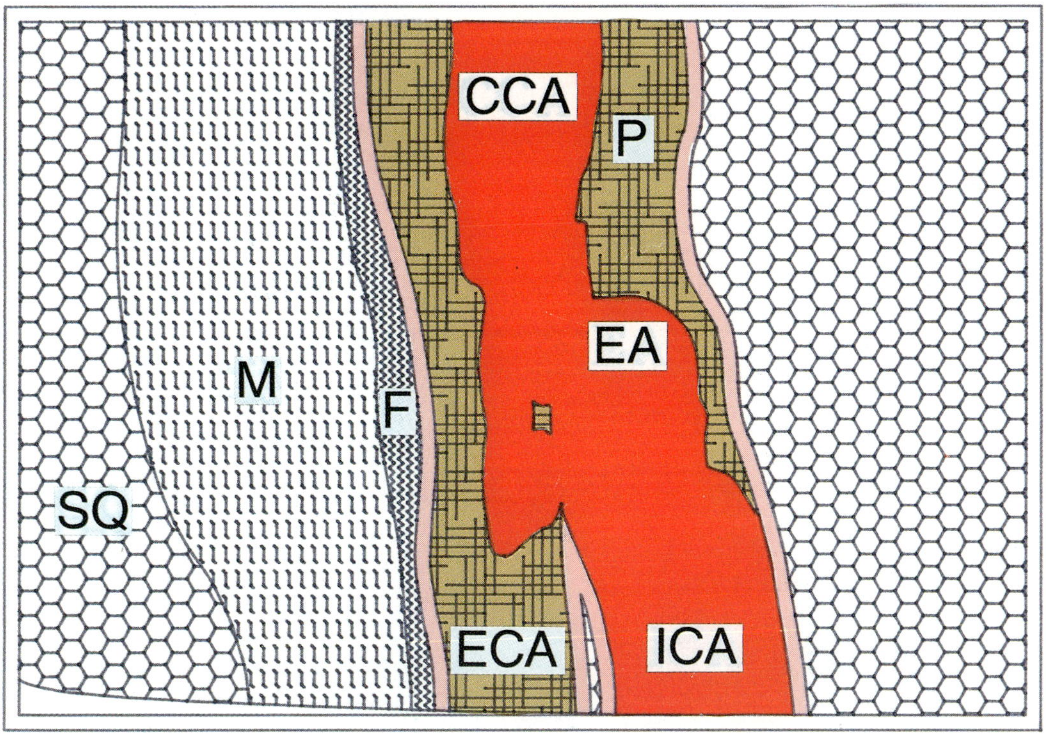
CCA
P
EA
M
F
SQ
ECA
ICA

Figure 112. COMMON CAROTID BEFORE ENDARTERECTOMY

This is a longitudinal view of the right common carotid artery (CCA) just proximal to the bifurcation. This scan was obtained immediately prior to an endarterectomy because of significant internal carotid stenosis. There are normal intimal margins with no plaque visible at this level. The maximum diameter of the artery equals 8.0 mm. The faint vertical streak passing through the deep portion of the carotid artery is due to "hard line" artifact from the probe and is not drawn (see Figure 158). Note the level at which this scan was taken, established by the relationship between the internal jugular vein (IJV) and a more superficial vein (V). SQ = subcutaneous tissue, M = sternocleidomastoid muscle, F = fascia.

HISTORY *This patient underwent a right carotid endarterectomy the following day because of the significant disease in the bifurcation above the level of this ultrasound scan.*

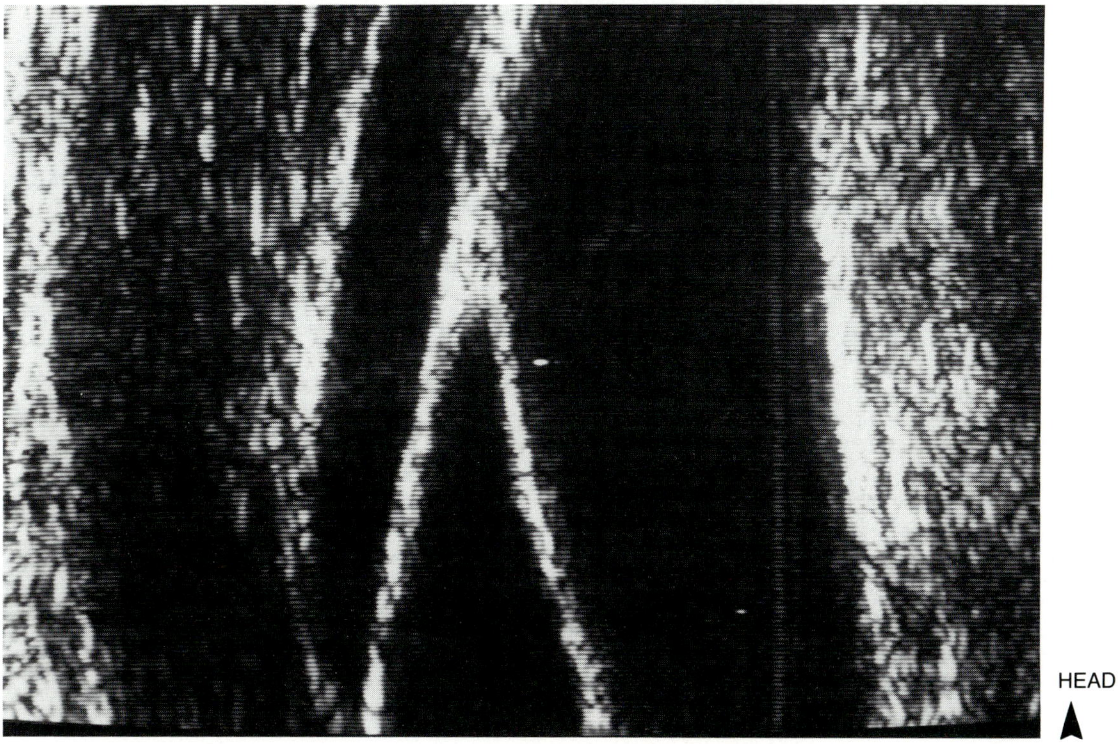
HEAD

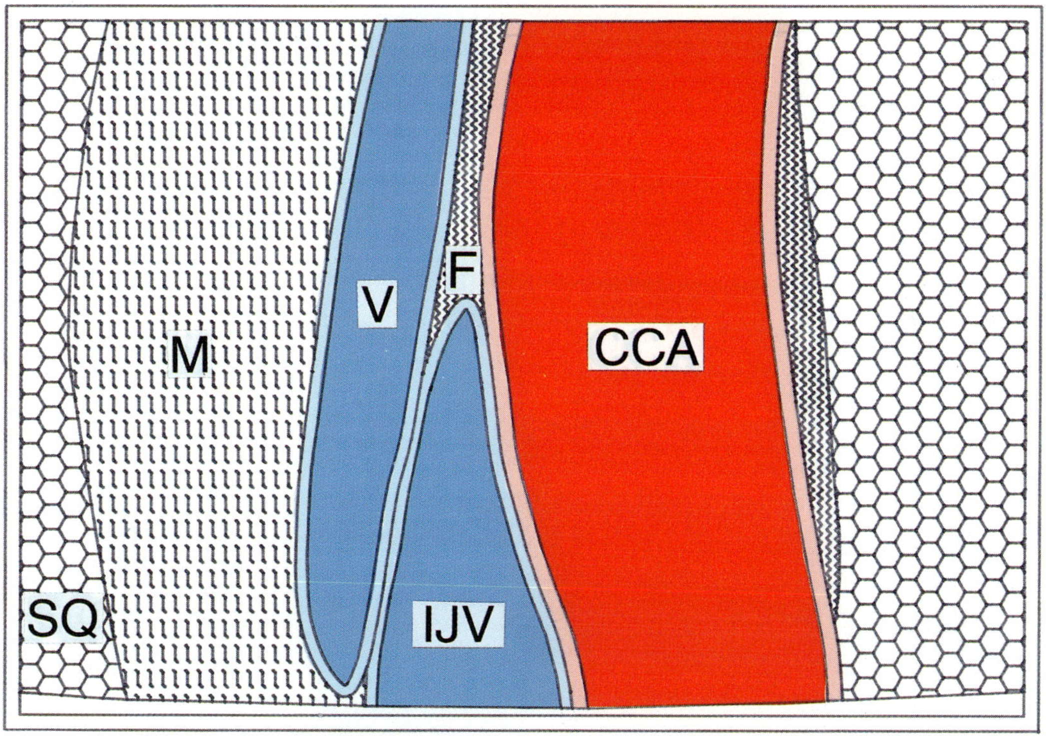
V
F
M
CCA
SQ
IJV

Figure 113. DILATATION AFTER ENDARTERECTOMY

This is a longitudinal view of the same common carotid artery (CCA) as in Figure 112 seen 2 months after the carotid endarterectomy. The endarterectomized portion of the artery has dilated to 11.0 mm in diameter down to the proximal endpoint of the suture line. The sutures themselves are not seen, being rotated slightly out of plane in this view. Note the similarity in levels between the two scans based upon the relationship of the superficial vein (V) with the internal jugular vein (IJV). This view was obtained at a slightly lower level. The patient has been followed for 26 months subsequent to these two scans, and there has been no further increase in the degree of dilatation. SQ = subcutaneous tissue, M = sternocleidomastoid muscle, F = fascia.

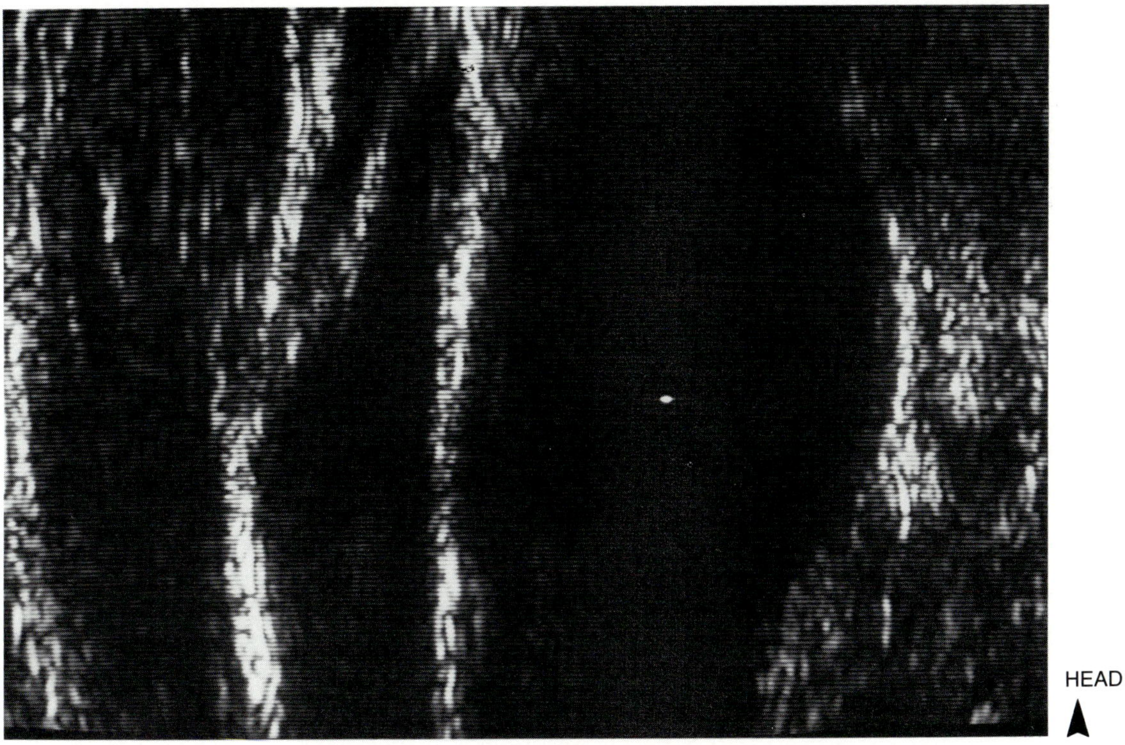
HEAD

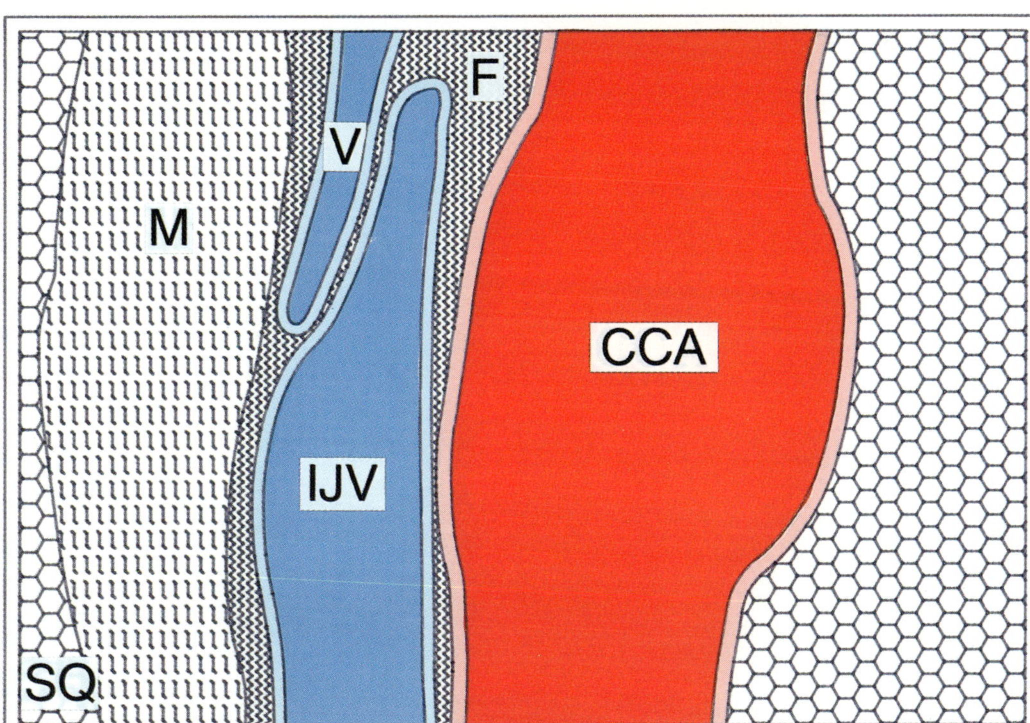
F
V
M
CCA
IJV
SQ

Figure 114. POST-ENDARTERECTOMY ANEURYSM

This is an example of a 16-mm diameter aneurysm (AN) of the distal common carotid artery (CCA) and base of the internal carotid artery (ICA), which developed following a carotid endarterectomy 2 years previously. There is a small amount of plaque (P) on the superficial wall. The ICA passes obliquely out of plane and is seen only at its origin. This view was obtained with the 8 MHz probe. S = skin, SQ = subcutaneous tissue, F = fascia (scar), M = muscle (sternocleidomastoid).

HISTORY *This 71-year-old male underwent carotid endarterectomy without patching of the artery 2 years prior to this scan.*

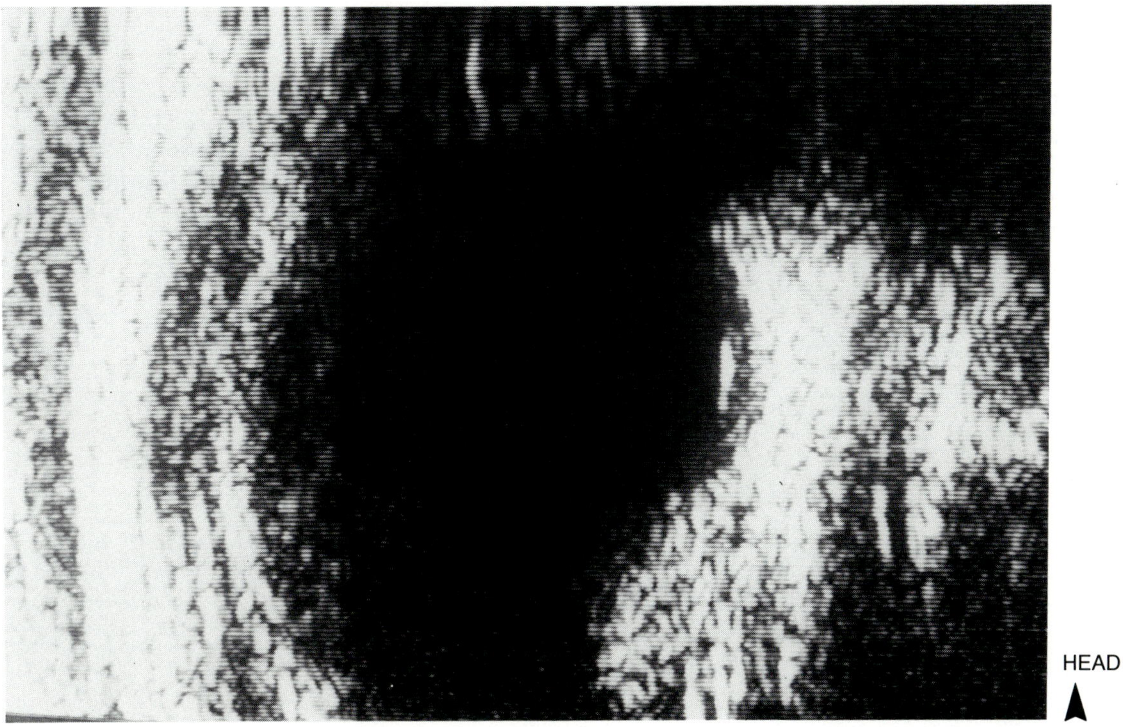
HEAD

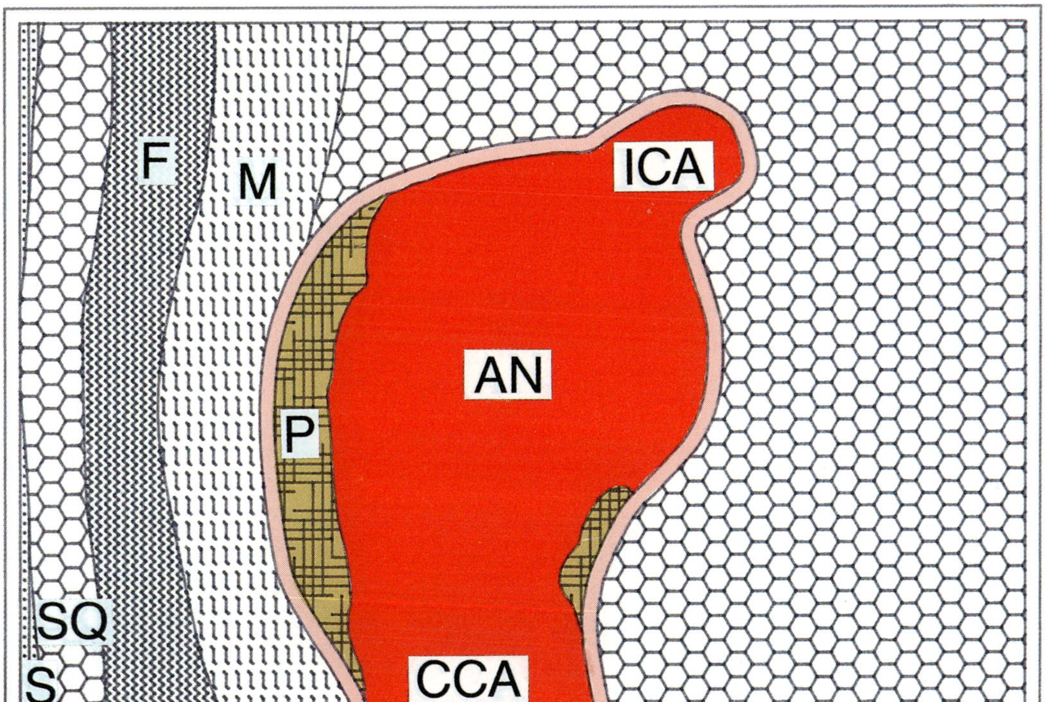
F
M
ICA
AN
P
SQ
S
CCA

Figure 115. POST-ENDARTERECTOMY ANEURYSM

This is a view of the same 16-mm diameter aneurysm as seen in longitudinal profile with the 4 MHz probe. The 4 MHz probe is occasionally useful for better visualization of the overall contours of large objects. The depth of field (from left to right) of this probe is 8 cm; however, the photograph has been cropped. S = skin, SQ = subcutaneous tissue, F = fascia, M = muscle (sternocleidomastoid), CCA = common carotid artery, ECA = external carotid artery, ICA = internal carotid artery (passing out of plane), AN = aneurysm.

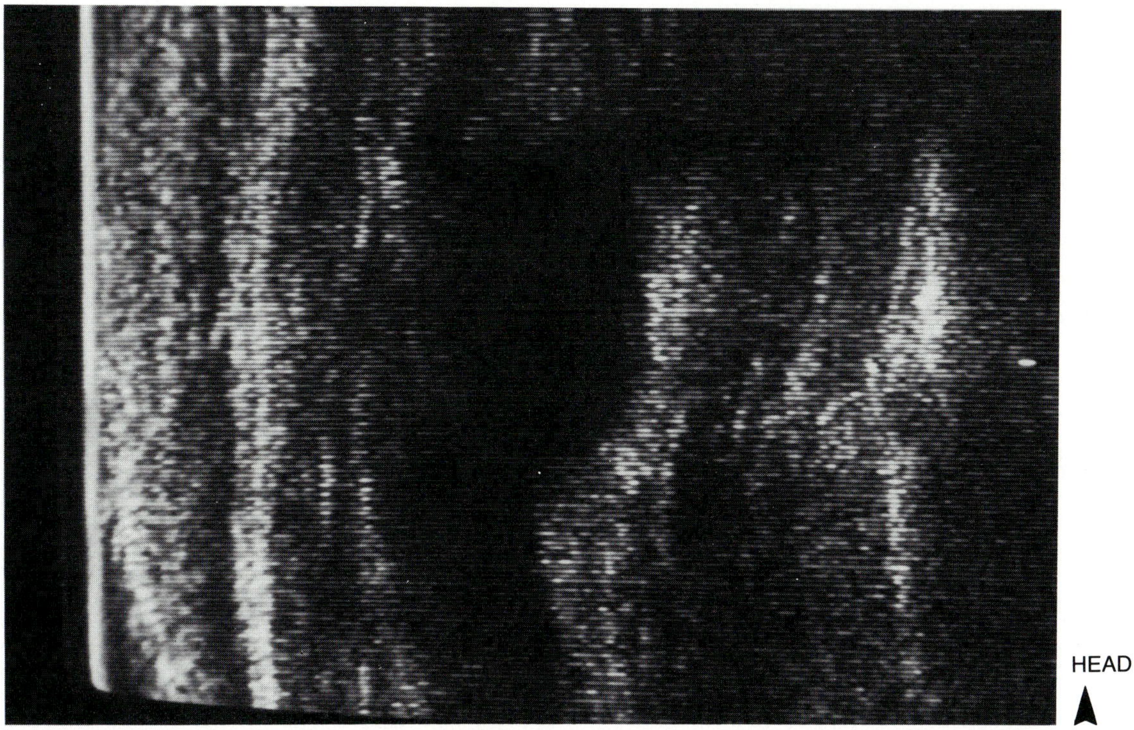
HEAD

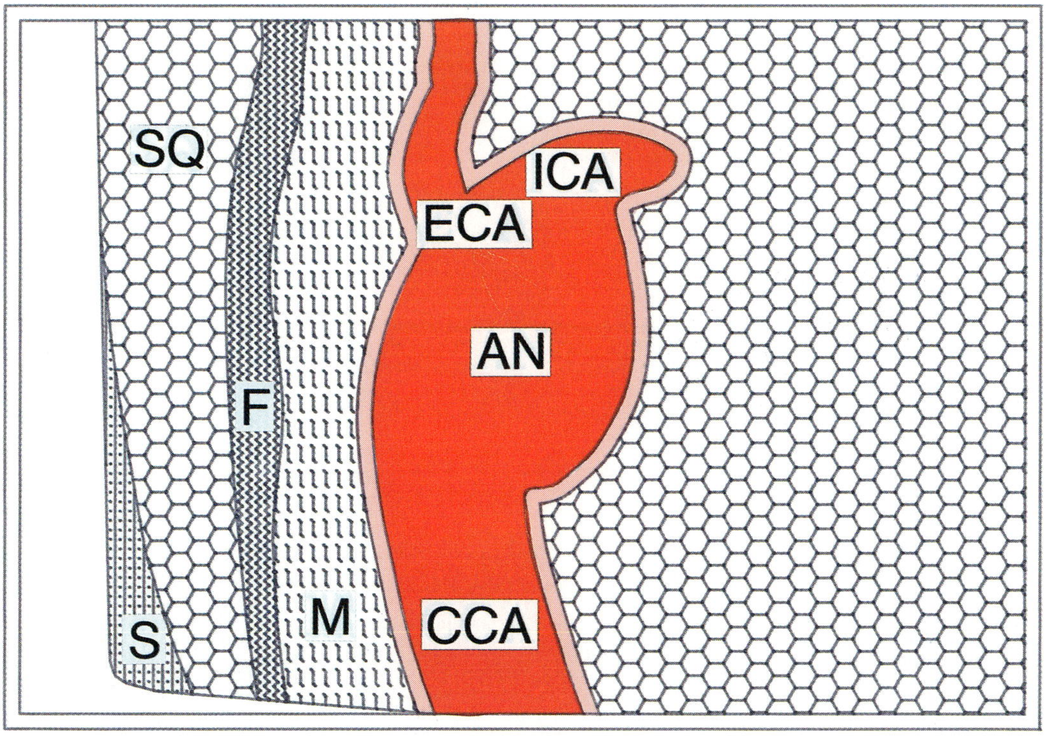
SQ
ICA
ECA
AN
F
S
M
CCA

Figure 116. VASCULAR CLAMP INJURY

This 67-year-old female had an endarterectomy $2\frac{1}{2}$ years prior to this scan. A flap of plaque (FP) in the proximal left common carotid artery (CCA) was fractured probably by the placement of a vascular clamp. The patient developed an immediate post-operative neurological deficit, consisting of hemiparesis on the opposite side that cleared prior to her discharge from the hospital. Flow in the carotid artery that goes from top to bottom in the scan caused the flap to bend out into center stream and to curl somewhat. Smooth plaque (P) extends up to this flap and is probably relatively new, filling in the gap left by the flap. SQ = subcutaneous tissue, M = sternocleidomastoid muscle.

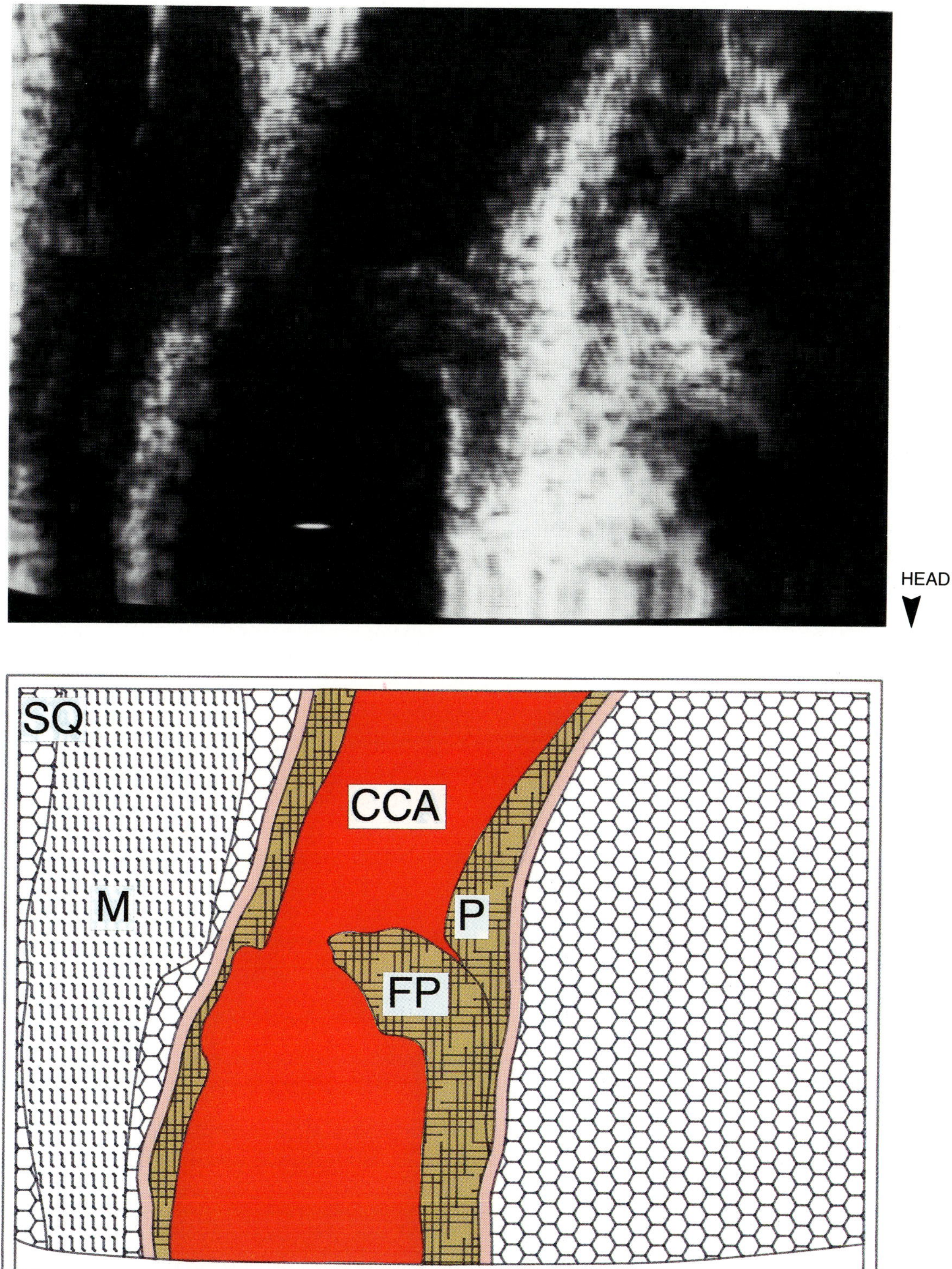
HEAD
SQ
M
CCA
P
FP

Figure 117. INTIMAL FLAP AFTER ENDARTERECTOMY

This is a transverse view of a right carotid bifurcation just below the point of separation of the internal carotid artery (ICA) and external carotid artery (ECA). A thin intimal flap (IF) protrudes from the bottom wall of the origin of the ICA. At its upper tip the flap is attached to some faintly echogenic thrombus (T) adherent to the superficial wall of the bifurcation. These findings were noted 3 months after performance of the endarterectomy. Intra-arterial defects have been reported in up to 30% of intra-operative ultrasound scans. These defects include intimal flaps, arterial thrombosis, residual stenosis, and narrowing of the artery by the suture line. We have noted these abnormalities less frequently among routine post-operative ultrasound scans. SQ = subcutaneous tissue, M = muscle (sternocleidomastoid), F = fascia.

HISTORY *This 61-year-old male had undergone a right carotid endarterectomy 3 months prior to the scan. He also had vertebrobasilar insufficiency with complaints of dizziness and double vision (diplopia) and has been maintained on warfarin sodium. Despite the finding of an intimal flap, the patient has not developed any localizing carotid territorial symptoms for $3\frac{1}{2}$ years.*

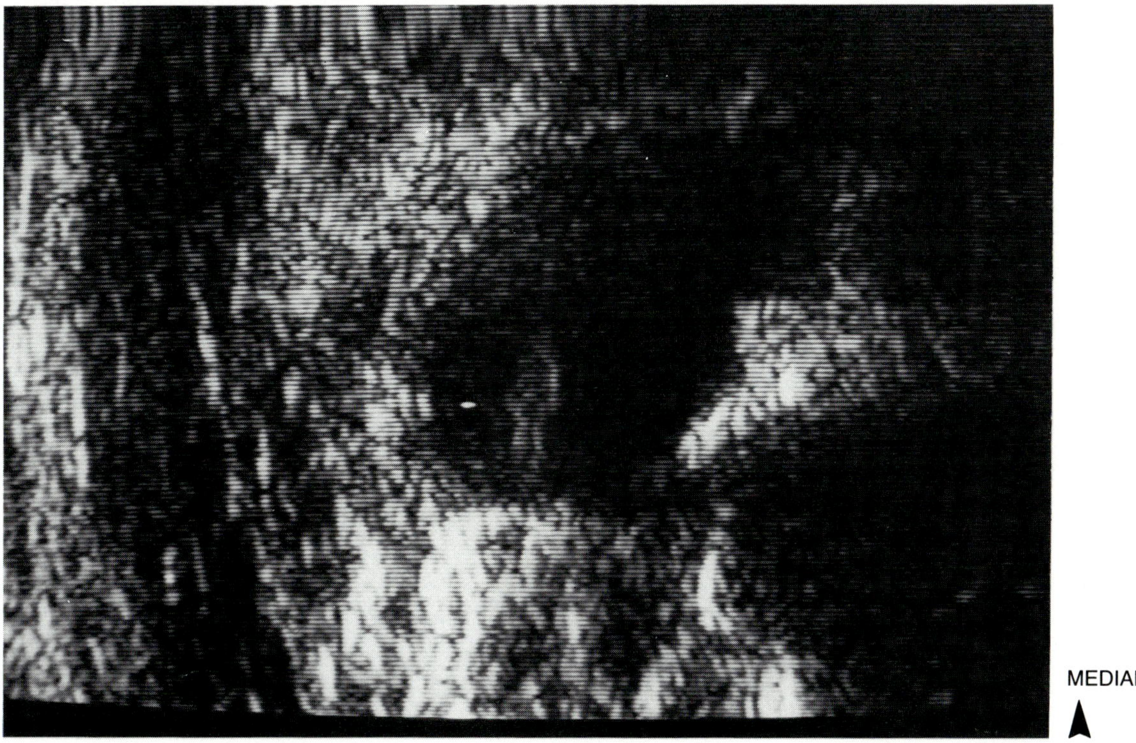
MEDIAL

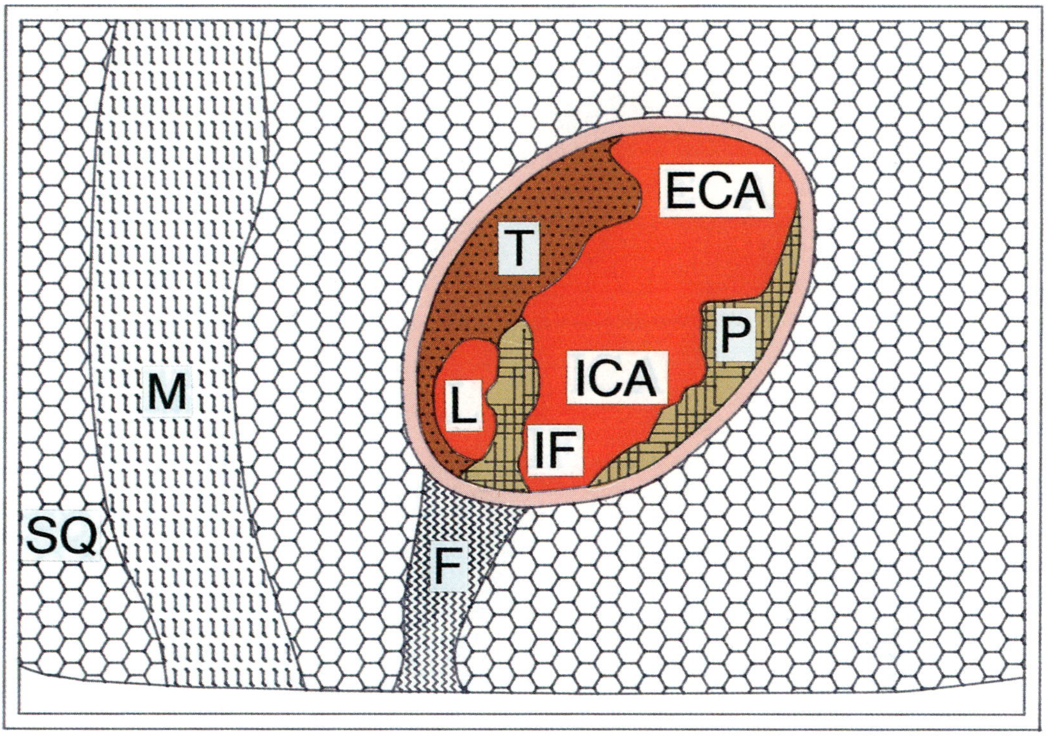
ECA
T
P
ICA
M
L
IF
SQ
F

Figure 118. POST-ENDARTERECTOMY THROMBUS

This is a transverse view through the right common carotid artery (CCA) of a patient who had undergone a carotid endarterectomy only a few days before. Note the faint round thrombus (T) seen just to the right of a small amount of residual plaque (P), leaving a crescent-like lumen of open artery above. Good quality ultrasound scans cannot always be obtained until a week post-operatively. In many cases, staples or tapes need to be removed because of the artifact they produce. Sometimes it is possible, however, to scan from a more anterior or posterior approach to obtain an adequate view. S = skin, M = platysma muscle, SQ = subcutaneous tissue, SCM = sternocleidomastoid muscle.

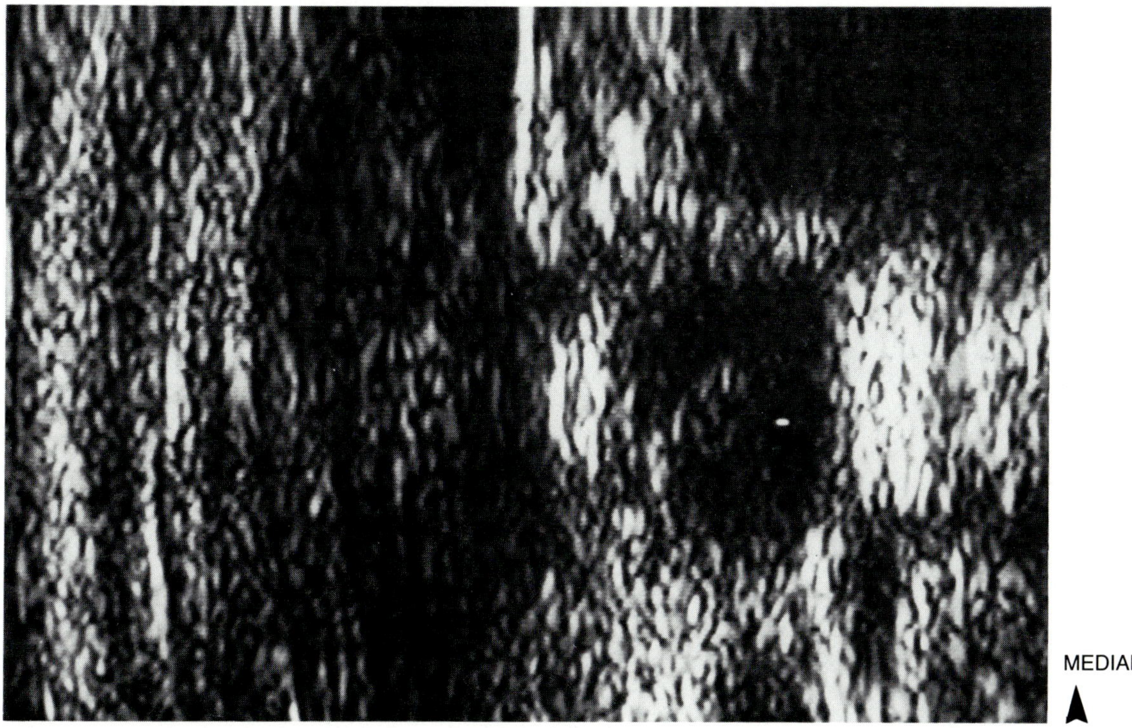
MEDIAL

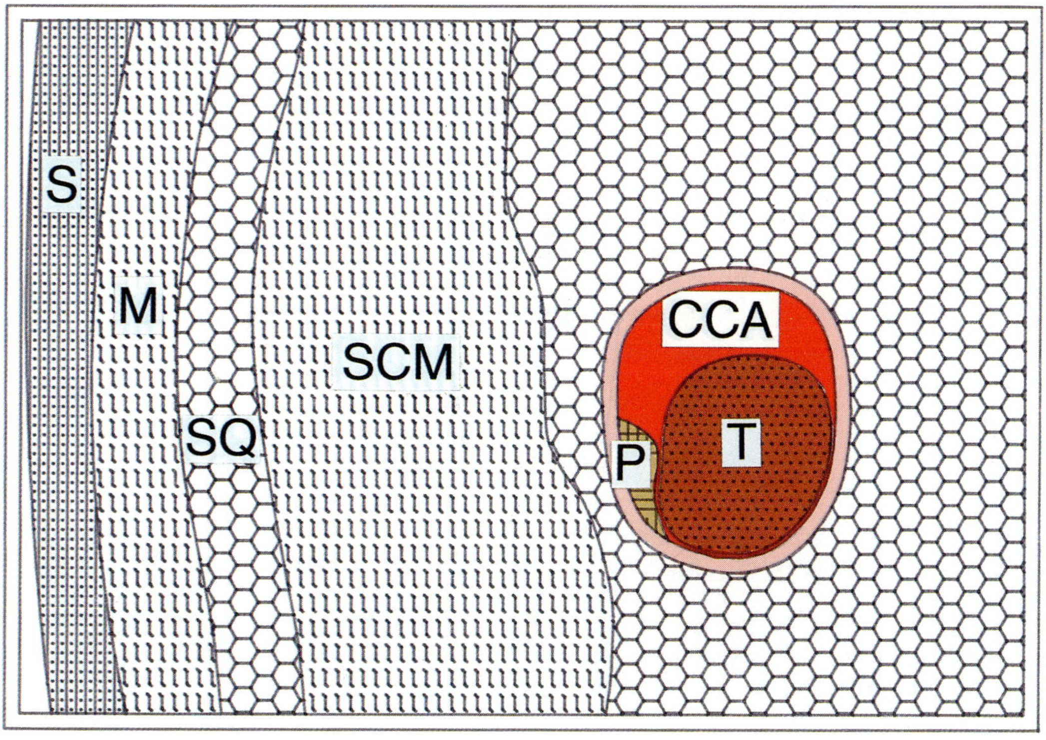
S
M
SQ
SCM
CCA
P
T

Figure 119. POST-ENDARTERECTOMY THROMBUS

This is a longitudinal view of the same artery as seen in Figure 118. One can now see the transition points (TP) between the untouched common carotid artery (CCA) toward the base of the neck and the endarterectomized portion above. The thrombus (T) is seen to line the entire endarterectomized portion of the artery along its superficial wall and to extend down onto the transition point of the endarterectomy. By putting these two views together, one can arrive at a three-dimensional perspective of this clot. It is a cylindrically shaped cord attached at its base. This is not a total thrombosis of the artery, as there remains an open lumen with a strong Doppler signal deep to the right of the clot. M = sterno-cleidomastoid muscle, SQ = subcutaneous tissue, IJV = internal jugular vein (oblique).

HISTORY *This 71-year-old female underwent right carotid endarterectomy. She did well until the fifth post-operative day when she became unresponsive. She had a persistent left hemiparesis. The ultrasound scan was done within 24 hours following her acute symptoms. A computed tomography scan 5 days following this duplex scan demonstrated infarction in the distribution of the right middle cerebral artery. Presumably, therefore, an embolized part of this thrombus was the event responsible for her delayed post-operative cerebrovascular accident (CVA).*

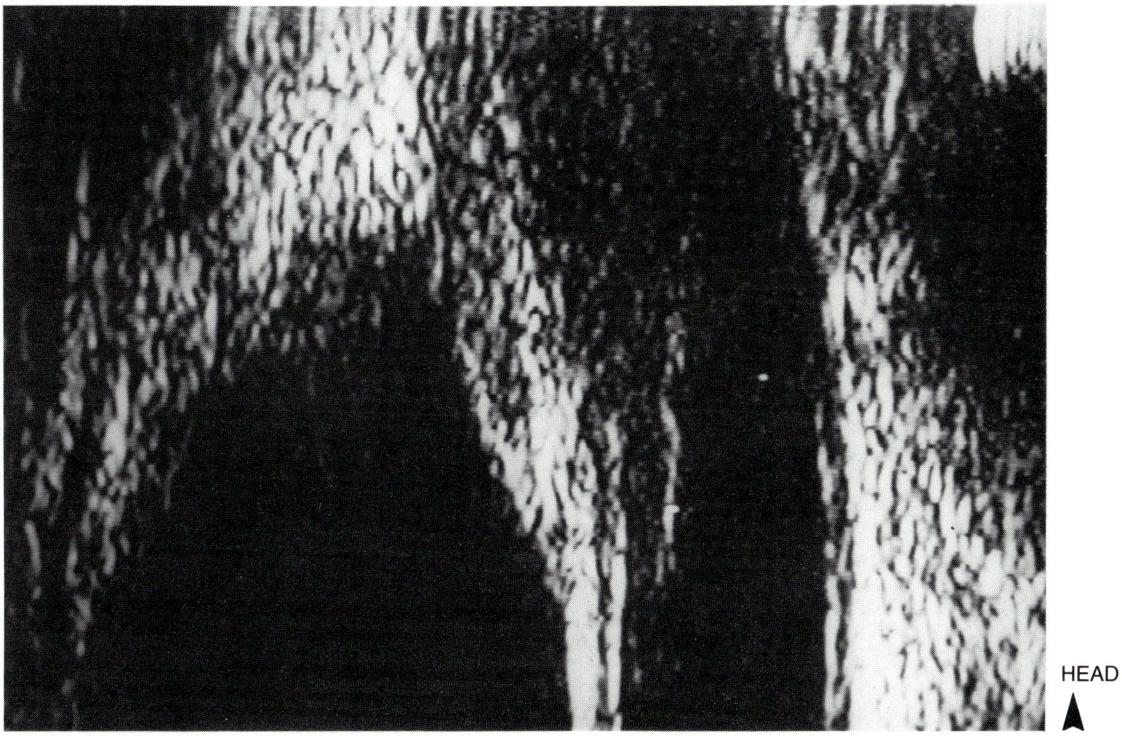
HEAD

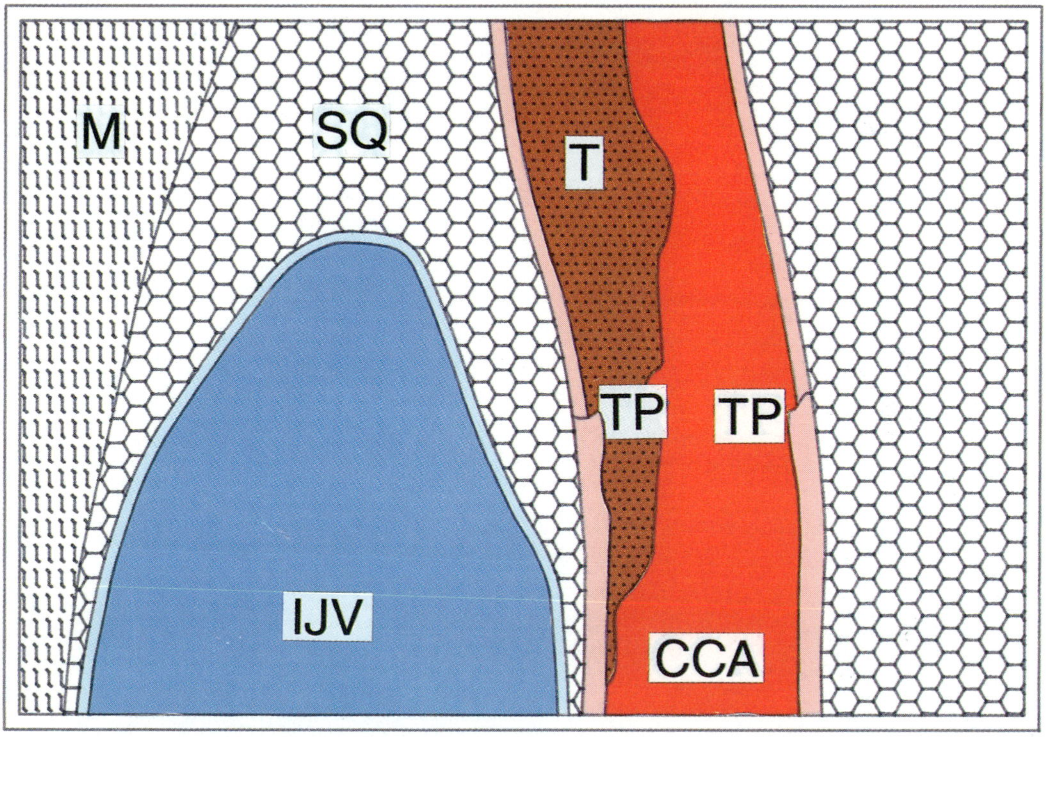
M
SQ
T
TP
TP
IJV
CCA

Figure 120. ACUTE POST-ENDARTERECTOMY THROMBOSIS

This is a longitudinal view of the left carotid bifurcation that demonstrates an acute total occlusion of the left internal carotid artery (ICA) at its origin by faint to moderately echogenic, slightly heterogeneous thrombus (T). This thrombus has the typical smooth concavity and up/down pulsatility of that associated with an acute occlusion. There is faintly visible "snow" within the common carotid (CCA) lumen due to visibility of the slowed blood, as it swirls within the blind pocket. Deep to the far right is seen one of the transverse cervical vertebral processes, which is not drawn. SQ = subcutaneous tissue, M = muscle, F = fascia.

HISTORY *This ultrasound scan was performed 13 months following a left carotid endarterectomy. The patient returned with right upper extremity weakness and expressive aphasia. This scan was obtained 9 days after the onset of symptoms. At operation 3 days after the scan, the acute occlusion was successfully reopened.*

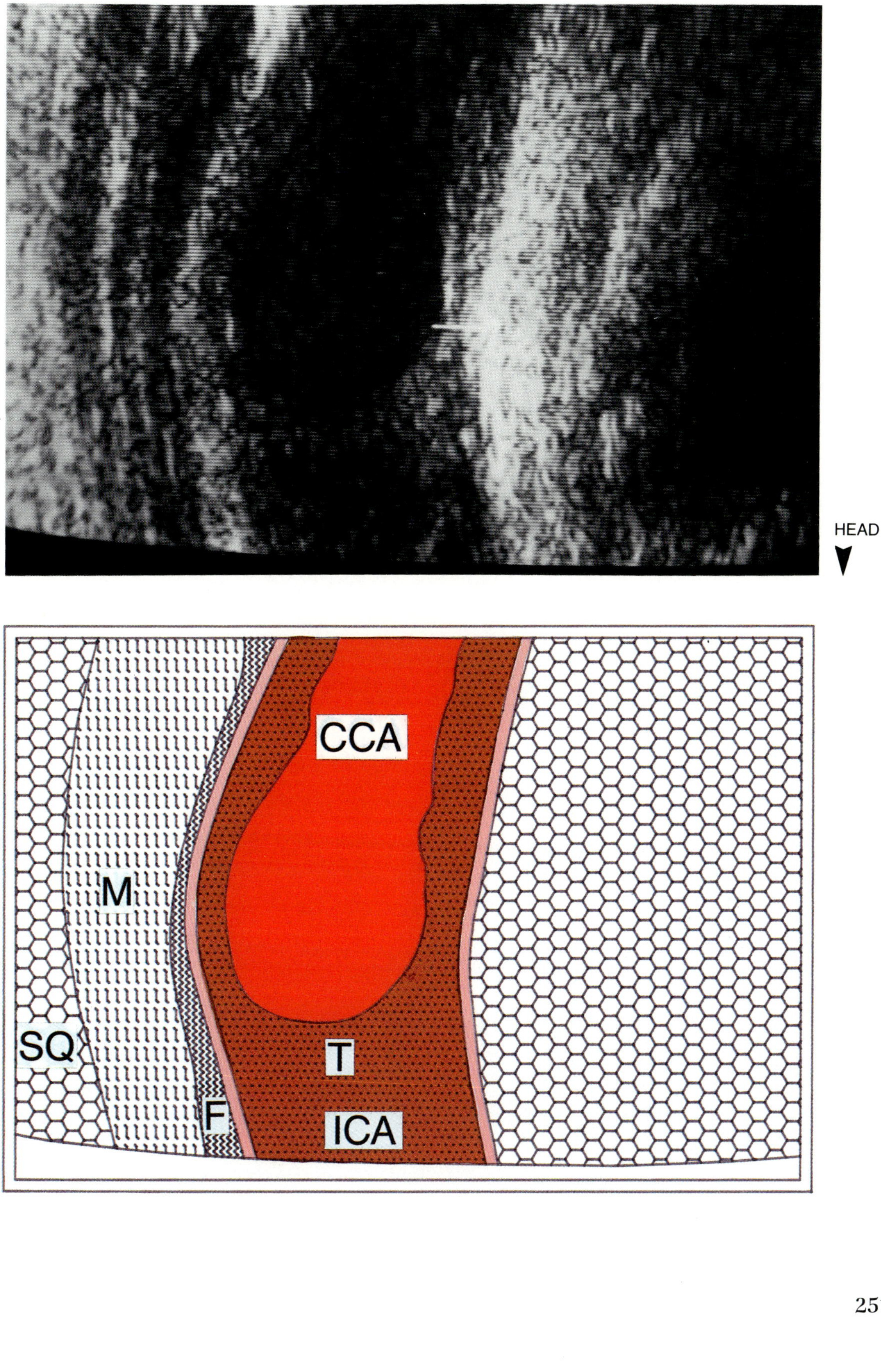
HEAD
CCA
M
SQ
T
F
ICA

Figure 121. INTERNAL CAROTID LIGATION

This is a longitudinal view of the right carotid bifurcation showing the common carotid artery (CCA) and external carotid artery (ECA). The suture line (SL) is seen along the superficial wall of the bifurcation. Opposite this level on the deep wall is an irregularity corresponding to closure of the orifice of the internal carotid. One cannot say whether the artery above is ICA or ECA utilizing this scan. In a scan such as this, the patient's history becomes an extremely important aid in identifying a single artery above the bifurcation. Doppler signal may be of some benefit in this case. One must also consider the possibility of a high bifurcation, but in this case the presence of the SL at this level assures the interpreter that the bifurcation corresponds to this level. The vertical streaks seen just to the right of the Doppler cursor (not drawn) are "hard-line" artifact (see Figure 158). This scan was obtained using the 8 MHz probe. G = gel, S = skin, SQ = subcutaneous tissue, M = sternocleidomastoid muscle.

HISTORY *This patient had previously undergone external carotid endarterectomy with ligation of a chronically occluded internal carotid artery.*

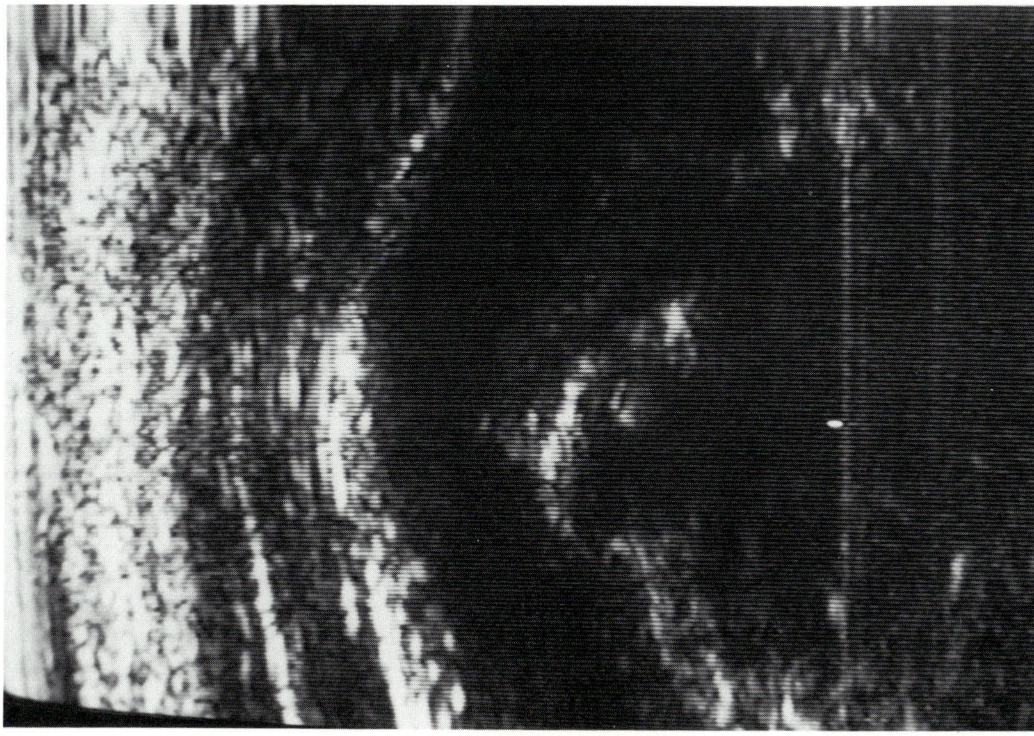

HEAD

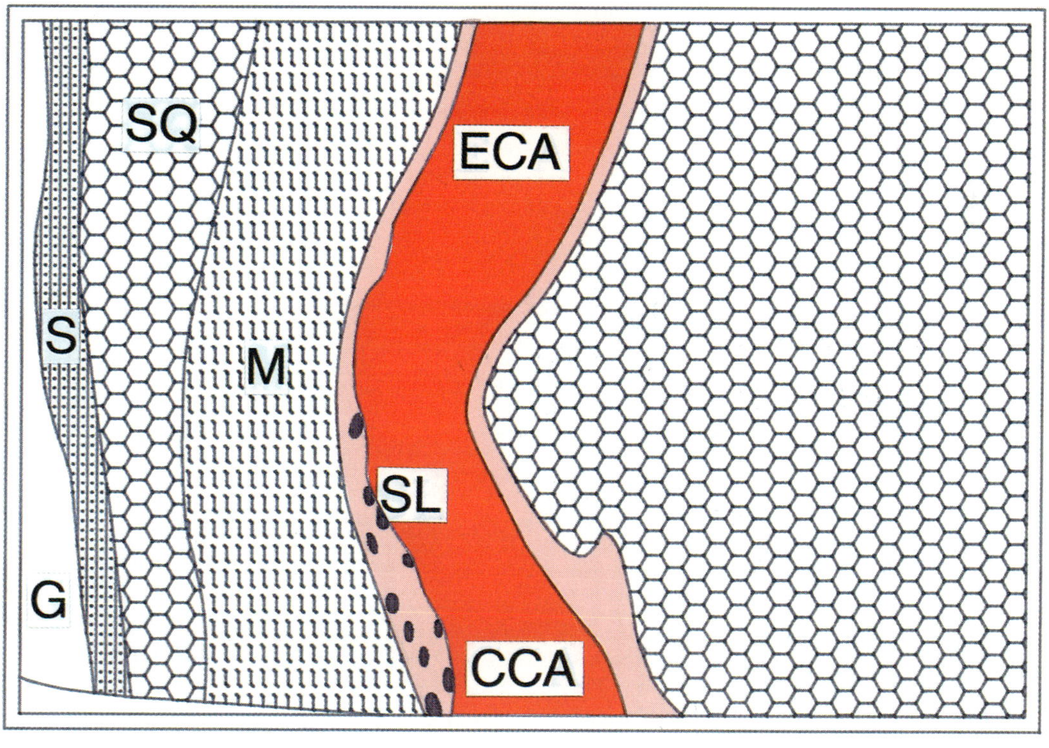

Figure 122. INTERNAL CAROTID LIGATION

This is another longitudinal view in orientation similar to that in Figure 121 but obtained with the 4 MHz probe. It shows the transition at the level of the Doppler cursor (not drawn) between the common carotid artery (CCA) and external carotid artery (ECA). At the top of the scan, the ECA measures 8 mm in diameter, which suggests compensatory dilatation (DIL). The chronically occluded internal carotid artery is not visualized. G = gel, S = skin, SQ = subcutaneous tissue, M = sternocleidomastoid muscle, F = fascia (carotid sheath).

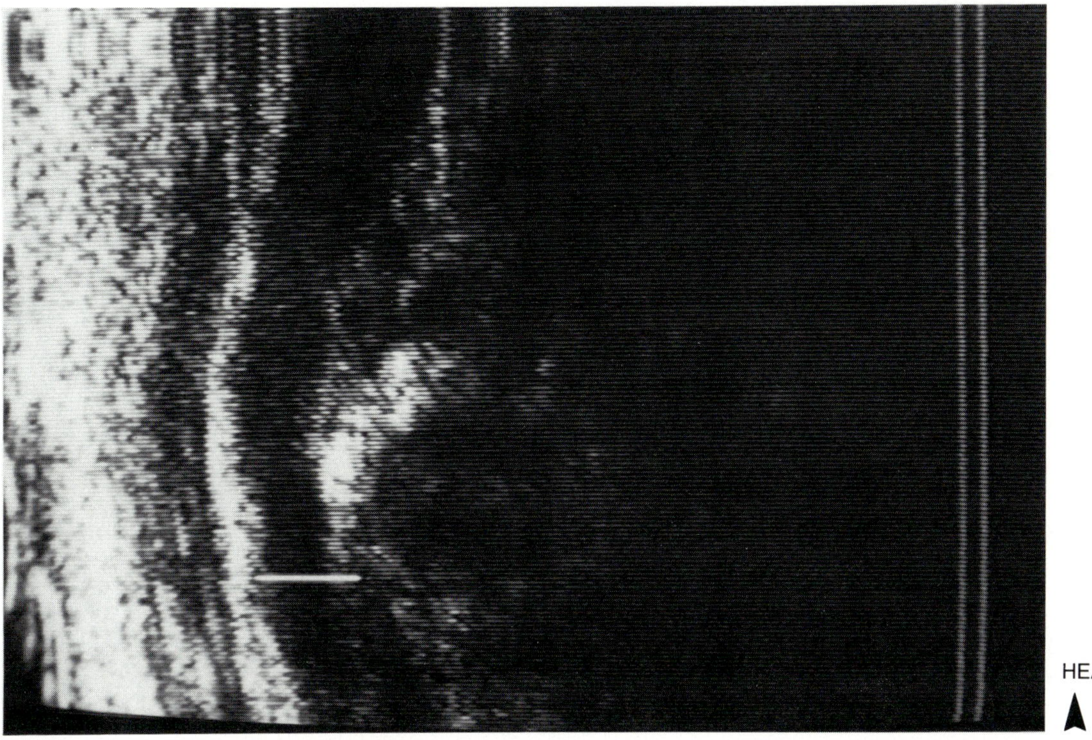
HEAD

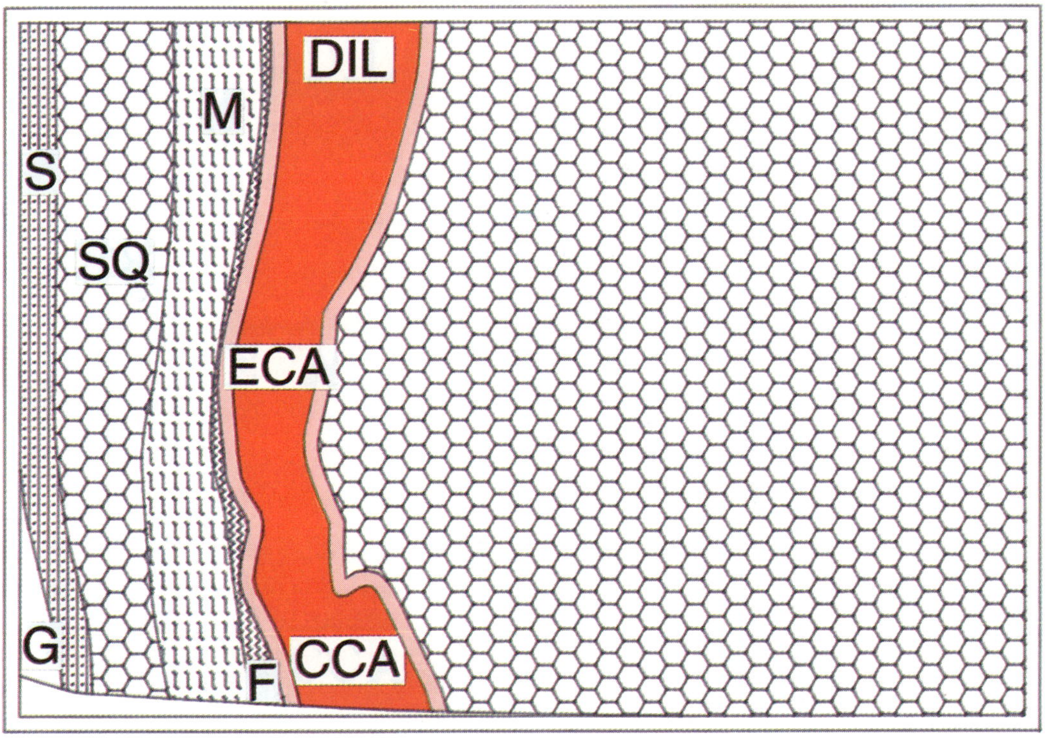
DIL
M
S
SQ
ECA
G
F
CCA

Figure 123. COMMON CAROTID VEIN PATCH

This ultrasound scan shows the typical appearance of a saphenous vein patch (VP) on a small common carotid artery (CCA). In this transverse view of the composite vessel near the lower end of the VP, the artery has not been endarterectomized and contains residual plaque (P). The native artery forms slightly more than half the circumference of the composite vessel. Note the "double pigtale effect" of shadowing from the side walls of the artery and the concentration of bright echoes deep to the artery. These are caused by the focusing effect of the artery on the ultrasound beam (see Figure 68). SQ = subcutaneous tissue, M = sternocleidomastoid muscle, F = fascia.

HISTORY *This scan was performed 18 months following patching of the CCA in a 67-year-old female.*

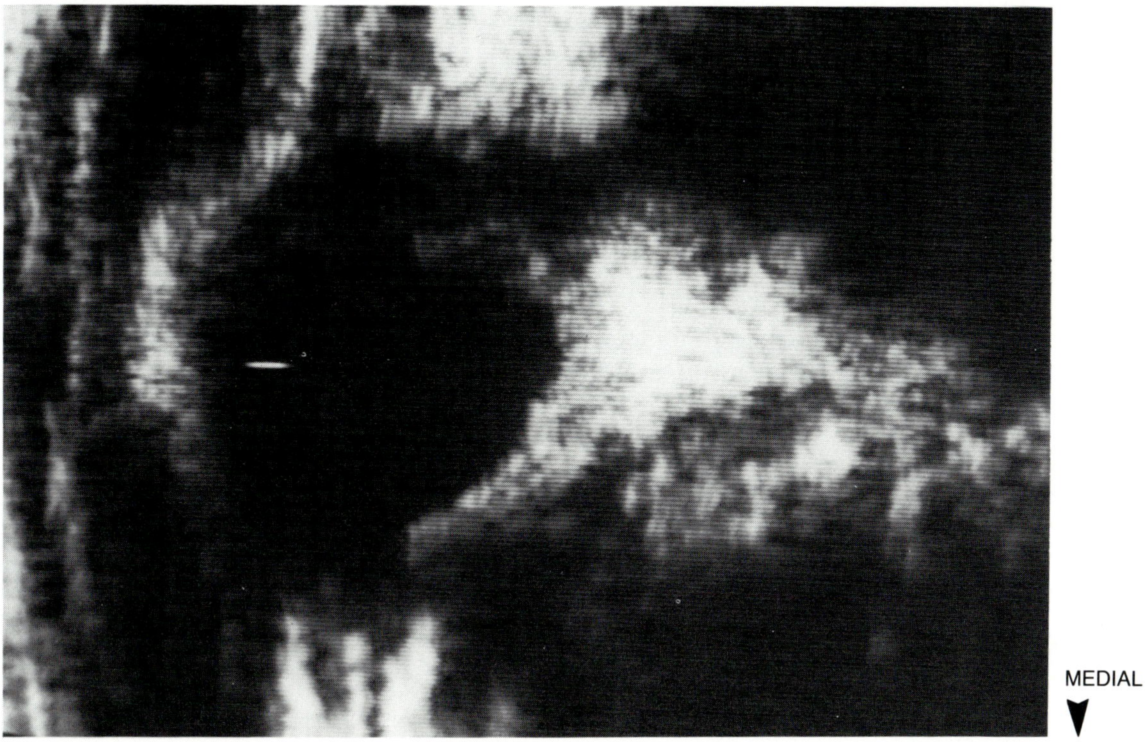
MEDIAL

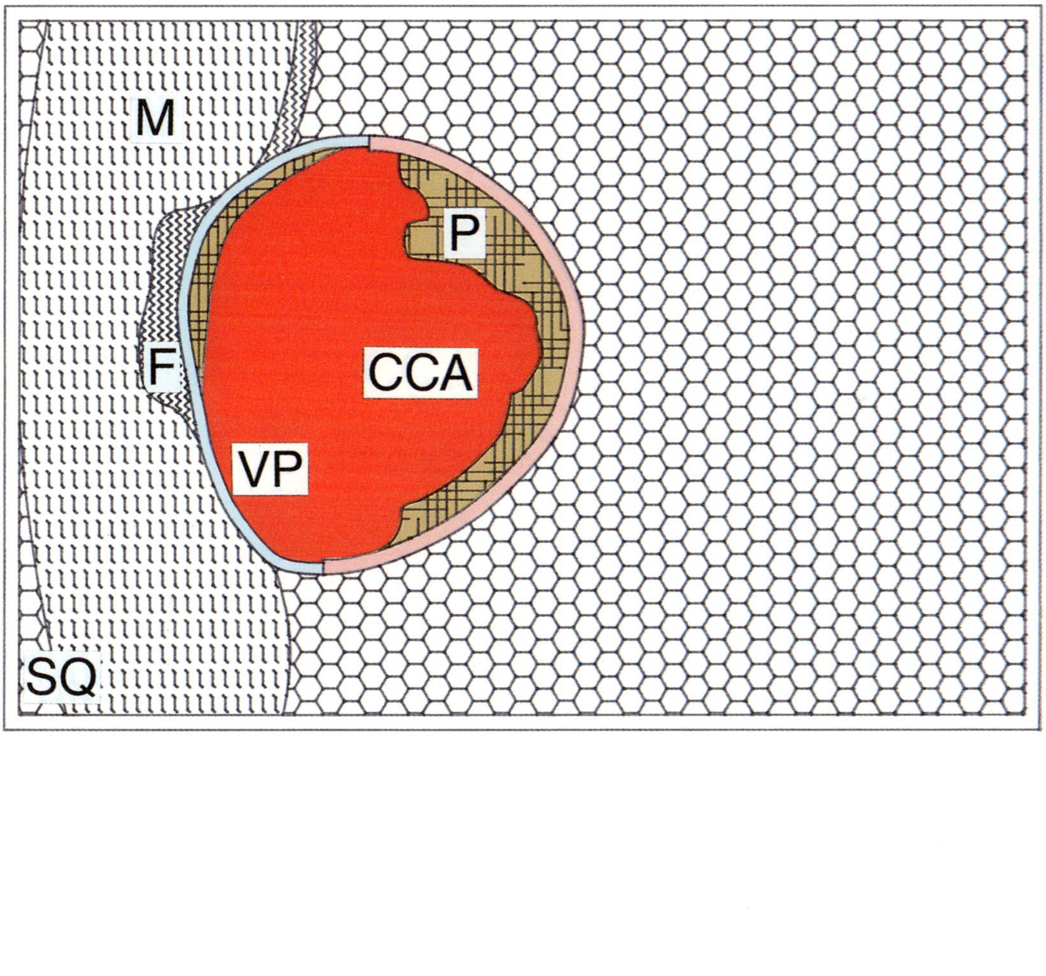
M
P
CCA
F
VP
SQ

Figure 124. CAROTID BIFURCATION VEIN PATCH

This is a longitudinal view of the left carotid bifurcation showing a vein patch (VP) on the superficial wall of the carotid bifurcation. The suture line (SL) at the proximal end of the vein patch is seen. Deep to this SL is the most significant projection of plaque (P), which is homogeneous and has moderate echogenicity consistent with neointimal hyperplasia. The plaque has a mildly irregular contour. The residual lumen at the level of the SL in this view measures 4.5 mm across, and the point of maximum dilatation of the vein patch (VP) measures 11.2 mm in diameter. SQ = subcutaneous tissue, M = sternocleidomastoid muscle, F = fascia, ICA = internal carotid artery (in the region of the bulb), CCA = common carotid artery.

HISTORY *This scan was performed 9 months after the second operation on this bifurcation for a recurrent stenosis of 75% within the CCA. This recurrent stenosis developed over $2\frac{1}{2}$ years subsequent to the patient's first endarterectomy. At the time of the second operation, the patient was found to have a fibrous type hyperplasia without a plane underneath the plaque that could be endarterectomized. Therefore, a VP was placed over the CCA stenosis, converting it from a 75% stenosis to a 25% stenosis.*

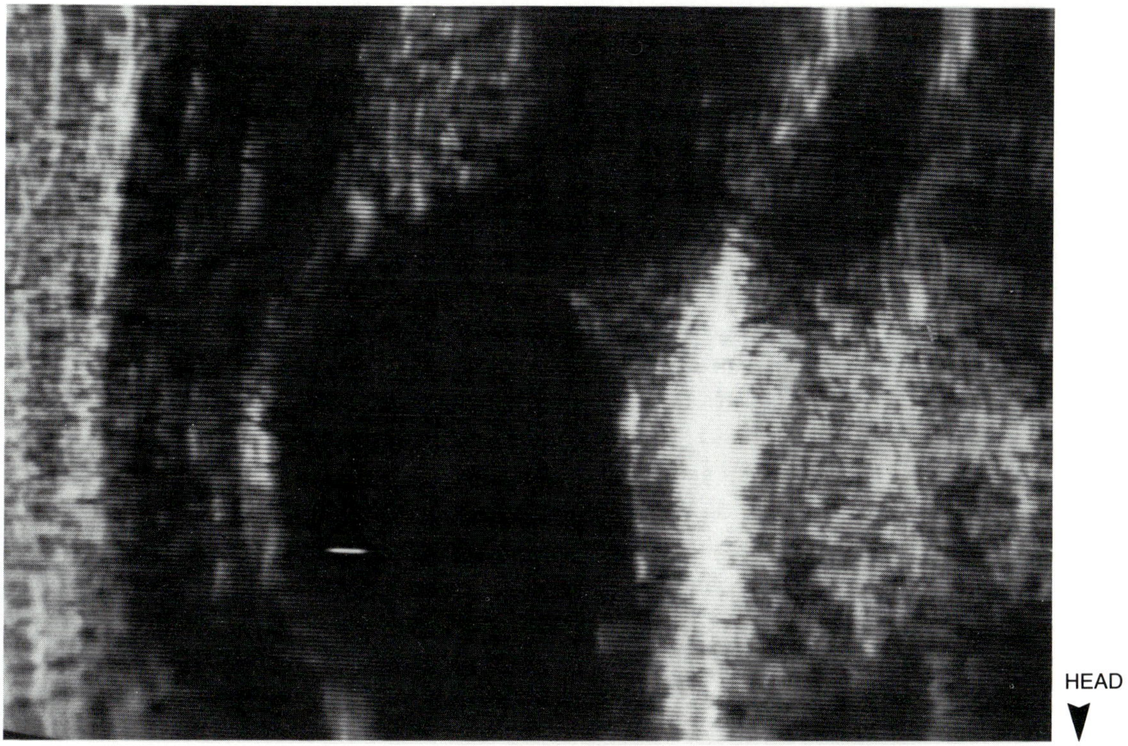
HEAD

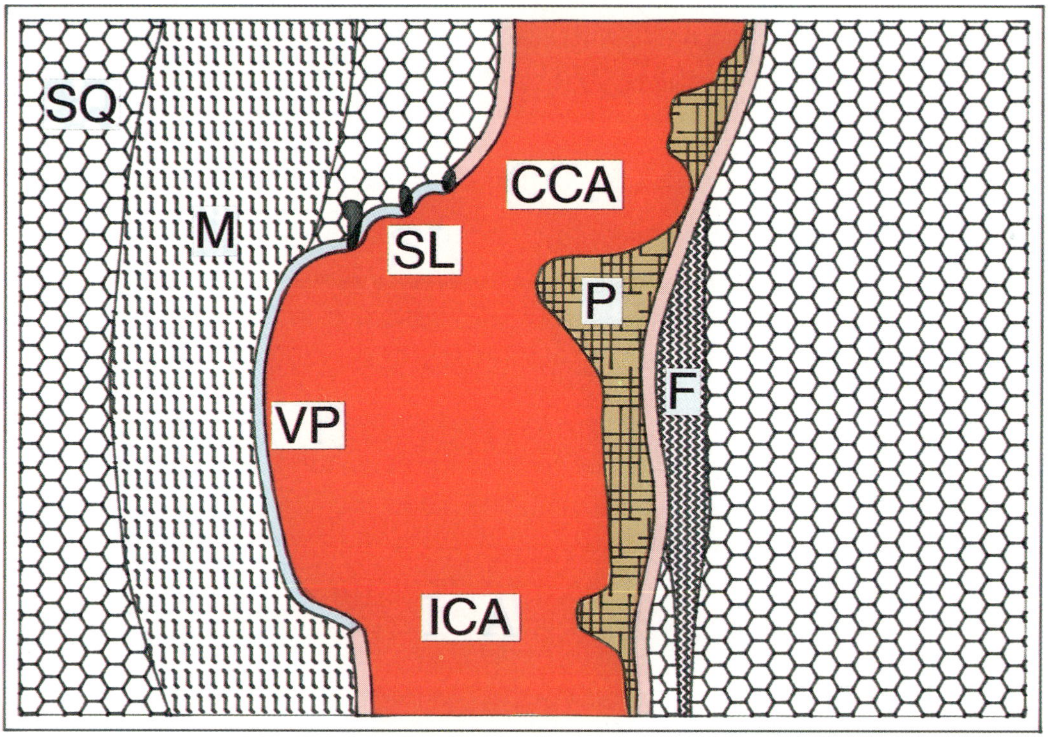
SQ
M
SL
CCA
P
VP
F
ICA

Figure 125. SAPHENOUS INTERPOSITION GRAFT

This is a 4 MHz view of the left carotid bifurcation following replacement of a portion of the internal carotid artery (ICA) by an end-to-end saphenous interposition graft (GSV). The common carotid artery (CCA) at the top of the scan measures 6 mm in diameter, and the distal ICA measures 4 mm in diameter. The mid section of the greater saphenous vein has dilated to 11 mm in diameter. SQ = subcutaneous tissue (including skin and platysmal muscle), M = sternocleidomastoid muscle.

HISTORY *History follows Figure 126.*

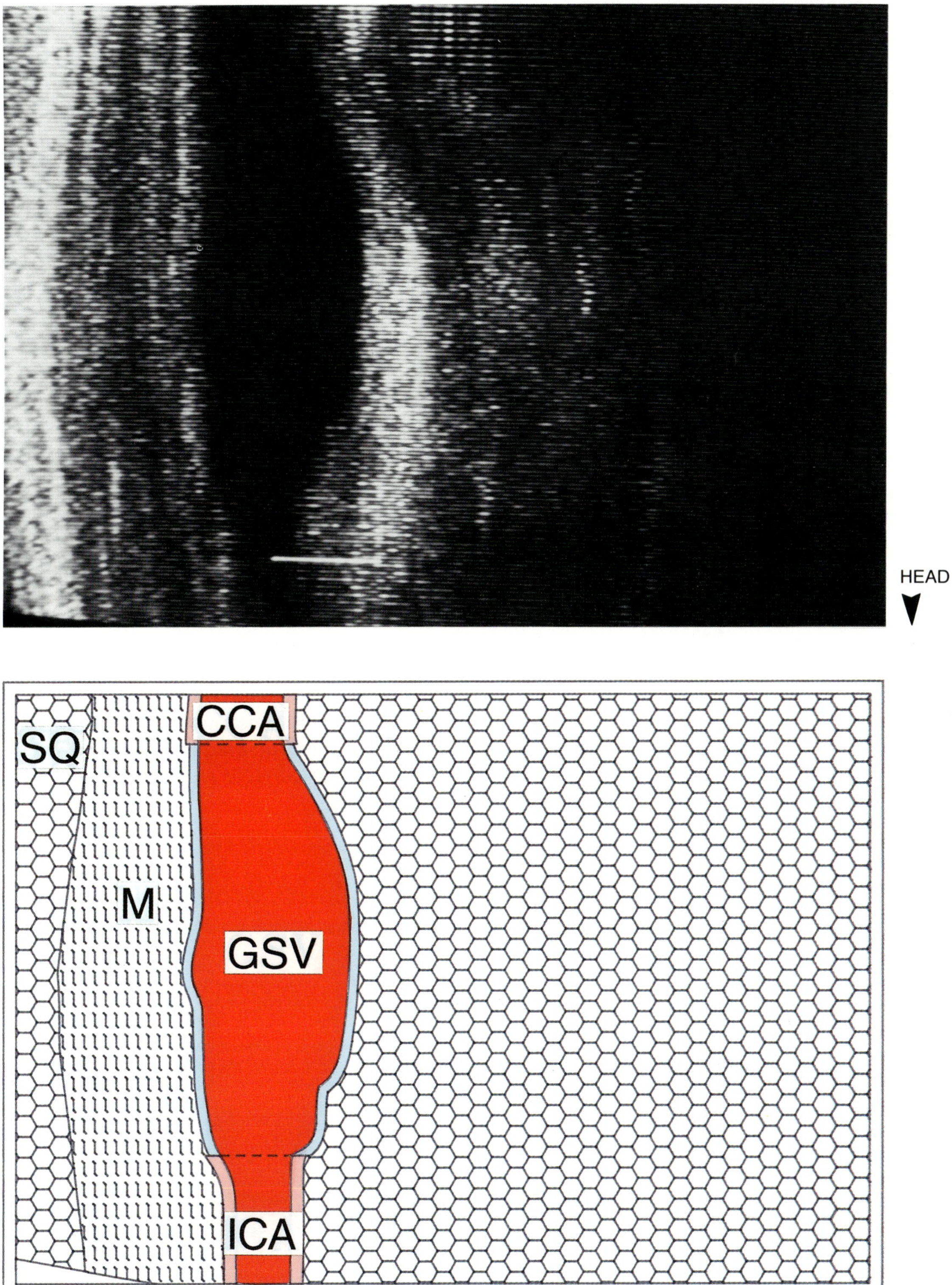
HEAD
CCA
SQ
M
GSV
ICA

Figure 126. SAPHENOUS PATCH GRAFT

In the same patient as presented in Figure 125, the internal carotid bulb was closed, following a right carotid endarterectomy, with an onlay patch graft of the greater saphenous vein. This ultrasound scan was also performed with the 4 MHz probe. In this view the onlay patch is seen face on, and the suture lines are not appreciated. The external carotid artery (ECA) is seen over several centimeters of its length, but the distal internal carotid artery (ICA) is not well seen beyond the upper end of the vein patch. The common carotid artery (CCA) has a well-visualized "intimal stripe" along the superficial wall and a very slight thickening of the "intimal stripe" on the deep wall caused by lipid plaque (P) immediately below the proximal endpoint of the endarterectomy. The cursor (not represented in the diagram) is located deep to the right of the patch graft and measures 4.5 mm in width. The reconstructed internal carotid bulb measures 9 mm in maximum diameter. Moderate dilatation of grafts and patches, as seen in this scan and the previous scan, is fairly common months to years following their placement. SQ = subcutaneous tissue, M = sternocleidomastoid muscle.

HISTORY *This 56-year-old male had bilateral carotid endarterectomies. He presented with a left hemispheric cerebrovascular accident (CVA) 13 months later. Both duplex scan and arteriogram showed a total occlusion of the left ICA. In addition, the patient had a recurrent 80% stenosis on the right side. He underwent a second left carotid endarterectomy and thrombectomy with interposition graft 10 days after the CVA. This procedure was successful as shown in Figure 125. Two months later, he underwent a second endarterectomy and patching on the right side. The patch was performed because at operation a marked narrowing of the artery was found with minimal recurrent atherosclerotic plaque. The scan shown in Figure 126 was obtained 2 months after the second right endarterectomy.*

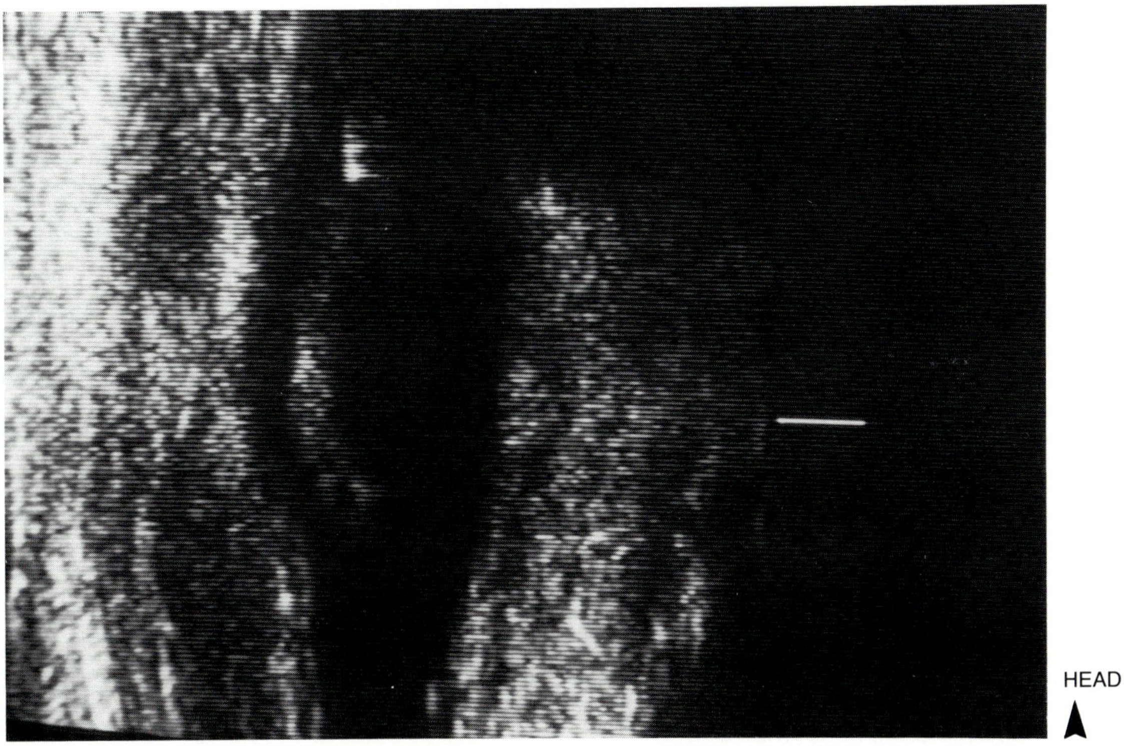
HEAD

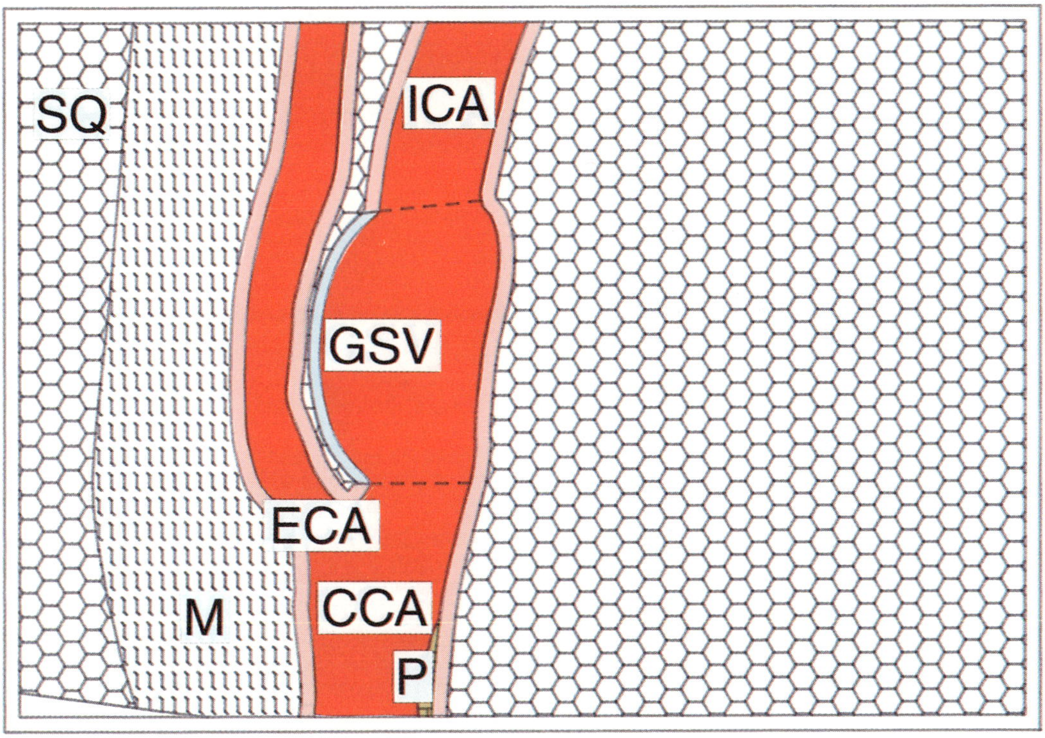
SQ
ICA
GSV
ECA
M
CCA
P

Figure 127. CAROTID-SUBCLAVIAN BYPASS

In this longitudinal view of the left common carotid artery (CCA) low in the neck, the proximal anastomosis of a carotid-subclavian bypass using greater saphenous vein (GSV) is seen. Except for a slight infolding of the proximal (PROX) end of the CCA at the anastomosis, there is no stenosis present. SQ = subcutaneous tissue, M = sternocleidomastoid muscle, F = fascia, DIST = distal.

HISTORY *This is of a 73-year-old male who underwent carotid-subclavian bypass for symptomatic, subclavian-steal syndrome with complaints of dizziness and visual blurring with use of the left arm. He had a 50-mm gradient between right and left arm blood pressures. The ultrasound scan was obtained 21 months following the bypass.*

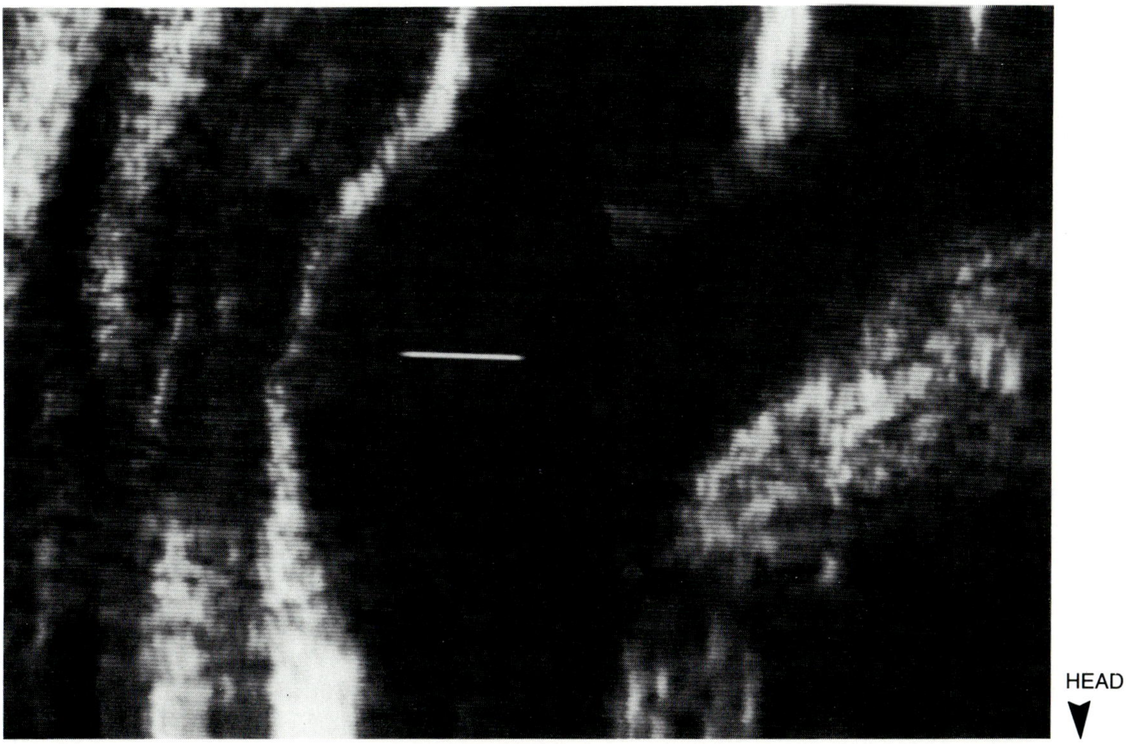
HEAD

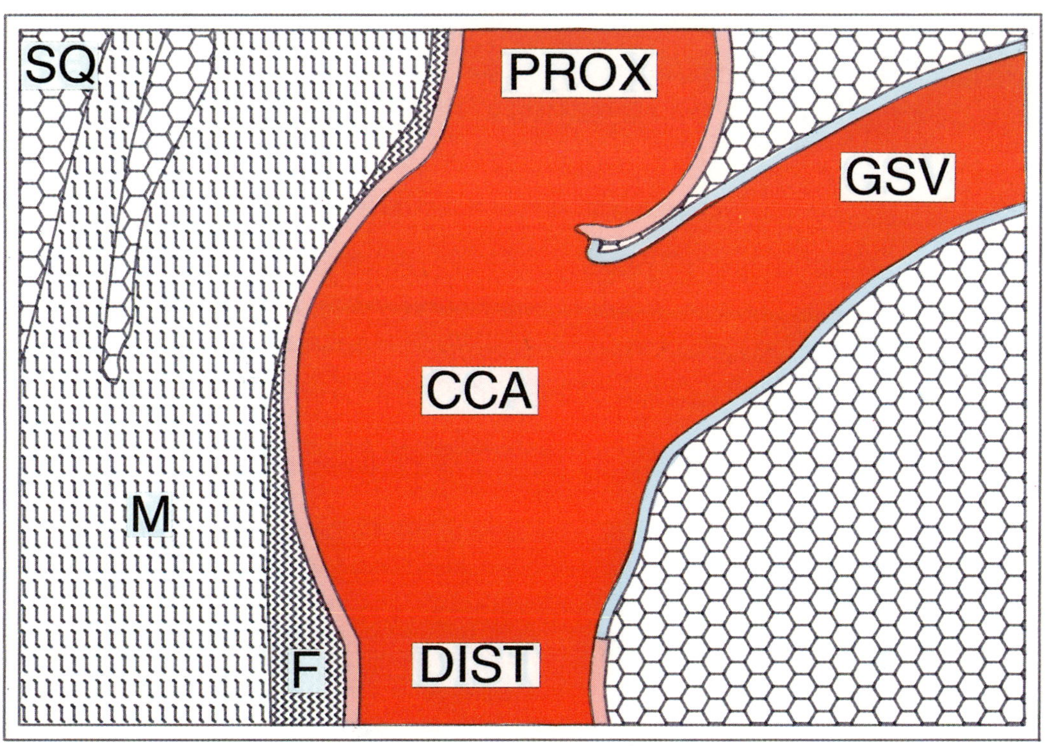
SQ
PROX
GSV
CCA
M
F
DIST

Figure 128. DACRON PATCH GRAFT

This longitudinal view of a left internal carotid artery (ICA) shows the ultrasonic appearance of corrugated Dacron (D) graft material. The deep wall of the ICA is native artery, not graft, but has a striped appearance extending into the deep tissues because of acoustical shadowing from the Dacron surface. The ICA distally (DIST) contains some homogeneous moderately echogenic plaque (P) on the deep wall, similar in brightness to some fascial thickening (F) to the right. The distal endpoint of the endarterectomy is located at the top of the plaque. There is some "fade-out" type artifact (AF) extending to the left of the superficial wall (see Figure 160). G = gel, S = skin, M = platysma muscle, SQ = subcutaneous tissue, SCM = sternocleidomastoid muscle, C = Doppler cursor, ? = tissue of uncertain composition, HL = "hard-line" artifact.

HISTORY *This is of a 75-year-old female who underwent a subclavian-to-internal carotid bypass graft 4 years prior because of persistent dizziness and episodes of syncope associated with a common carotid occlusion at that time. As the internal and external arteries were open, an 8-mm knitted Dacron graft was inserted from the subclavian artery to the internal carotid bulb. This distal anastomosis is end-graft to side-artery. Post-operatively she experienced severe headaches, but otherwise has been asymptomatic over the past 4 years with an untreated 45% stenosis on the opposite side that has remained stable by yearly scans.*

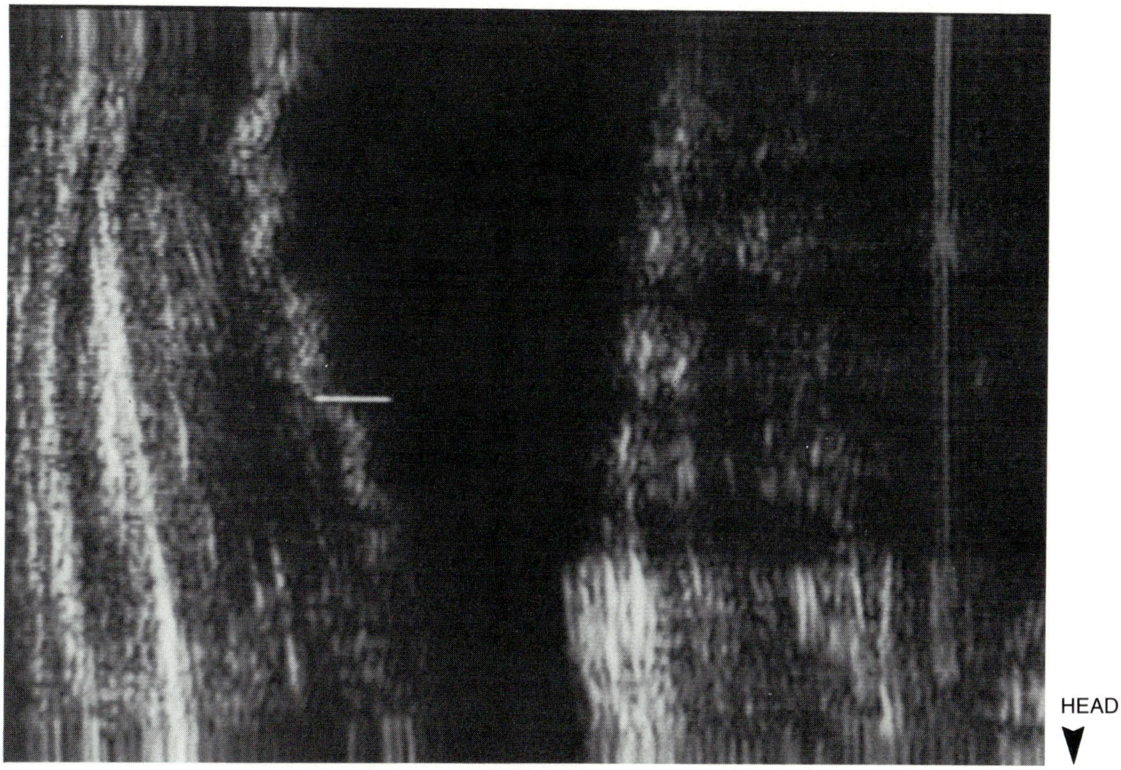
HEAD

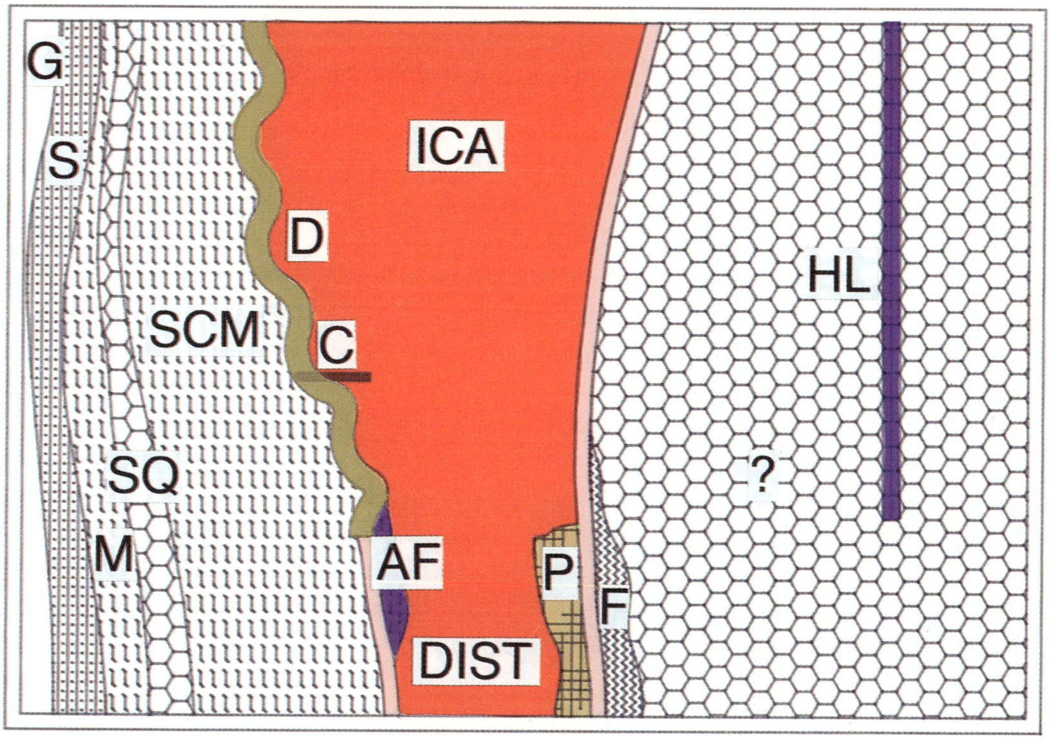
G
S
ICA
D
HL
SCM
C
SQ
?
M
AF
P
F
DIST

CHAPTER 7

OTHER FINDINGS

Figure 129. INTERNAL CAROTID CURLS

These two sketches (Examples A and B) are included to assist the reader in understanding the three-dimensional configuration of internal carotid curls as seen in the following sets of ultrasound images. Example A refers to Figure 130, and Example B refers to Figure 131.

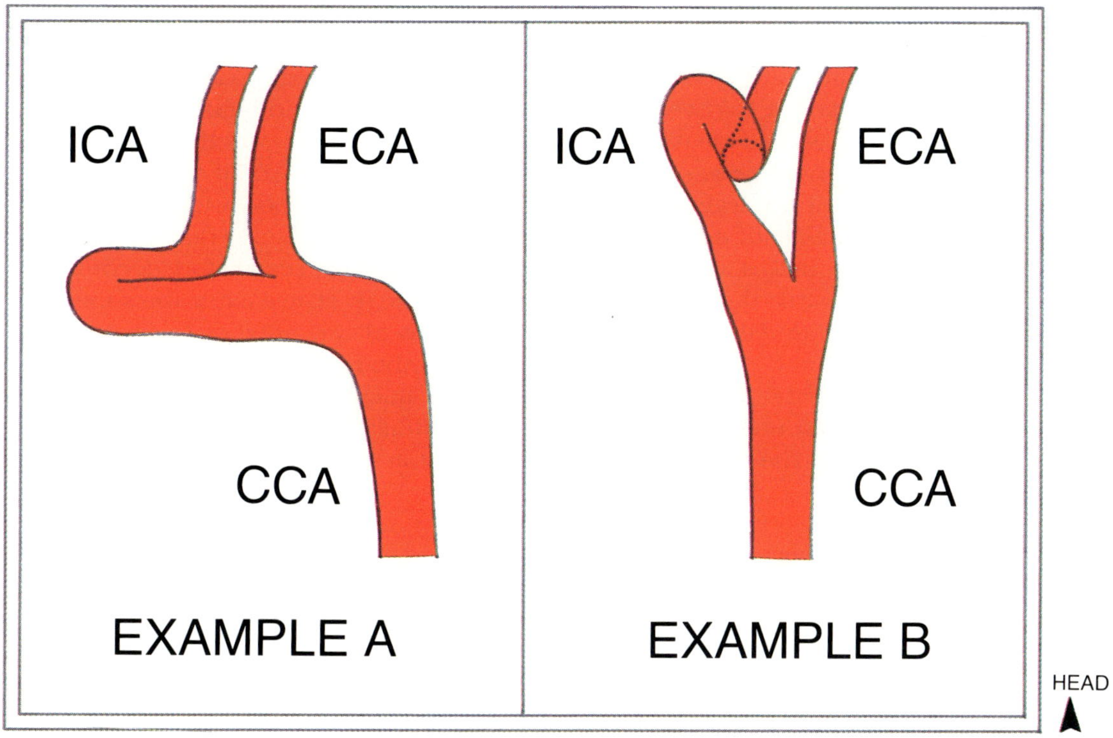
ICA
ECA
CCA
EXAMPLE A
ICA
ECA
CCA
EXAMPLE B
HEAD

Figure 130. INTERNAL CAROTID CURL

This is the first rather bizarre example of tortuosity of the right carotid bifurcation. This is actually a transverse view of the neck. The carotid bifurcation has been tipped over on its side (see Figure 129). A longitudinal view of the bifurcation is seen in this transverse plane. The external carotid artery (ECA) curves back into a longitudinal plane almost immediately. The internal carotid artery (ICA) is fairly straight initially but doubles back on itself and then appears to reach a dead end as the artery makes a right angle out of the plane of the scan before curving back up to go towards the head. There is some plaque (P) visible along the superficial wall of the internal carotid bulb. Note that this plaque appears to cause a 40% stenosis of the ICA relative to its diameter at the level of the plaque. However, because of distal tapering of the artery, this qualifies as only a 25% diameter stenosis when one compares the residual lumen with the cross-sectional diameter of the ICA, as it curves out of plane at its most distal extent.

HISTORY *This 65-year-old diabetic female was admitted with unstable angina and subsequently underwent coronary artery bypass grafting. This ultrasound scan was performed as part of her pre-operative evaluation. She was asymptomatic with respect to dizziness on turning the head and other cerebrovascular symptoms.*

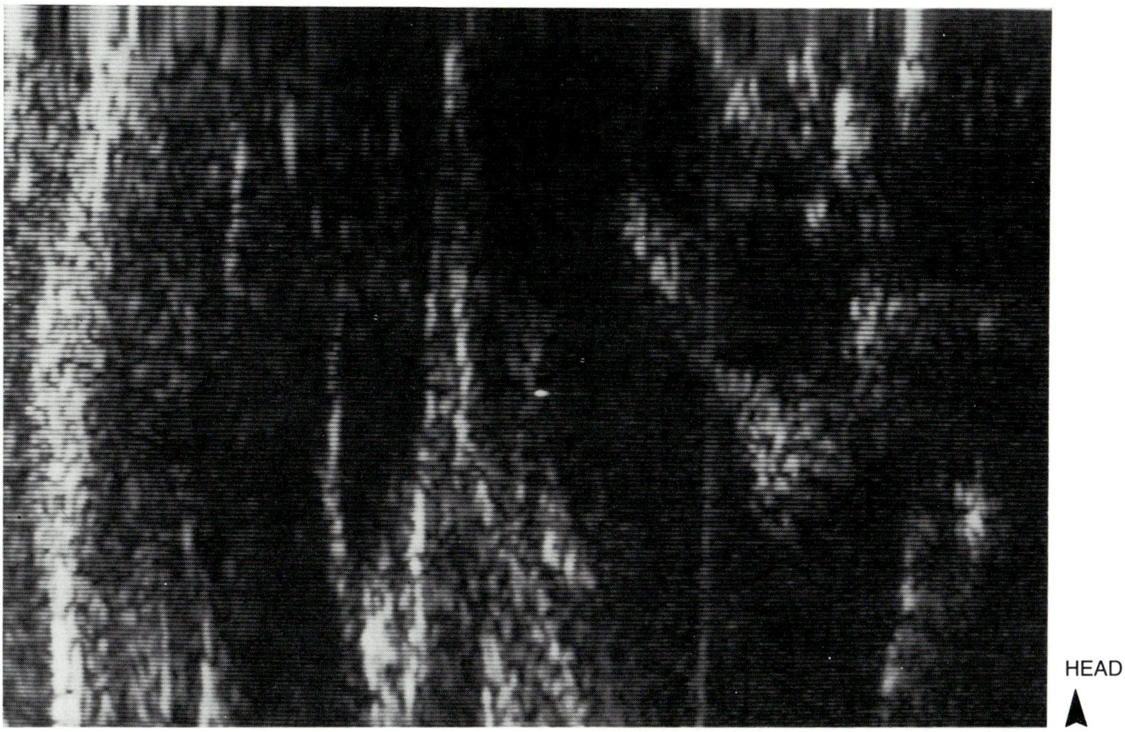
HEAD

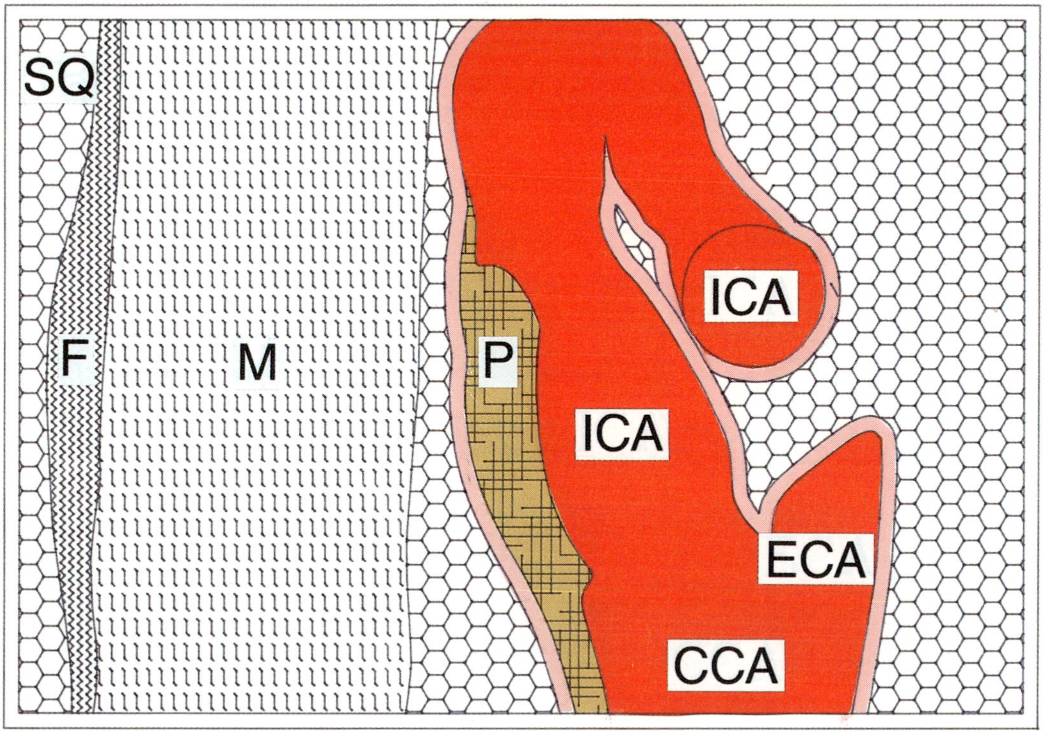
SQ
F
M
P
ICA
ICA
ECA
CCA

Figure 131. INTERNAL CAROTID 180-DEGREE CURL

This is the second example of a 180-degree curl that the distal (DIST) internal carotid artery (ICA) makes before it disappears out of plane (see Figure 129). There appears to be a slight reduction of the arterial diameter as a result of the kink. Doppler signal spectrum can be improperly interpreted, if one does not know the exact angle the blood flow makes with respect to the ultrasound beam. With a configuration such as this, a high velocity Doppler signal at the point of kinking is to be expected and does not prove the presence of plaque or even significant stenosis. This is one of the reasons why image quality is important. S = skin, SQ = subcutaneous tissue, M = sternocleidomastoid muscle.

HISTORY *This is of an 88-year-old female who had a left hemispheric cerebrovascular accident (CVA) 3 years previously with mild residual right hemiparesis. She presented with complaints of several episodes of falling while at home, without loss of consciousness, for a week prior to this scan. On the opposite side she had no kink or curl, but she did have a 45% stenosis with possibly ulcerated plaque. It remains unclear whether her symptoms were due to kinking of this artery or to overmedication with an antihypertensive agent.*

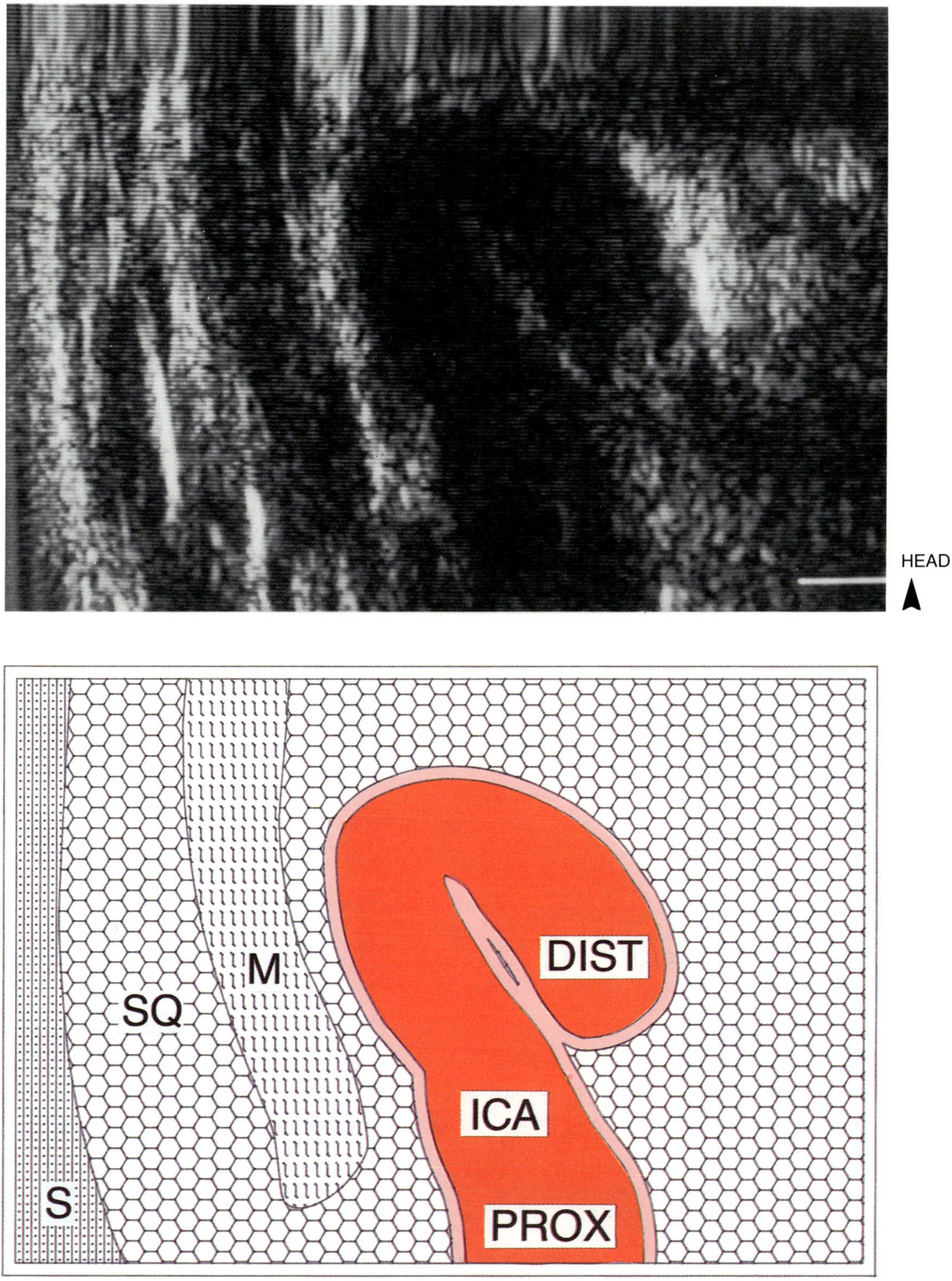
HEAD
S
SQ
M
DIST
ICA
PROX

Figure 132. CAROTID CURL—LONGITUDINAL

This scan is a longitudinal view of the neck in the same patient as in Figure 131. However, the internal carotid artery (ICA) appears as two vessels seen in cross section. The artery forms a tortuous loop bent over at right angles to the long axis of the neck. One sees the artery at two points along its length as the blood is coming and going. To re-emphasize, arterial tortuosity requires a very careful tracing of the path of the vessel. The probe is held in multiple orientations so as to arrive at a three-dimensional concept of the path. This is necessary to properly identify the vessel and correctly assess the Doppler signals and apparent visible narrowings of the artery, as it passes to and fro within the plane of the scan. G = gel, S = skin, M = muscle, SQ = subcutaneous tissue, F = fascia.

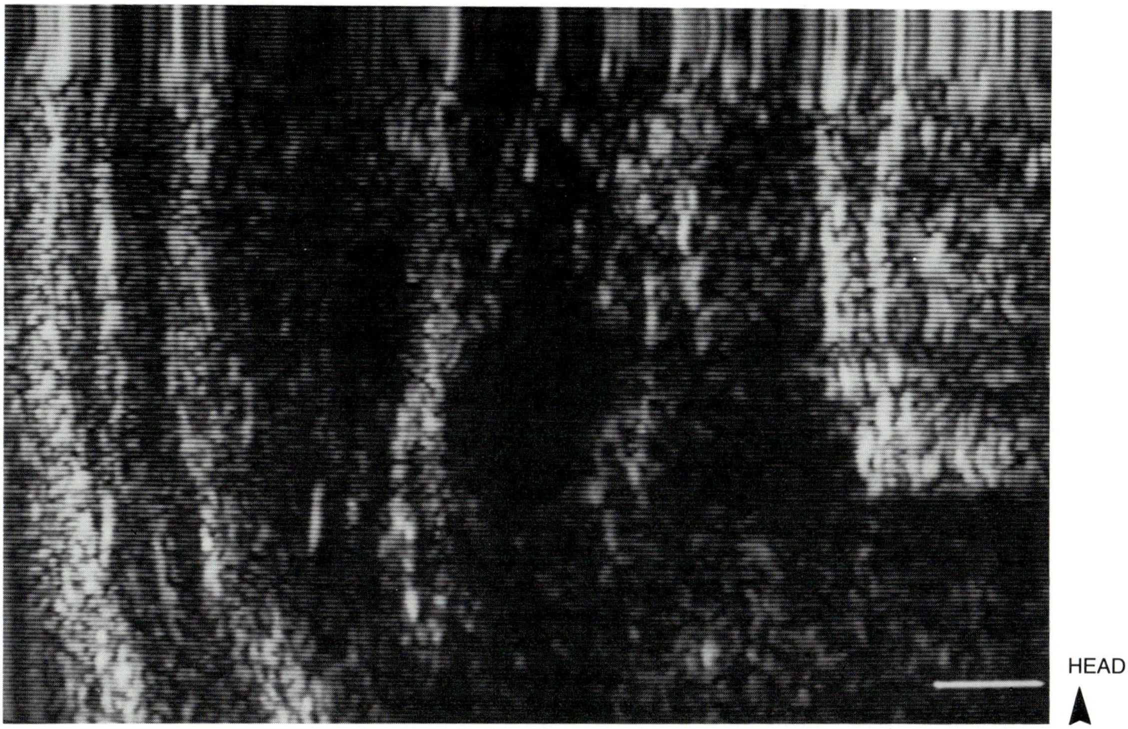
HEAD

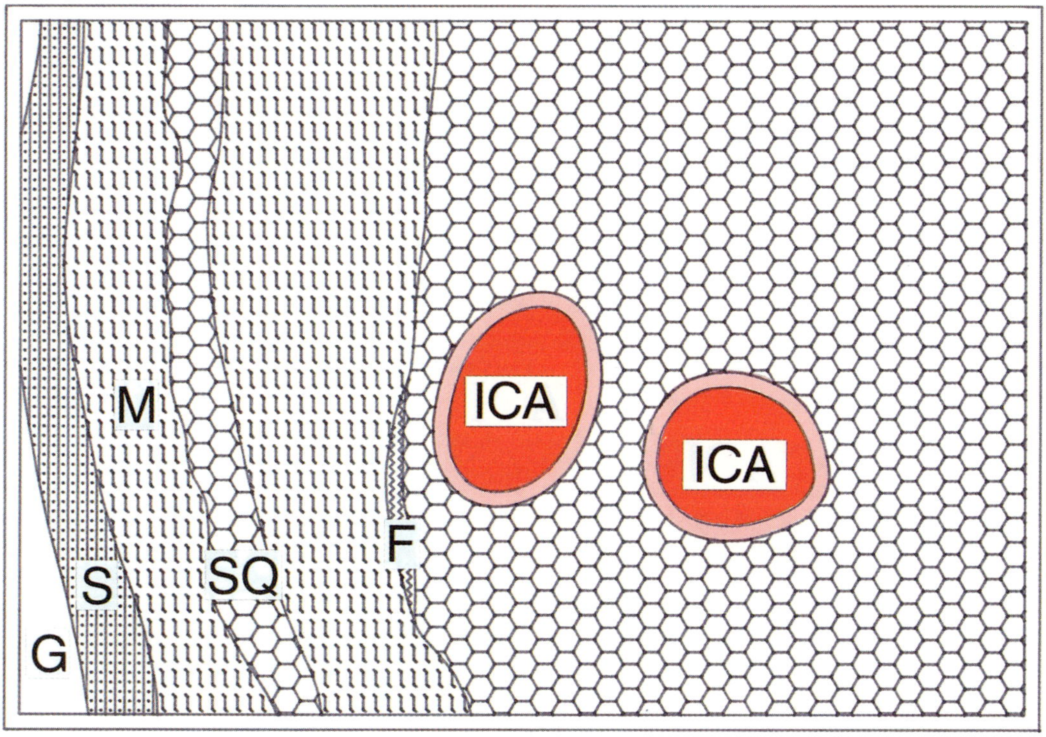
M
ICA
ICA
F
S
SQ
G

Figure 133. 360-DEGREE CAROTID LOOP

This third example is another bizarre form of carotid anatomy. This is a longitudinal view of the left internal carotid artery (ICA) with the head toward the bottom of the screen. The ICA makes a complete 360-degree loop, passing alongside itself before straightening out to a well-visualized distal artery. Note the well-demarcated intimal margins of the artery at the bottom of the screen. These intimal margins are not well seen in the curved position of the artery where the orientation of the vessel does not allow a 180-degree reflection of the incoming beam directly back out toward the probe. The deep wall of the internal jugular vein (IJV) is indented by the ICA loop. Note also the single "pigtail" effect of acoustical shadowing produced by the bottom edge of the loop in this scan (see Figure 68). CCA = common carotid artery, M = muscle.

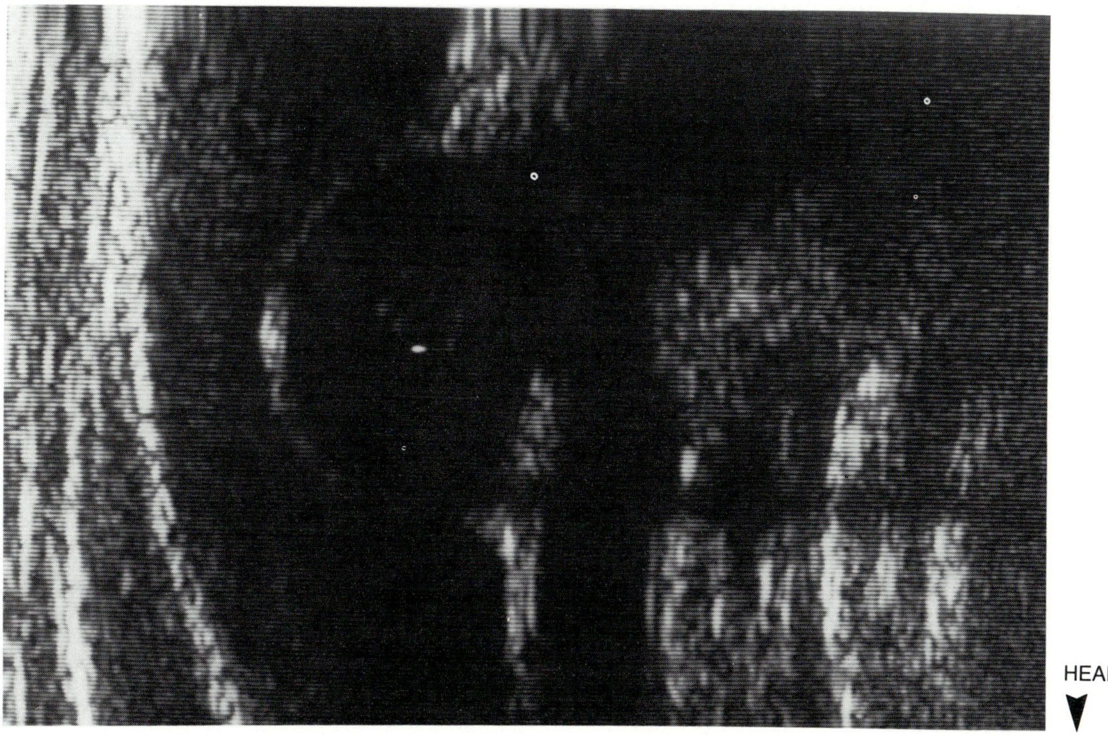
HEAD

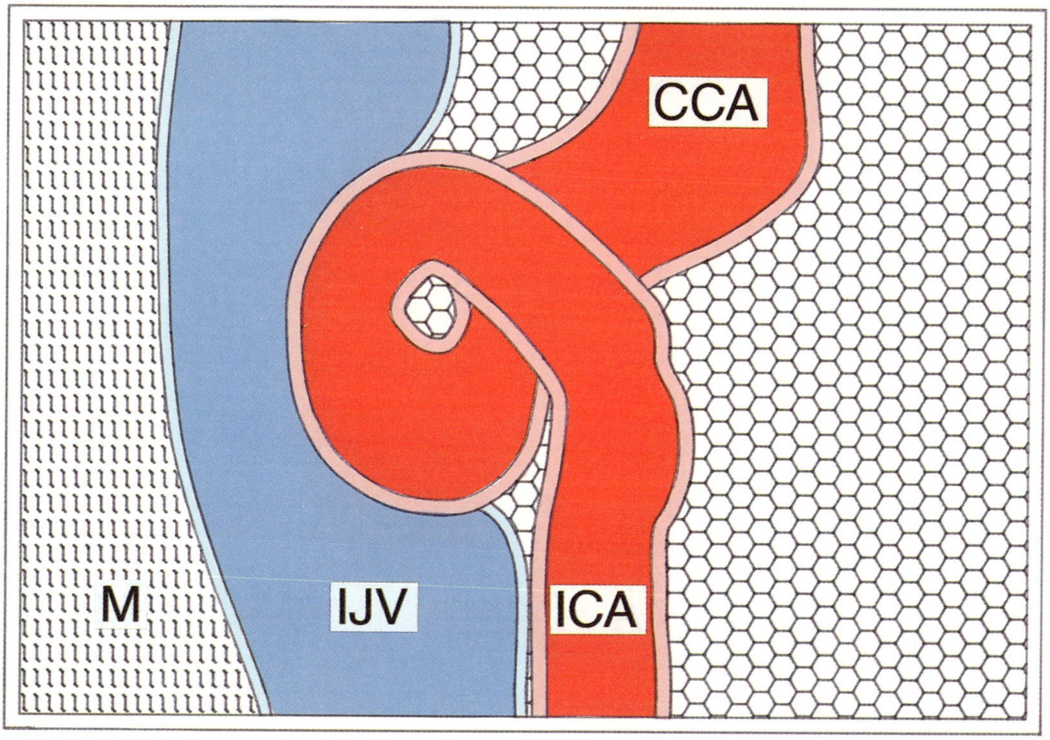
CCA
M
IJV
ICA

Figure 134. NATIVE CAROTID ANEURYSM

This is a longitudinal view of a native aneurysm (AN) of the right carotid bifurcation with the common carotid artery (CCA) toward the bottom of the scan and the internal carotid artery (ICA) above. The aneurysm has a maximum diameter of 15 mm. Note the eccentric shape of this aneurysm with a bulge only in the superficial wall of the artery. It is this portion that is filled with thrombus (T) as indicated by the Doppler cursor (not drawn). There is a small amount of plaque (P) on the deep wall and at the origin of the ICA. The residual lumen measures 7.0 mm in diameter. Given the presence of thrombus filling the aneurysmal portion of the artery, it would not be possible to detect this lesion by arteriography. SCM = sternocleidomastoid muscle, F = fascia, SQ = subcutaneous tissue, IJV = internal jugular vein (compressed against the aneurysm), ? = tissue of uncertain composition, HL = "hard-line" artifact (note that this artifact is seen only in the dark portions of the deep field).

HISTORY *This 69-year-old female presented with transient ischemic attacks consisting of left upper extremity and facial paresis. She underwent a right carotid endarterectomy 1 week following this scan. A "2-cm aneurysm" of the lateral aspect of the CCA at the bifurcation was found. This was not suspected on the basis of pre-operative contrast media–studies. She also had a 4.5-cm abdominal aortic aneurysm but no other peripheral aneurysms.*

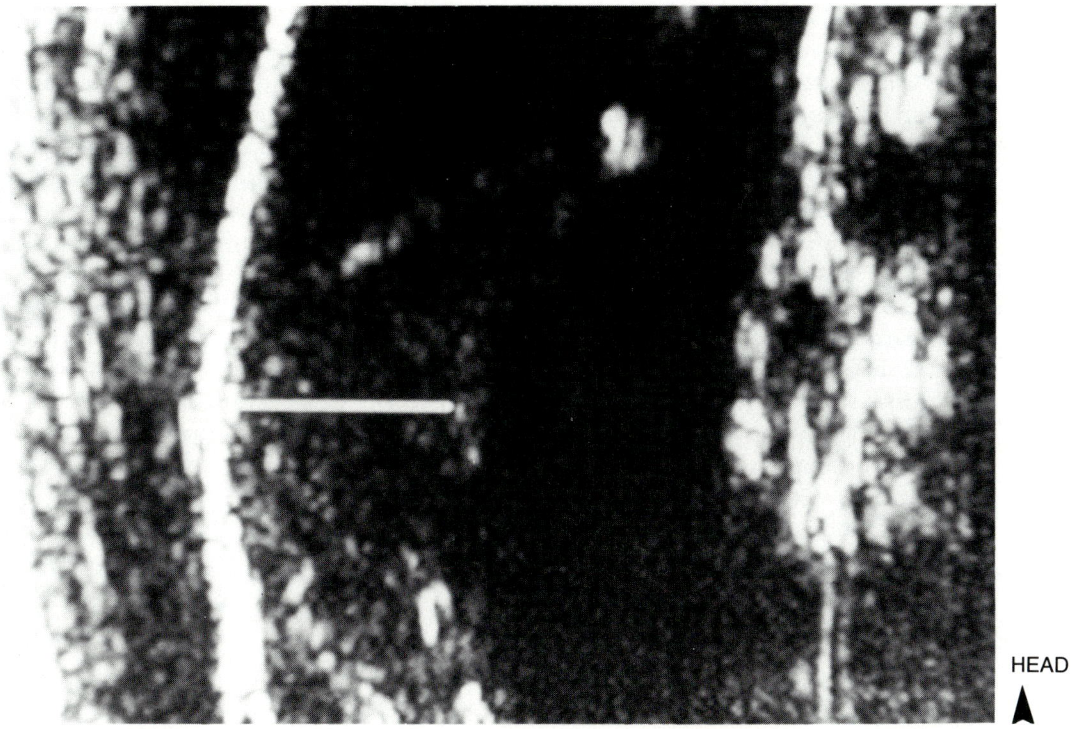
HEAD

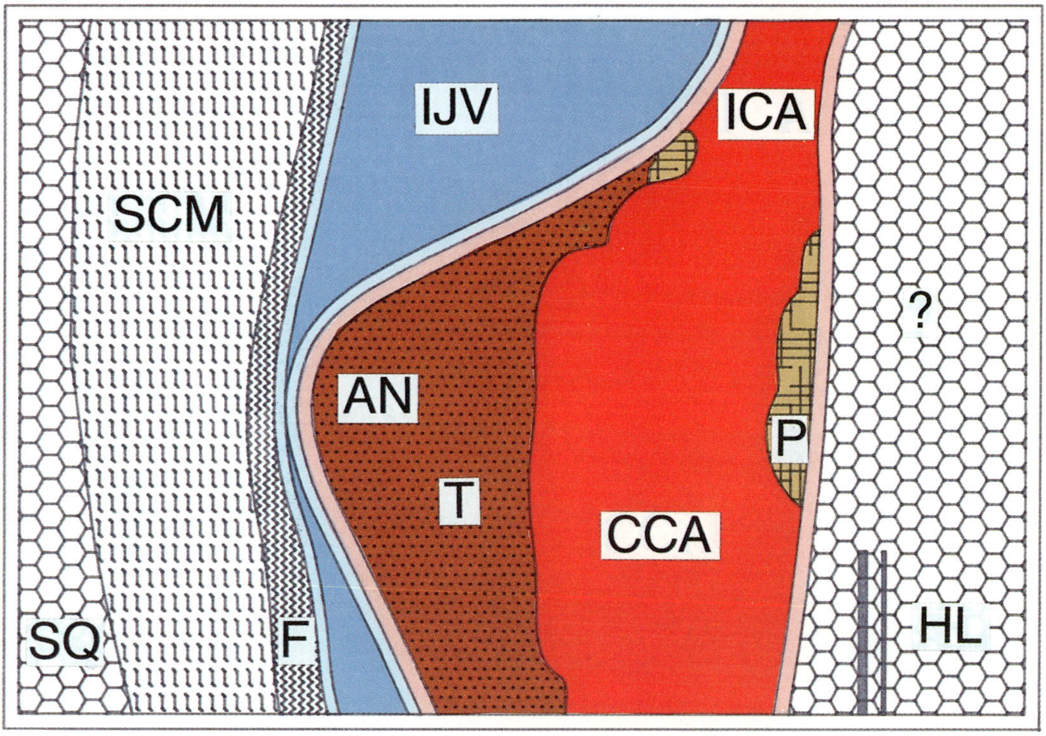
IJV
ICA
SCM
?
AN
P
T
CCA
SQ
F
HL

Figure 135. NATIVE CAROTID ANEURYSM

When seen in transverse orientation, this native carotid aneurysm (AN) is seen to have a rather peculiar saccular shape arising from the superficial and posterior walls of the common carotid artery (CCA) at the bifurcation. There is a slight amount of plaque (P) on both sides of the artery, but for the most part the aneurysmal cavity is filled with thrombus (T). It is not uncommon to see large CCA diameters at the bifurcation reaching 12 mm or more. However, this is the only case encountered with the discrete saccular bulge from one side of the artery not caused by operation. One might think from this projection that this is the division of internal and external carotid arteries. In fact, the external carotid artery arises at the 12-o'clock position relative to the internal carotid artery and does so at a higher level than the plane of this scan. The coarse (high contrast) appearance is due to the camera settings and does not appear on the original video tape. These settings were used to demonstrate the thrombus that was very faintly echogenic. SCM = sternocleidomastoid muscle, F = fascia, SQ = subcutaneous tissue, V = internal jugular vein, ? = tissue of uncertain composition.

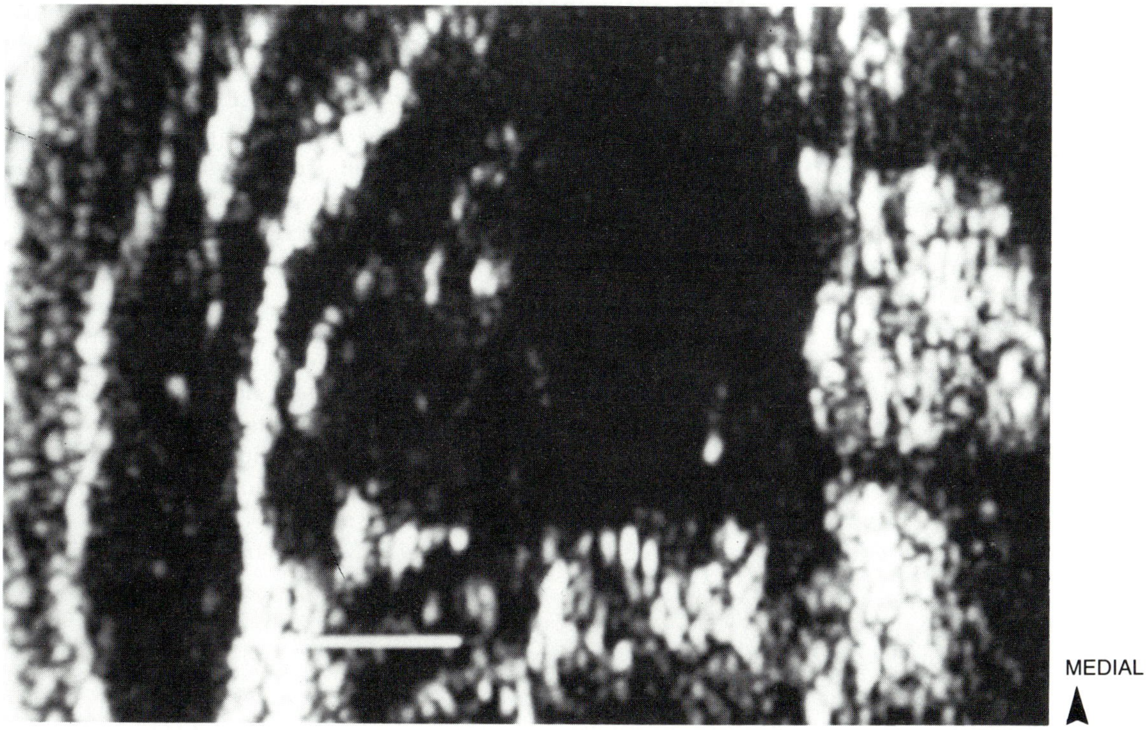
MEDIAL

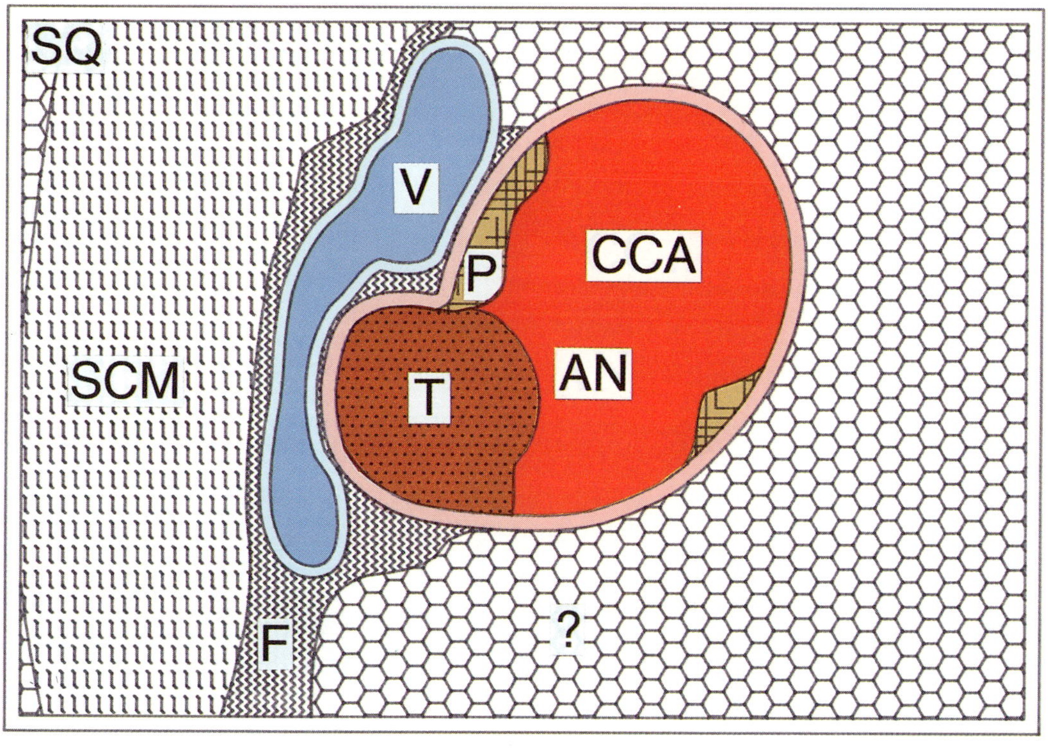
SQ
V
P
CCA
AN
T
SCM
F
?

Figure 136. CAROTID BODY TUMOR

This is an example of a carotid body tumor. These tumors can be distinguished by their location in the crotch of the carotid bifurcation. As is seen in this scan, the tumor causes splaying of the internal carotid artery (ICA) and external carotid artery (ECA). Note the very homogeneous but very faintly echogenic composition of the tumor itself. The ECA does not stay completely in the plane of this scan, and some back wall (BW) echoes are seen in its mid section. G = gel, S = skin, M = sternocleidomastoid muscle, SQ = subcutaneous tissue, CCA = common carotid artery.

HISTORY *This is a 51-year-old female with a neck mass on the left, enlarging over the span of 7 years. She had previously undergone resection of a chemodectoma on the right side but suffered a post-operative stroke and so declined to have the tumor on this left side removed. The presence of chemodectoma on this side was confirmed by arteriography, which revealed the tumor blush of a mass 2.5 cm in diameter and 5 cm in length, extending toward the base of the skull.*

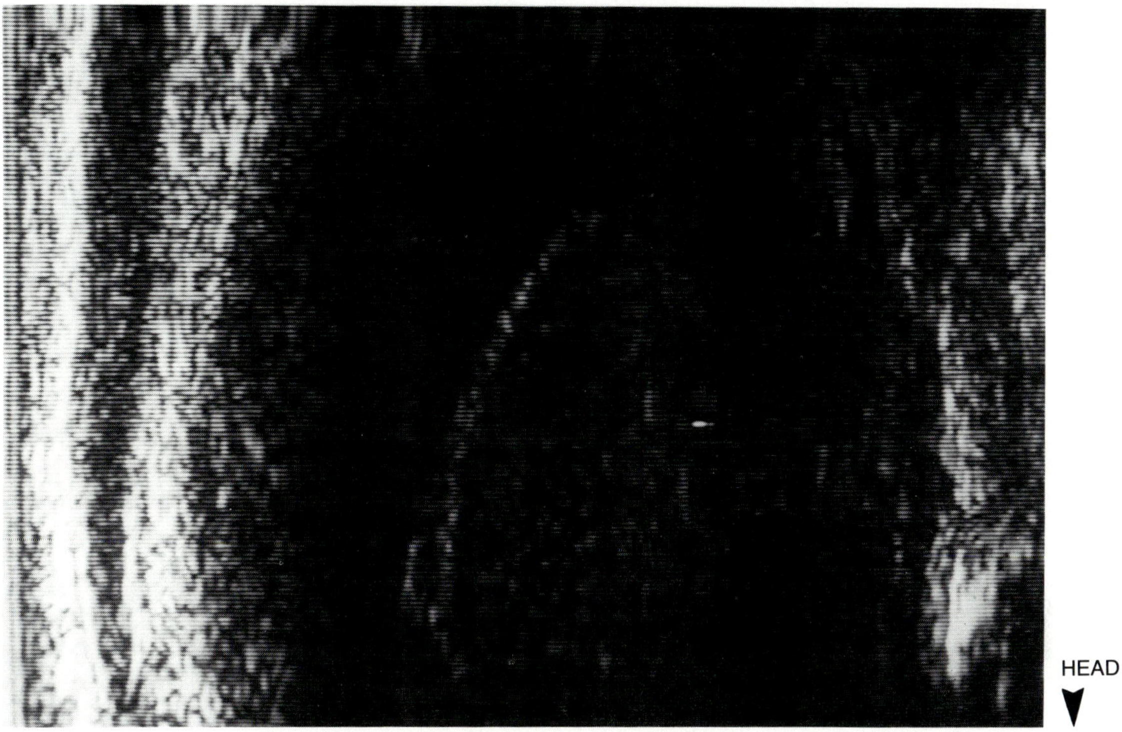
HEAD

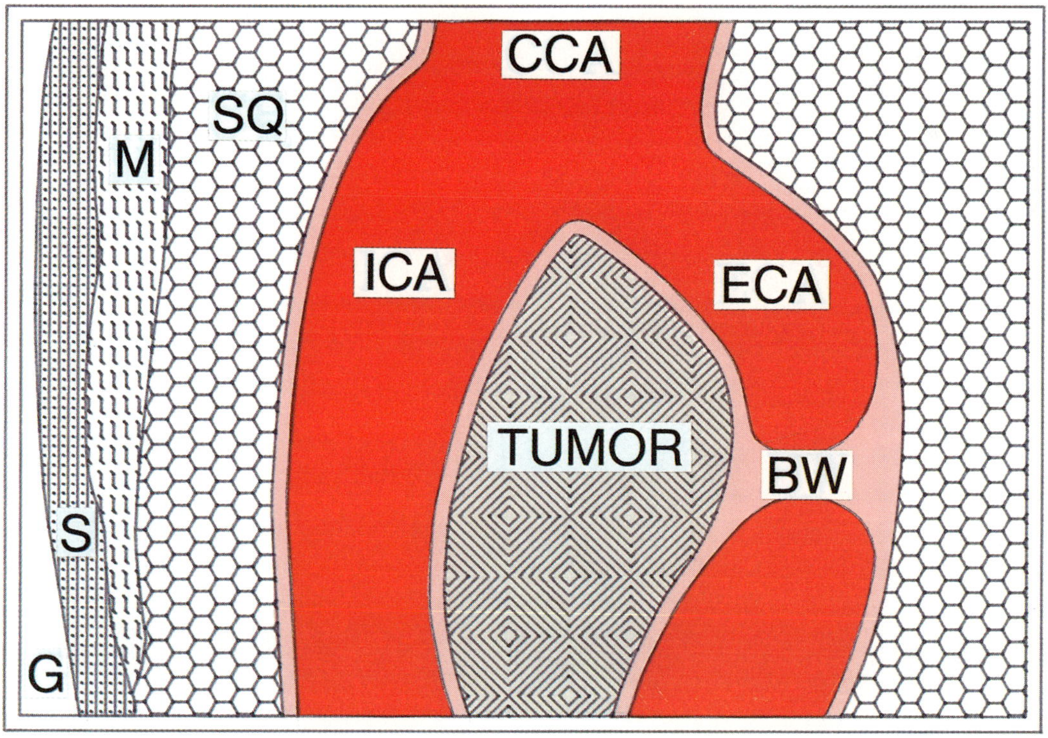
CCA
SQ
M
ICA
ECA
TUMOR
BW
S
G

Figure 137. CAROTID BODY TUMOR

This is a transverse view of the same left-sided carotid body tumor as in Figure 136. Again, one can see that the tumor in the crotch of the bifurcation partly surrounds the internal and external carotid arteries. The tumor itself has a very dark homogeneous appearance. The tumor measures 20 mm in transverse diameter in this view. S = skin, M = sternocleidomastoid and platysma muscles, SQ = subcutaneous tissue, ICA = internal carotid artery, ECA = external carotid artery, ? = tissue of uncertain composition.

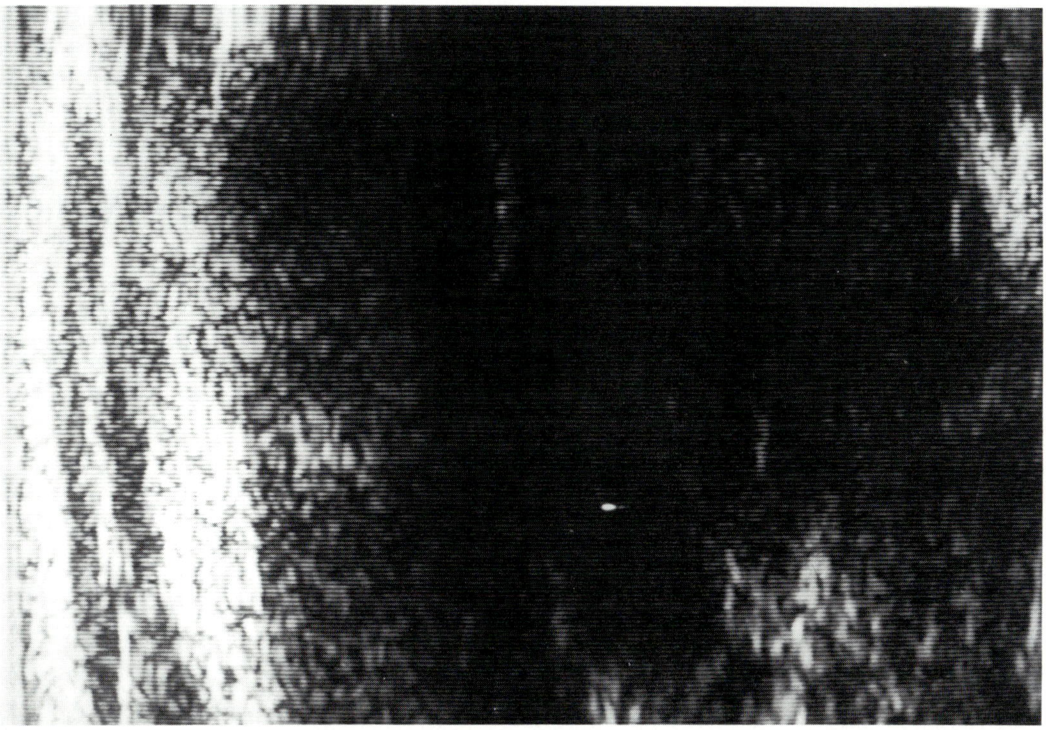
MEDIAL

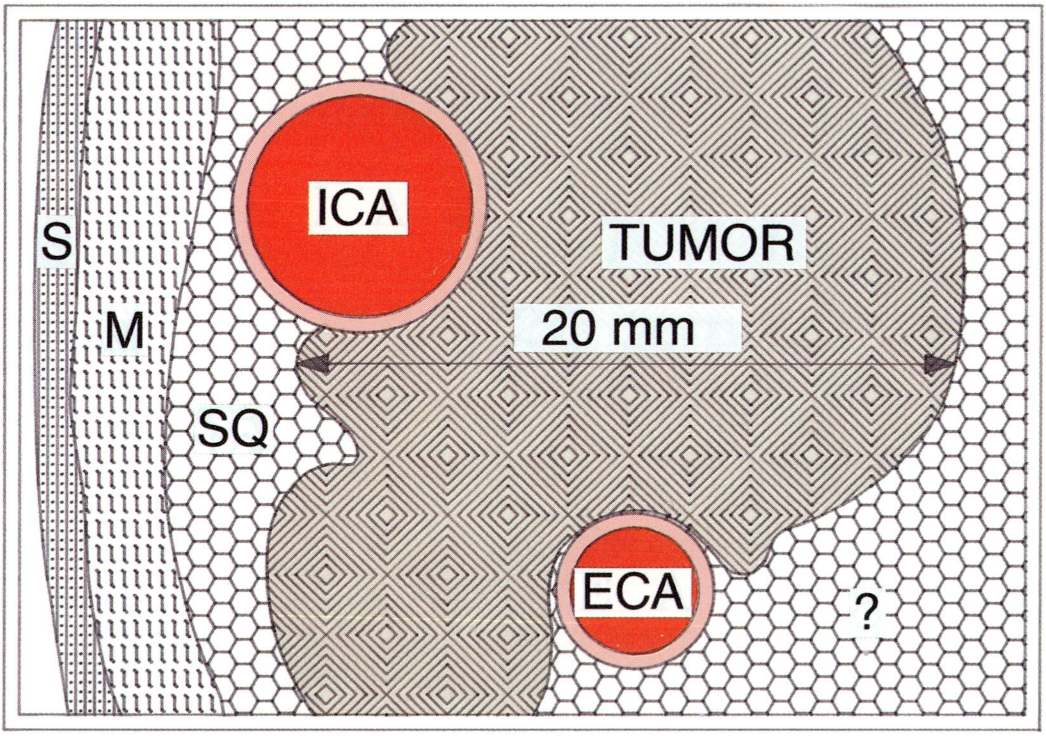
S
M
SQ
ICA
TUMOR
20 mm
ECA
?

Figure 138. VERTEBRAL ARTERY—MID SECTION

This is a good view of the right vertebral artery (VA) that is obscured in its mid section by the transverse process of the 6th cervical vertebra (B). Note the loss of definition of the arterial wall at this level although the contour of the bone is not well seen. This scan and the one following are abutting sections of the same vertebral artery. SQ = subcutaneous tissue, M = muscle (sternocleidomastoid and others), F = fascia.

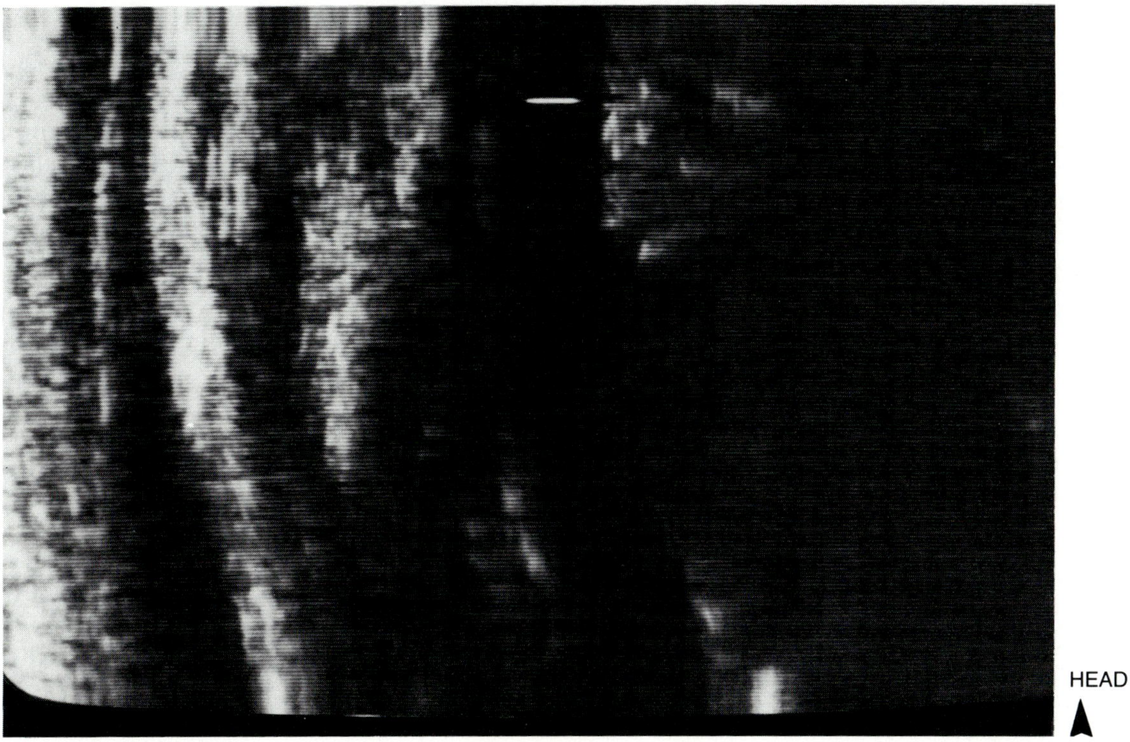
HEAD

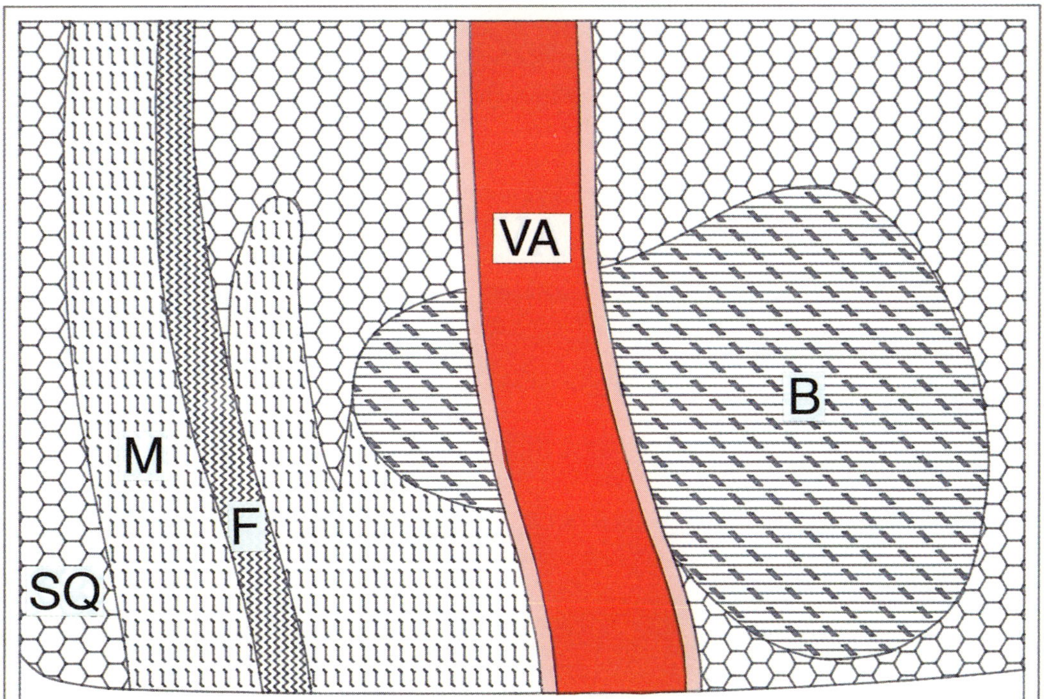
VA
B
M
F
SQ

Figure 139. VERTEBRAL ARTERY ORIGIN

This is an exceptionally clear longitudinal view of the same right vertebral artery (VA) as it originates from the subclavian artery (SCA), which is seen in transverse view. Usually the subclavian artery is hidden behind the clavicle. Note how narrow the "intimal stripe" is as seen on the deep wall of the typically thin-walled subclavian artery. The bone (B) is a transverse cut of the first rib, which is sandwiched between the transverse vertebral processes above and below. SQ = subcutaneous tissue, F = fascia, M = muscle (sternocleidomastoid and anterior scalene).

HISTORY *This 21-year-old female patient had a particularly high course of the subclavian artery, which allowed visualization of the vertebral artery at the base of the neck. She presented with complaints of syncope, but there was no evidence of carotid or vertebral stenosis by scan. She did have a seizure disorder.*

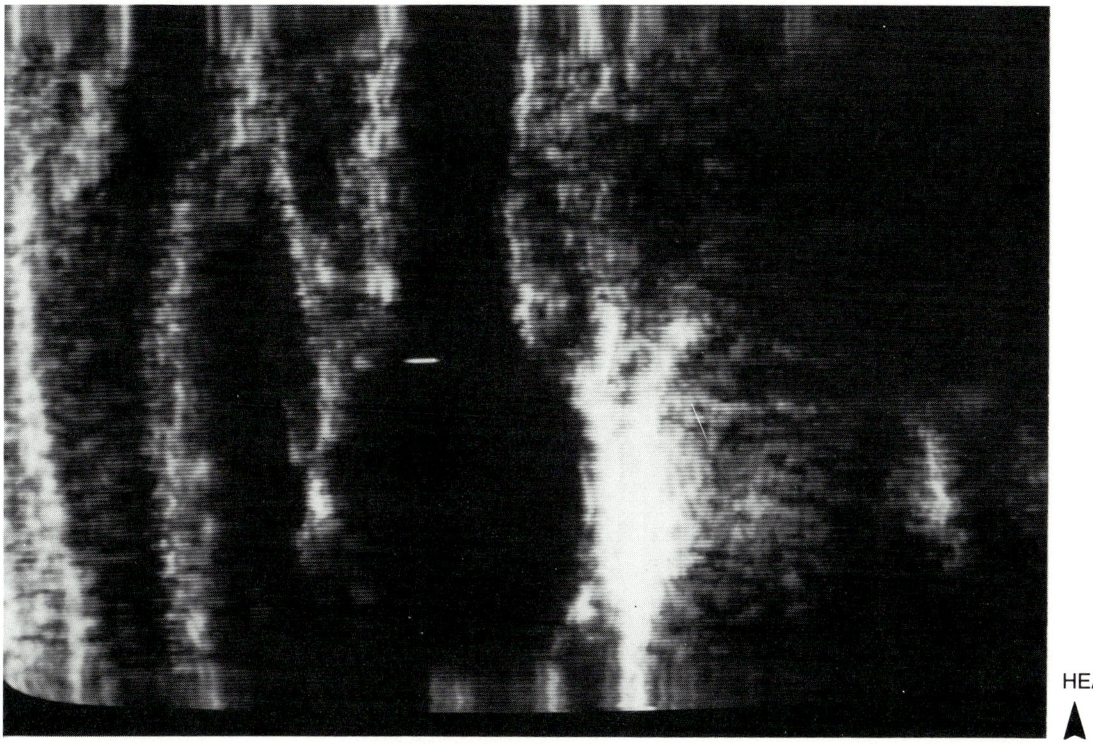
HEAD

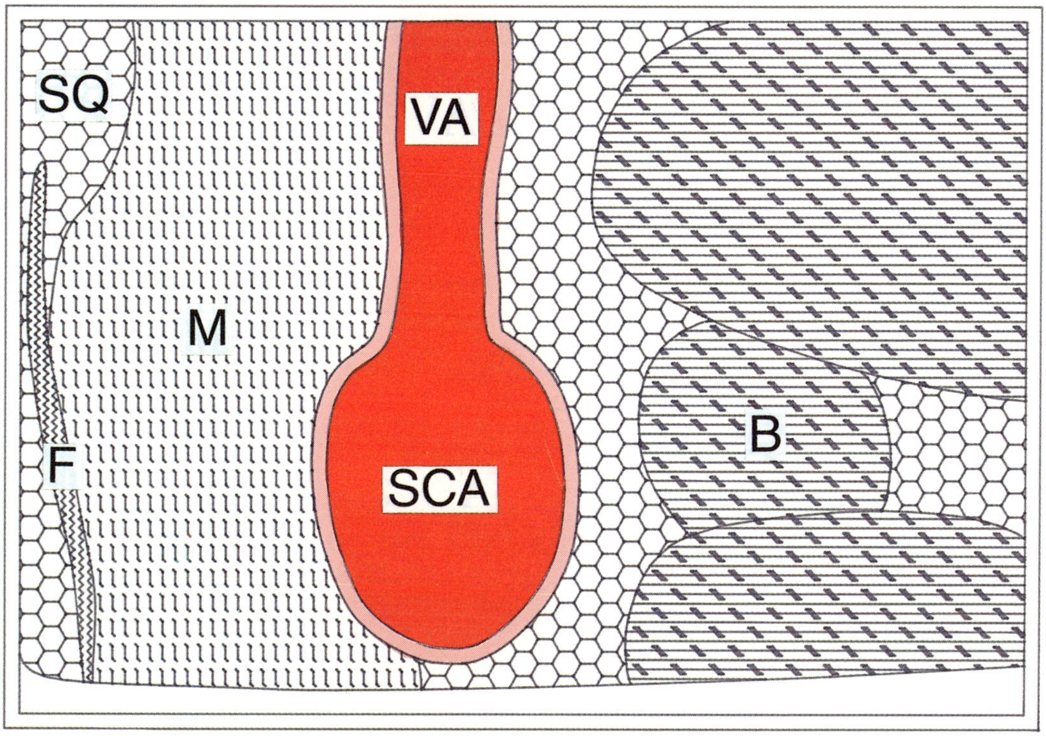
SQ
VA
M
B
F
SCA

CHAPTER 8

ARTIFACT

This chapter is included to assist the reader in two respects as follows: to help the person who performs the scan in recognizing commonly encountered artifacts so as to improve the image quality of the scan and to make the interpreting physician aware of these possible sources and characteristics of artifact because artifact can, in some cases, be mistaken for plaque and other forms of pathology.

Figure 140. GOOD GEL CONTACT

Certainly the most common and most important artifact is that caused by gel separation. The following series of scans is an experiment to demonstrate changes in image quality, as the nature of contact between the probe and skin is changed. The first scan represents the ideal view obtained when, after the application of sufficient gel, the probe is applied so that the probe membrane (M) makes close contact with the skin (S) along the entire image.

In previous scans we have somewhat loosely indicated the parts of the probe-skin interface, and these are examined here in greater detail. The clear black area at the left edge of the scan is actually the water within the probe itself. The position of the membrane-skin interface is slightly offset from the left edge of the image and corresponds to the green stripe in the diagram. The manufacturer has intentionally included some of the probe components in the image so that the skin edge can always be seen. The probe membrane is so thin that it is not actually seen as a discrete entity. The skin typically appears as a tissue thickness of medium gray bounded by two brighter layers. The bright zone on the left of the skin edge is a composite of membrane, gel, and skin surface and in this scan is only 0.1 mm or 0.2 mm in thickness and of the same brightness as the deeper skin boundary. These features are very important in indicating good gel contact. Deep to the skin is subcutaneous tissue (SQ), which has nearly the same brightness as the skin itself. The sternocleidomastoid muscle (SCM) has the typical darker appearance. The internal jugular vein is almost out of plane in this view and shows some of its back wall (BW) toward the bottom half of the image. A thin layer of fascia (F) separates the vessels. The common carotid artery (CCA) is very clearly seen. In the portion of the artery that is most perpendicular to the skin the superficial and deep intimal margins are clearly defined. The deep edge of the Doppler cursor (C) cuts into the deep "intimal stripe" slightly. The thyroid gland is seen to have a finely mottled but intermediate shade of gray, which darkens to the right as signal strength is lost in the deep field. Note the lack of any dark bands passing from left to right through the scan. Note that although the sternocleidomastoid muscle is quite dark, some echoes can still be seen arising from it.

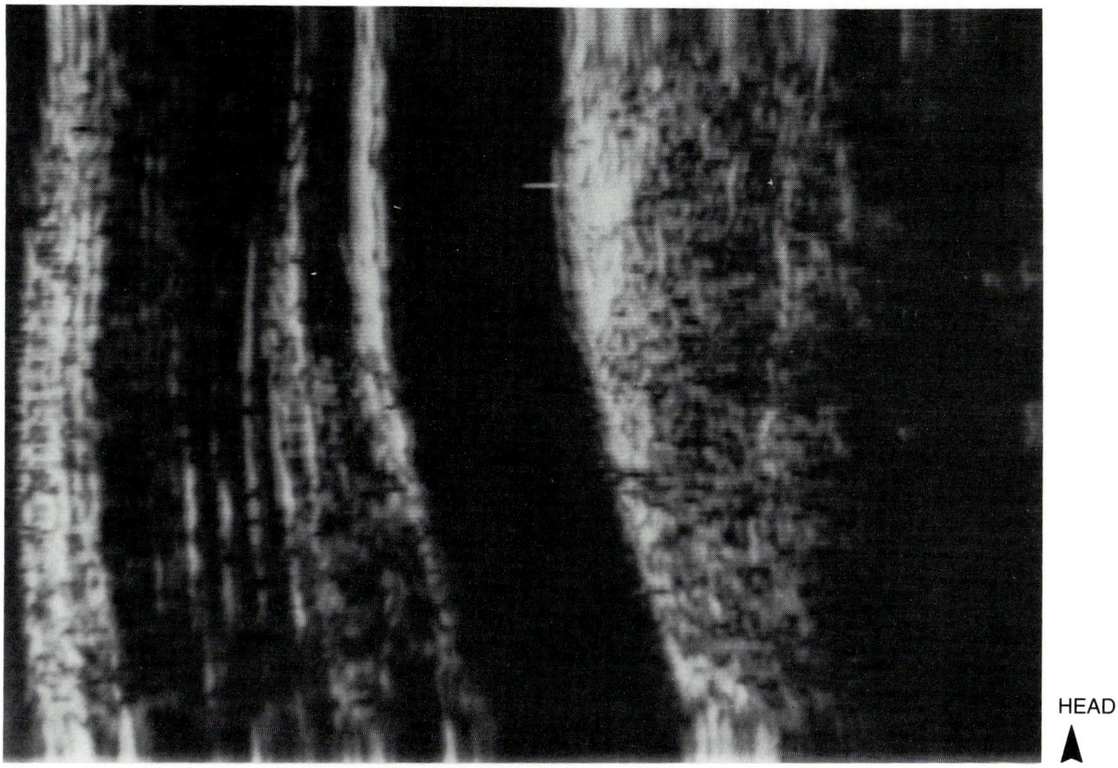
HEAD

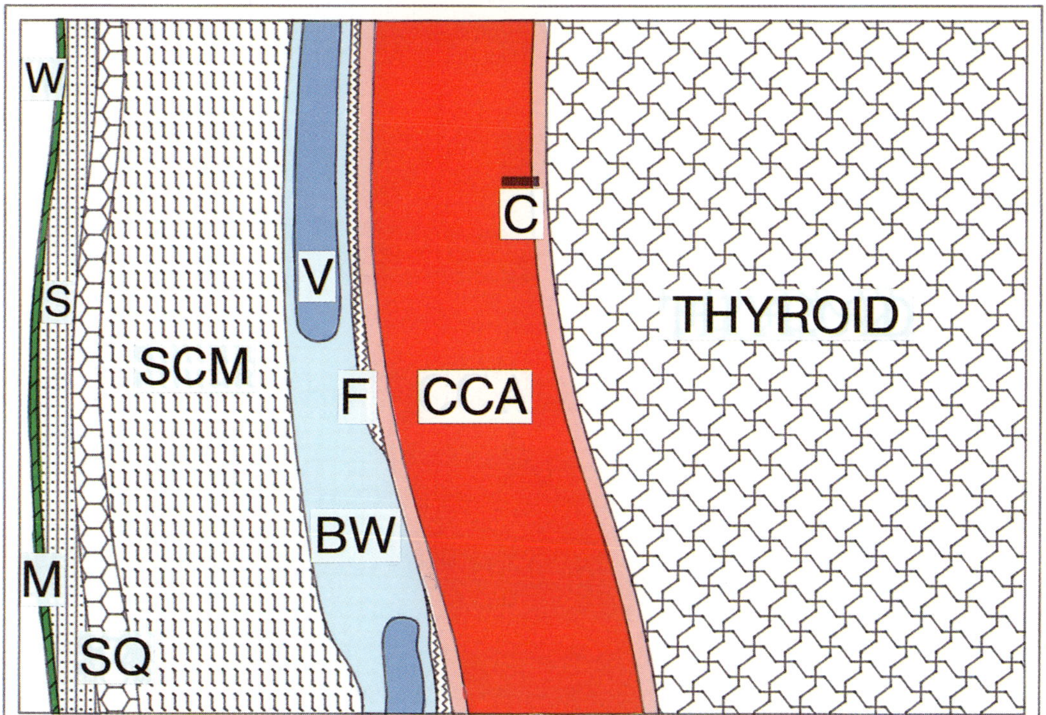
W
S
SCM
V
F
CCA
C
THYROID
BW
M
SQ

Figure 141. LATERAL GEL SEPARATION

As the right hand edge of the probe is lifted off the skin, gel separation appears and is apparent in two ways. The first and most obvious is the loss of the bottom half of the image by a dark zone created by the gel separation (GS). Secondly, a very bright wedge-shaped thickening of echoes due to poor gel contact (G) is seen along the skin surface. The brightness of the normal tissues is in inverse proportion to the brightness of this gel interface, which causes so much echo reflection at the bottom of the screen that no deeper tissues can be seen.

There are two additional but more subtle findings with poor gel contact. These are the loss of resolution of tissue elements in the top half of the image and loss of visualization of deep field structures. These are discussed in more detail in Figure 143. The purple area corresponds to the total loss of image whether due to gel separation in the bottom half or due to lack of deep tissue penetration in the top half of the scan. SQ = subcutaneous tissue, SCM = sternocleidomastoid muscle, V = internal jugular vein, F = fascia, CCA = common carotid artery, C = Doppler cursor, VN = vagus nerve, T = thyroid.

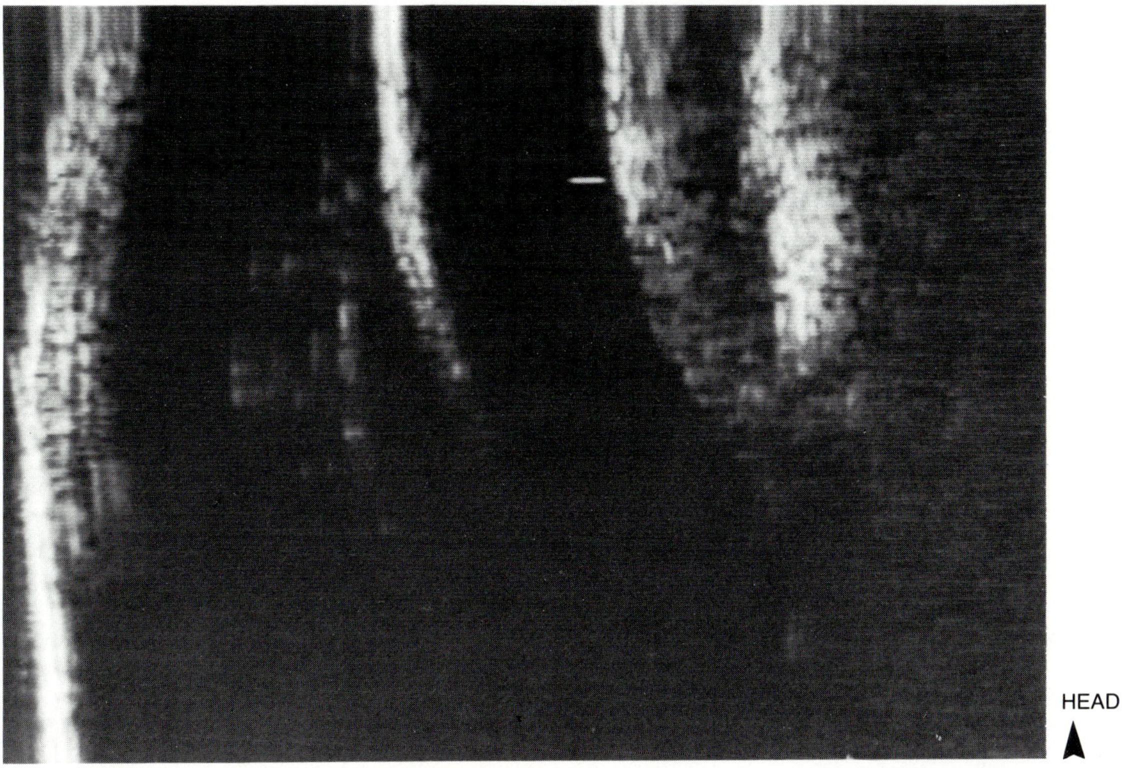
HEAD

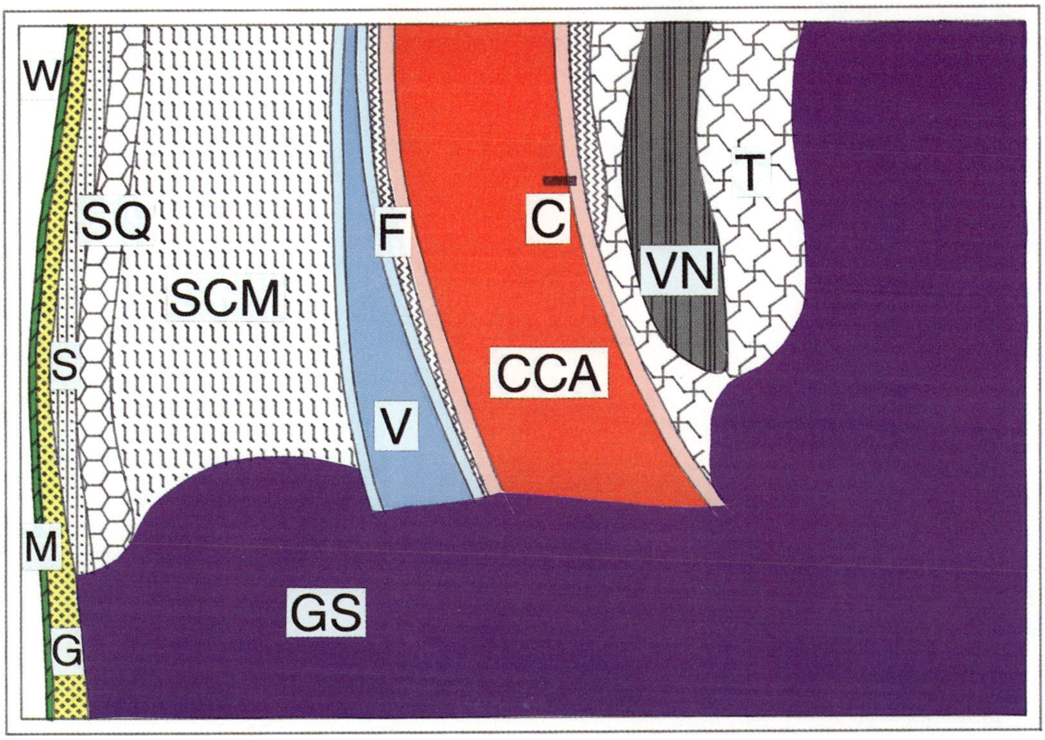
W
SQ
SCM
S
M
G
F
V
C
CCA
VN
T
GS

Figure 142. LATERAL GEL SEPARATION

In this view the probe is rocked the other way on the skin with the right side of the probe making better contact and the left side of the probe lifted up. Note the appearance of gel separation (GS) now in the top half of the scan. Observe that because of this rocking effect the arteries seem to have slanted the other side of vertical. Note that the areas of brightest echo reflection at the membrane-skin interface caused by poor contact of gel (G) are associated with the greatest tissue shadowing. W = water (within the probe), M = membrane, S = skin, SQ = subcutaneous tissue, SCM = sternocleidomastoid muscle, HL = "hard-line" artifact, F = fascia, CCA = common carotid artery, C = Doppler cursor, VN = vagus nerve, T = thyroid.

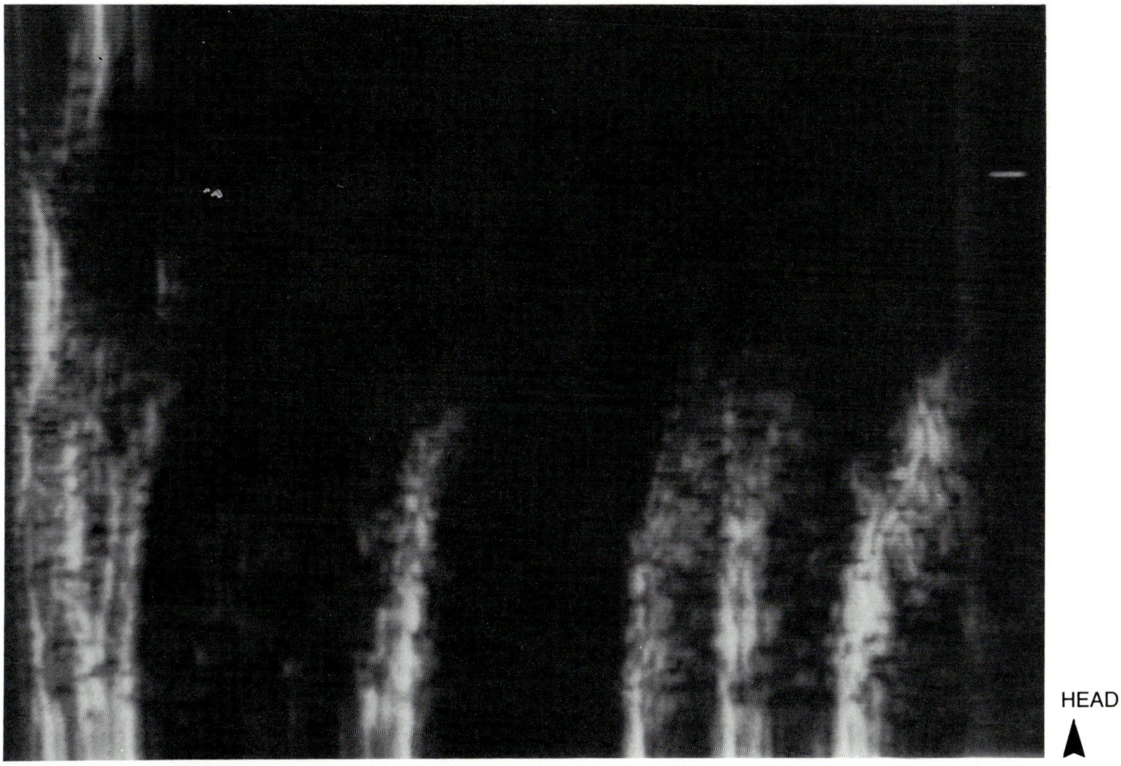
HEAD

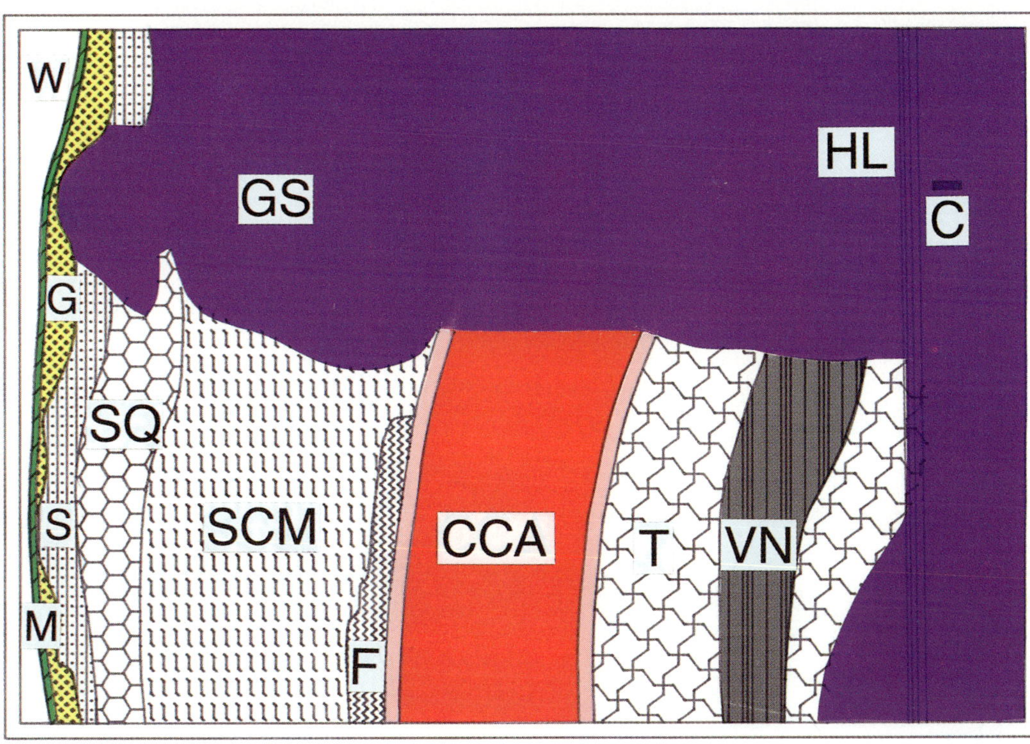
W
GS
HL
C
G
SQ
S
SCM
CCA
T
VN
M
F

Figure 143. NO GEL

Prior to this scan, all gel was wiped away until the skin and probe were completely dry. Nevertheless, a fairly good image is obtained because the probe was "rubbed" against the skin surface so as to obliterate any air pockets and required considerably more pressure than when gel was used. Furthermore, in this region corresponding to the mid neck, the skin is fairly flat and can accommodate the probe surface. Actually, there is a slight degradation in the quality in the image when compared with Figure 140. The superficial line (G) of skin contact is somewhat brighter than in the previous figure, and there are some subtle differences in the deeper tissues. Note the lack of fine echoes within the sternocleidomastoid muscle (SCM). Also note the lack of a visible "intimal stripe" that on the deep wall of the common carotid artery (CCA) overlaps the mid section of the Doppler cursor (C). In this somewhat degraded image one would be inclined to measure from adventitial margin to adventitial margin rather than the true inner luminal diameter of the artery. Many trainees make this error. One must learn to allow for the "intimal stripe" in a poorer quality image, if one is to obtain true measurements of arterial diameters. There is a loss of image in the deep field corresponding to the purple area on the diagram, which is also associated with poor gel contact. This loss is due to relative attenuation of the beam in the deep field, using the same gain settings (compare with Figure 140). W = water (within the probe), M = probe membrane, S = skin, SQ = subcutaneous tissue, V = internal jugular vein, F = fascia, VN = vagus nerve, T = thyroid gland, AF = reverberation artifact, NV = non-visualized deep tissues.

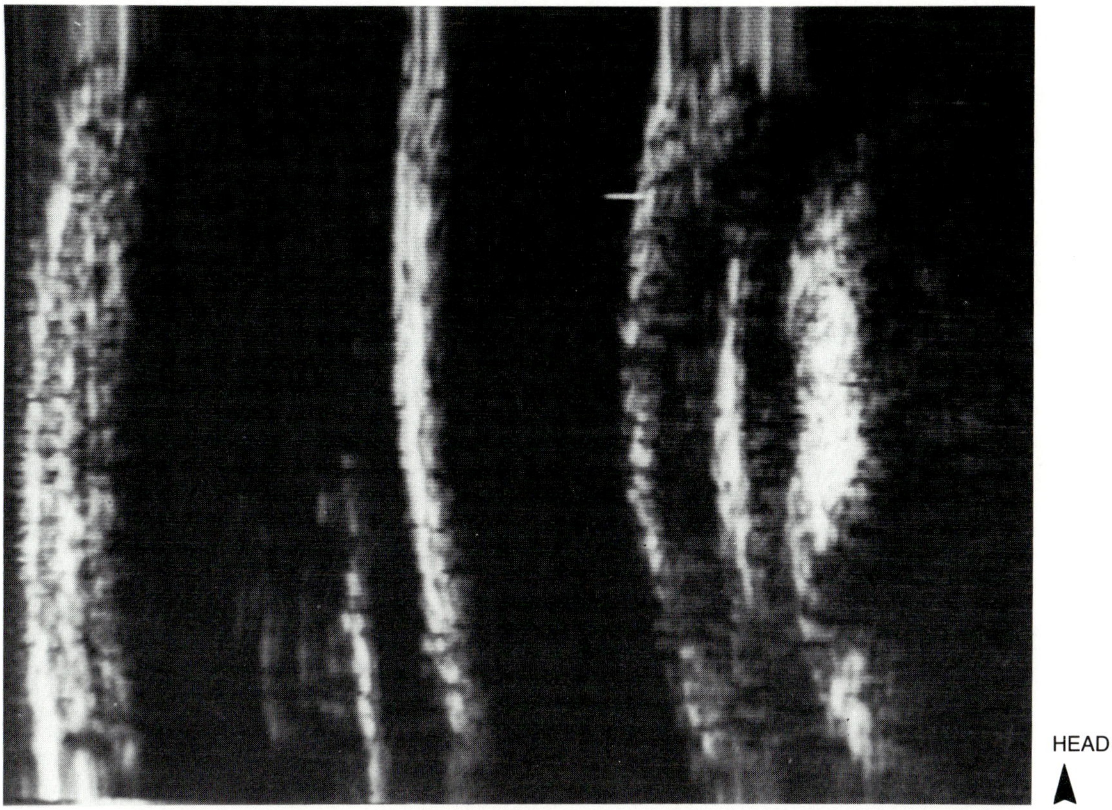
HEAD

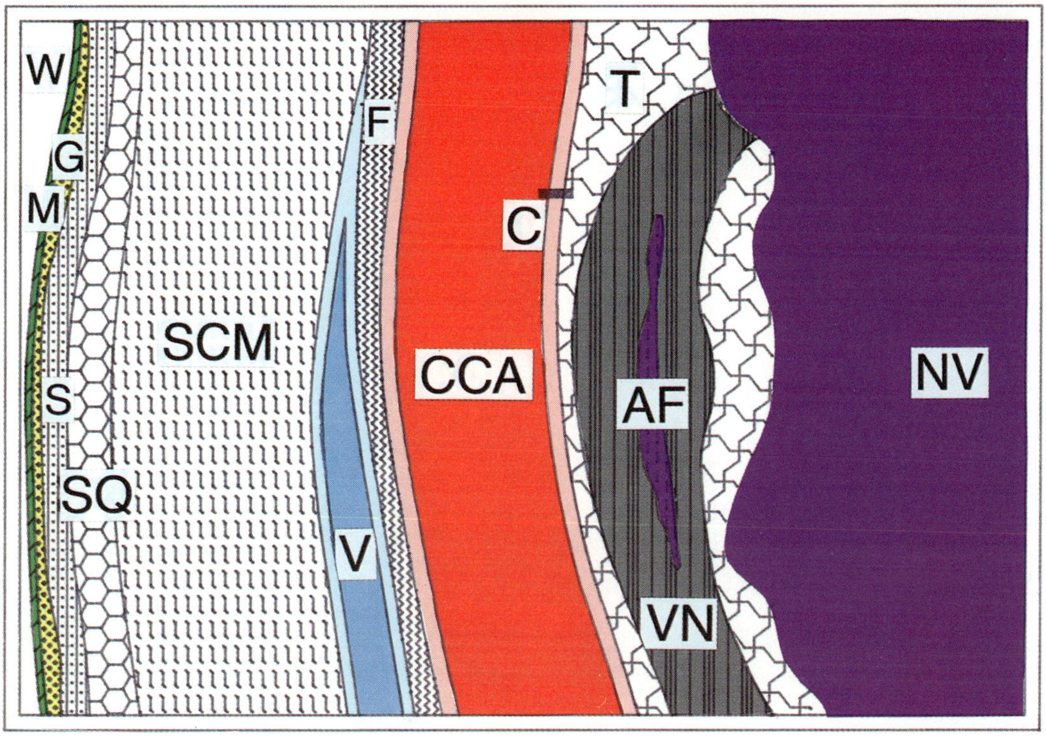
W
G
M
S
SQ
SCM
F
V
CCA
C
T
AF
VN
NV

Figure 144. CENTRAL GEL SEPARATION

On occasion it is possible to cause gel separation (GS) in the center of the image. This GS can come about as a result of a gap in the applied gel, a large air pocket, or a concavity of the tissues, which prevents full contact with the flat surface of the probe. The second situation can be encountered in the hollow under the mandible, if insufficient gel is applied. Some of the other ultrasound scans in this atlas have these same bands of gel separation, which have not been drawn (see Figures 147, 148, and 149). W = water (within the probe), M = probe membrane, G = gel, S = skin, SQ = subcutaneous tissue, CCA = common carotid artery, SCM = sternocleidomastoid muscle, C = Doppler cursor, T = thyroid gland, VN = non-visualized deep tissues (due to gain settings), AF = reverberation artifact.

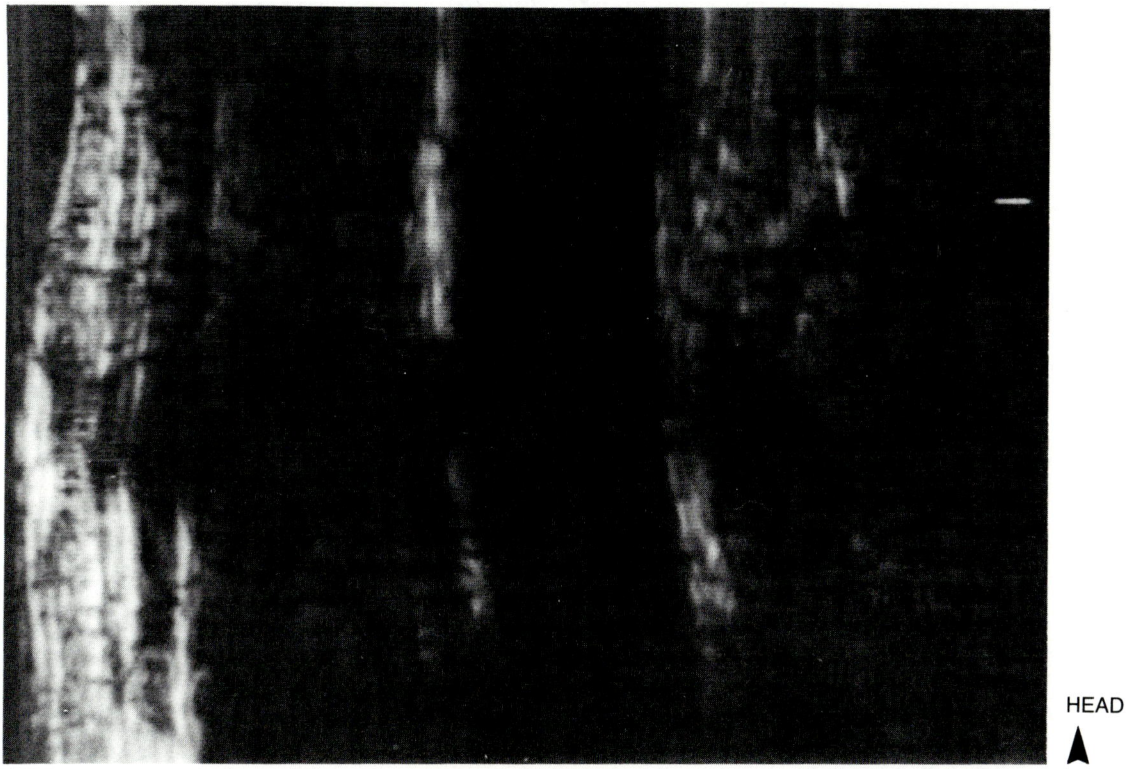
HEAD

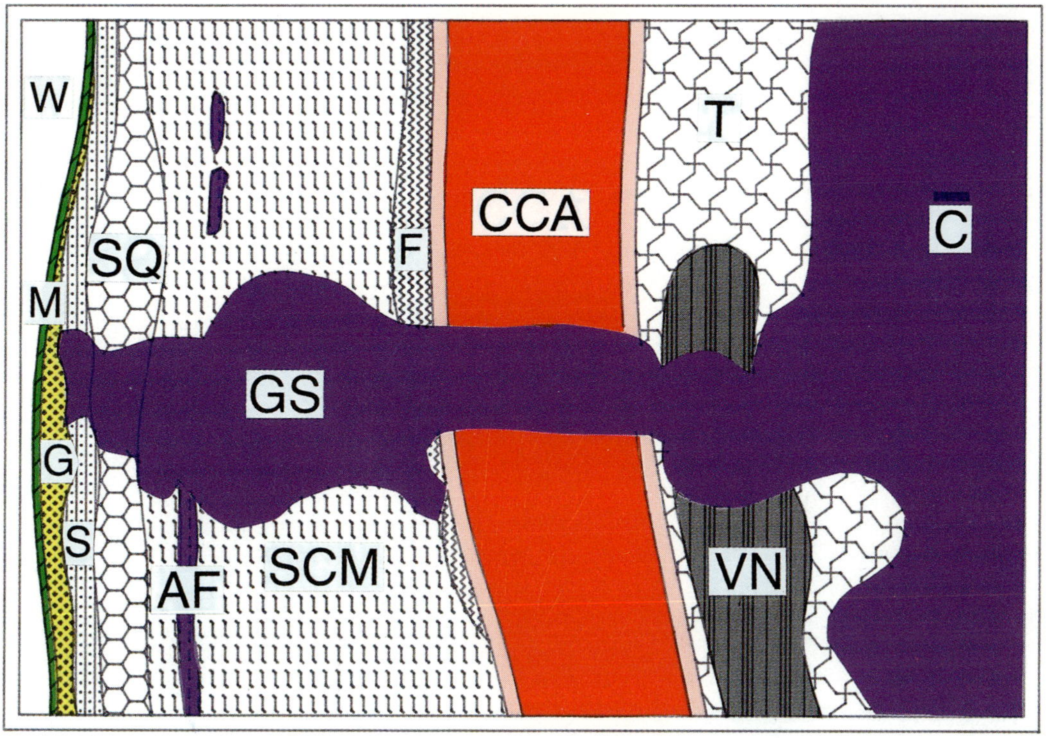
W
SQ
M
G
S
AF
SCM
GS
F
CCA
T
C
VN

Figure 145. INTENSIVE CARE UNIT (ICU) ENVIRONMENT ARTIFACT

This is an example of various artifacts (AF) encountered in an ICU environment. In this case there appear to be two different patterns of artifact in the deep field. The first is the presence of diagonal bands of short fine lines of uniform length. In addition to this pattern is the presence of short bright streaks of varying length in a more random pattern. Note that both these artifacts are more prominent in the deep field and fade out at about center screen. Both of these types of artifact have the appearance of electrical interference from an external source. If a good quality image is to be obtained, one must attempt to localize the offending electrical interference. What follows is a controlled experiment using the example of a normal common carotid artery (CCA). S = skin, M = platysma muscle, SQ = subcutaneous tissue, SCM = sternocleidomastoid muscle, IJV = internal jugular vein, C = Doppler cursor, ? = tissue of uncertain composition.

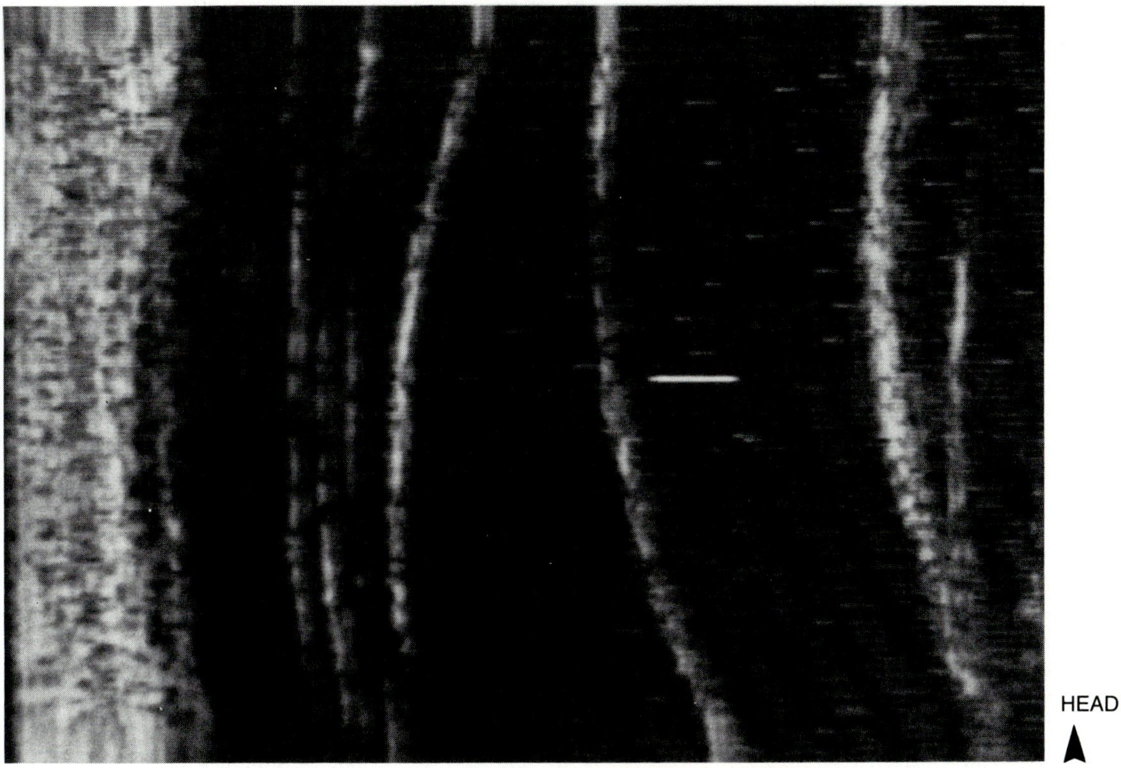
HEAD

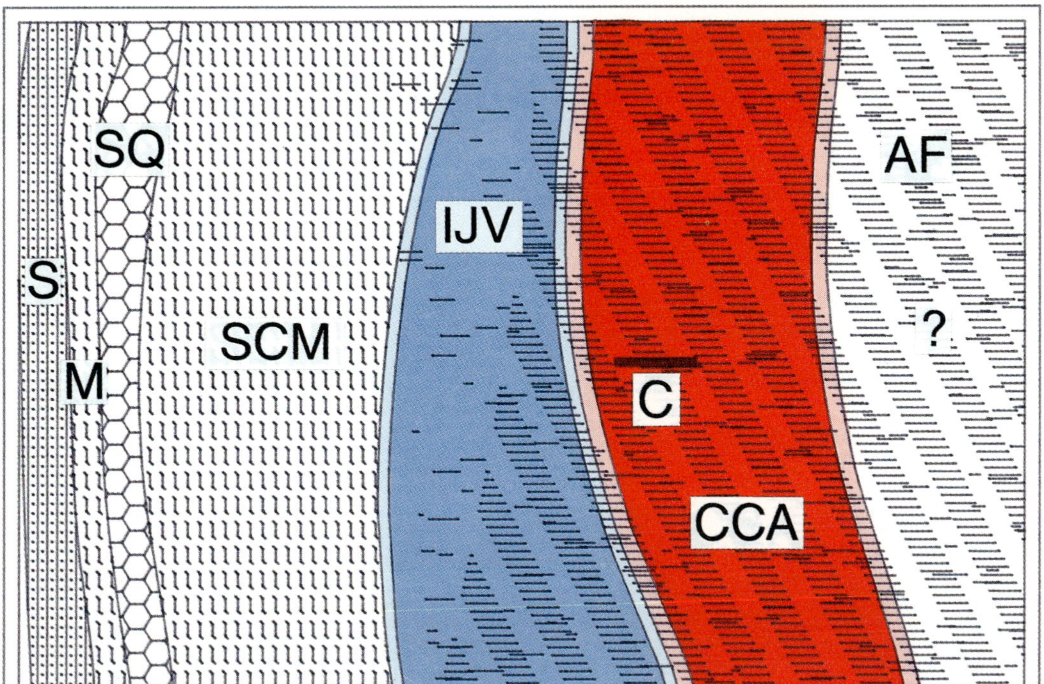
SQ
AF
IJV
S
SCM
?
M
C
CCA

Figure 146. 60-HZ POWER SUPPLY ARTIFACT

The diagonal striated bands of artifact (AF) arising from the electrical outlet become even more prominent after an electrocardiogram monitor is turned off. Despite the incorporation of electrical "noise" filters within the power supply circuitry within the scanner it is possible for very "dirty" wall outlets to overwhelm the noise suppression. The source of electrical noise conducted through the power supply can sometimes be elusive. The chief offender in our hospital is in the ICU when the scanner is plugged into the customized electrical "headboard" that supplies power to ventilators, intravenous (IV) pumps, and other equipment. Some of the older IV pumps can be sources of noticeable noise. Since noise is most often conducted through the power supplies, it is of great help to be able to plug the scanner into an independent power source if one is available. S = skin, SQ = subcutaneous tissue, M = platysma muscle, SCM = sternocleido-mastoid muscle, IJV = internal jugular vein, CCA = common carotid artery, C = Doppler cursor, F = fascia.

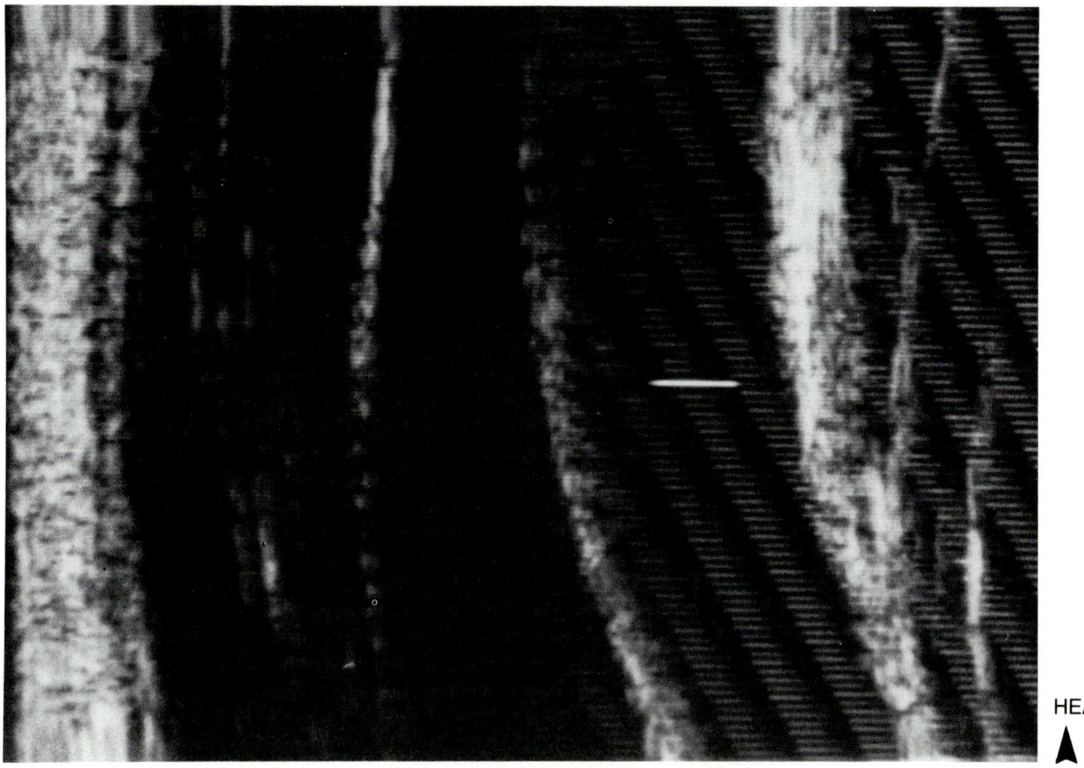
HEAD

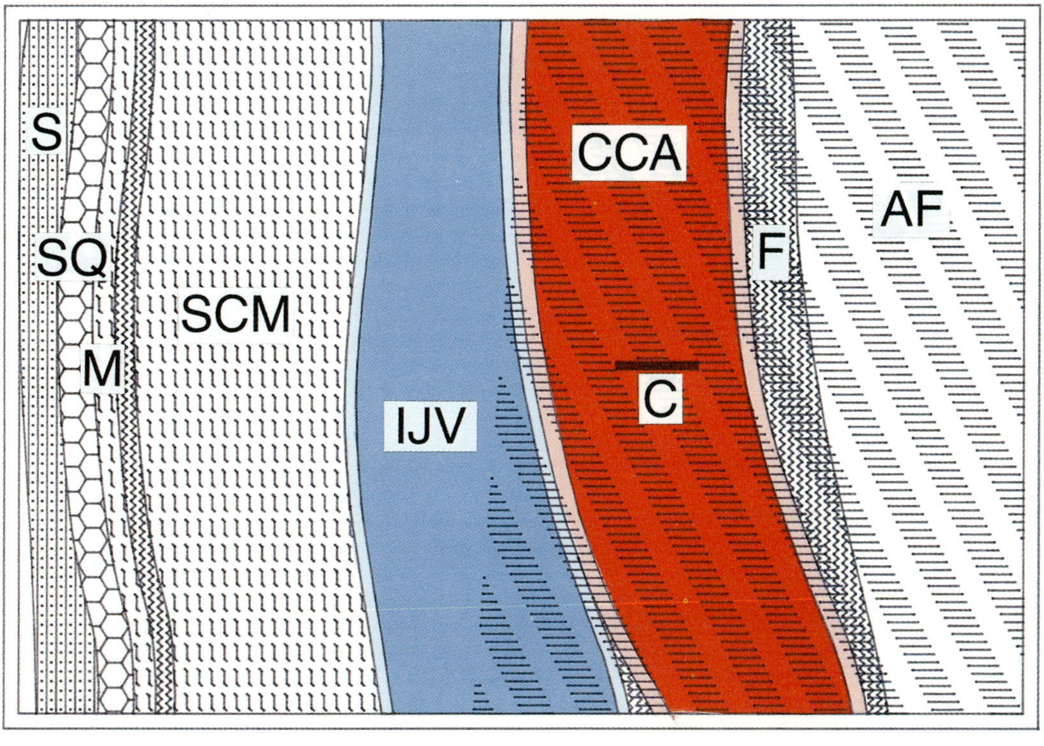
S
SQ
M
SCM
IJV
CCA
C
F
AF

Figure 147. ELECTROCARDIOGRAM MONITOR ARTIFACT

While holding the probe motionless, the scanner is turned off, and the power supply is disconnected from the intensive care unit (ICU) headboard and connected by an extension cord to a distant wall outlet. Note the disappearance of the diagonal bands seen in the previous view, confirming the fact that the power supply artifact is conducted electrically and not by means of electromagnetic interference. What remains is the artifact (AF) seen in this scan that is arising from electromagnetic interference from the electrocardiogram (ECG) monitor. This present artifact fades as the subject is moved many feet away from the monitor. SCM = sternocleidomastoid muscle, F = fascia, IJV = internal jugular vein, C = Doppler cursor, CCA = common carotid artery, ? = tissue of uncertain composition.

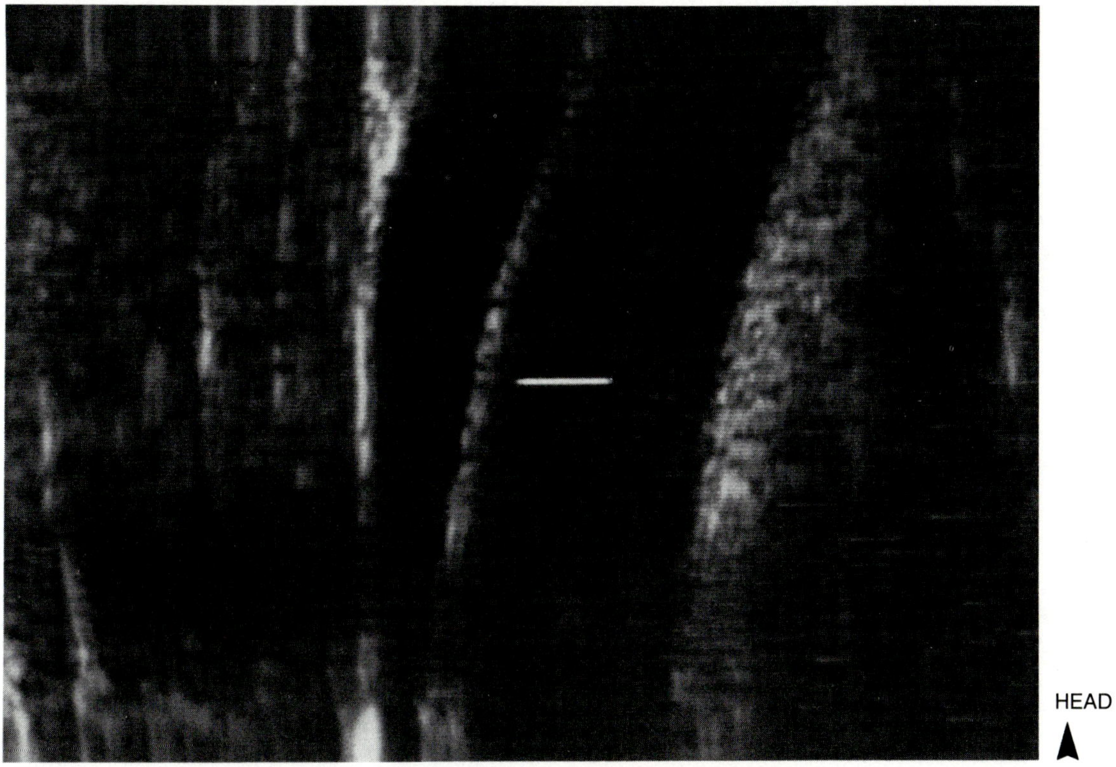
HEAD

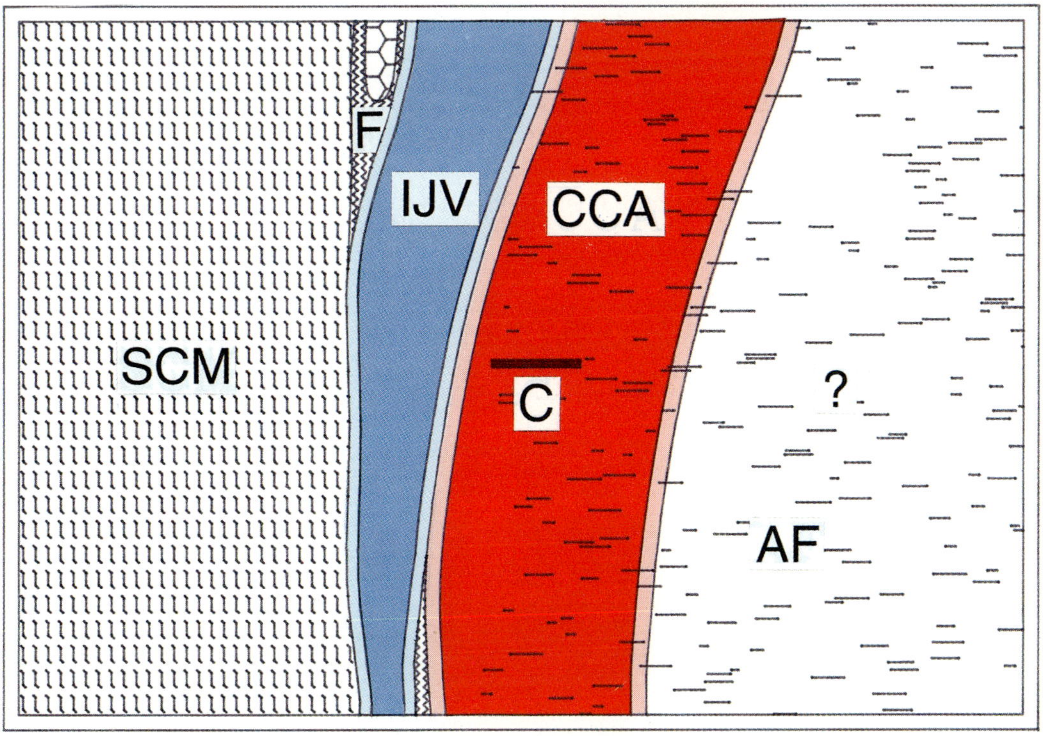
F
IJV
CCA
SCM
C
?
AF

Figure 148. ELECTROCARDIOGRAM "OFF"

After turning the electrocardiogram (ECG) monitor off, in addition to switching the power supply source, all electrical interference is abolished. Far-field details can now be successfully imaged. Under controlled circumstances, we have disconnected ventilators, IVAC pumps, and the like for short periods when interference presents an insurmountable obstacle to imaging a deep artery or vein. In addition to the visual aspects, electrical interference can add a particularly unpleasant whine to a weak Doppler signal, thereby obscuring it. SCM = sternocleidomastoid muscle, F = fascia, IJV = internal jugular vein, C = Doppler cursor, CCA = common carotid artery, ? = tissue of uncertain composition.

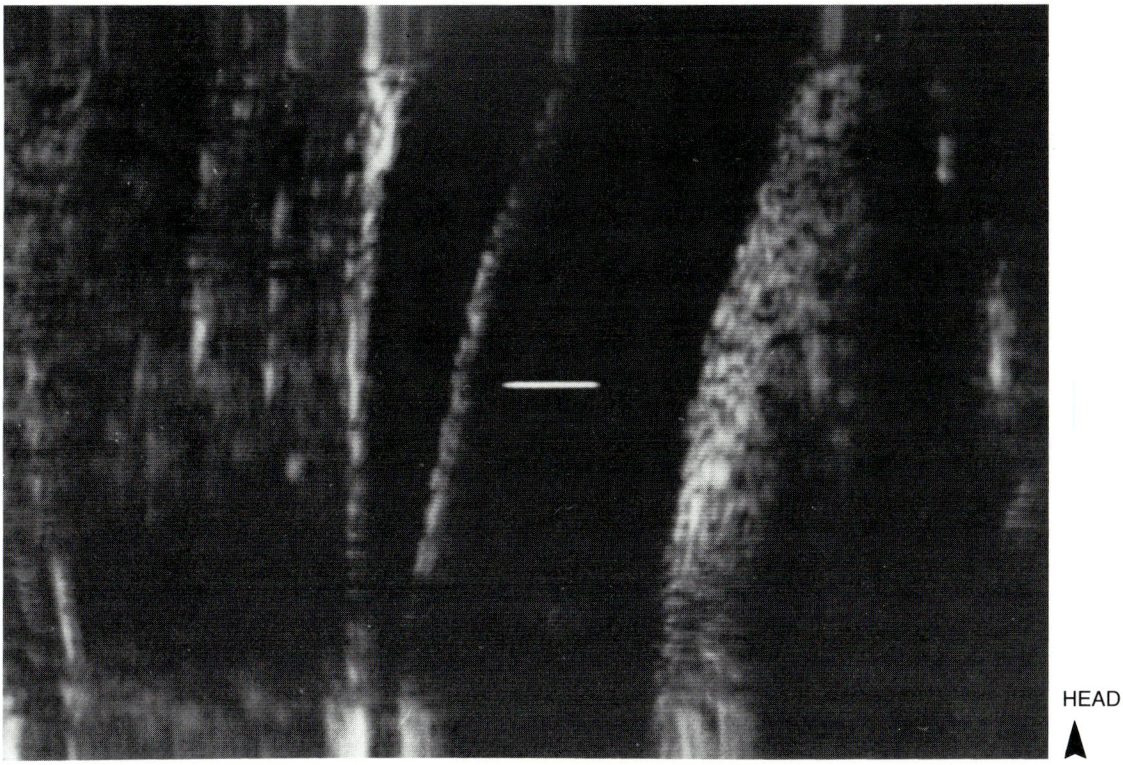
HEAD

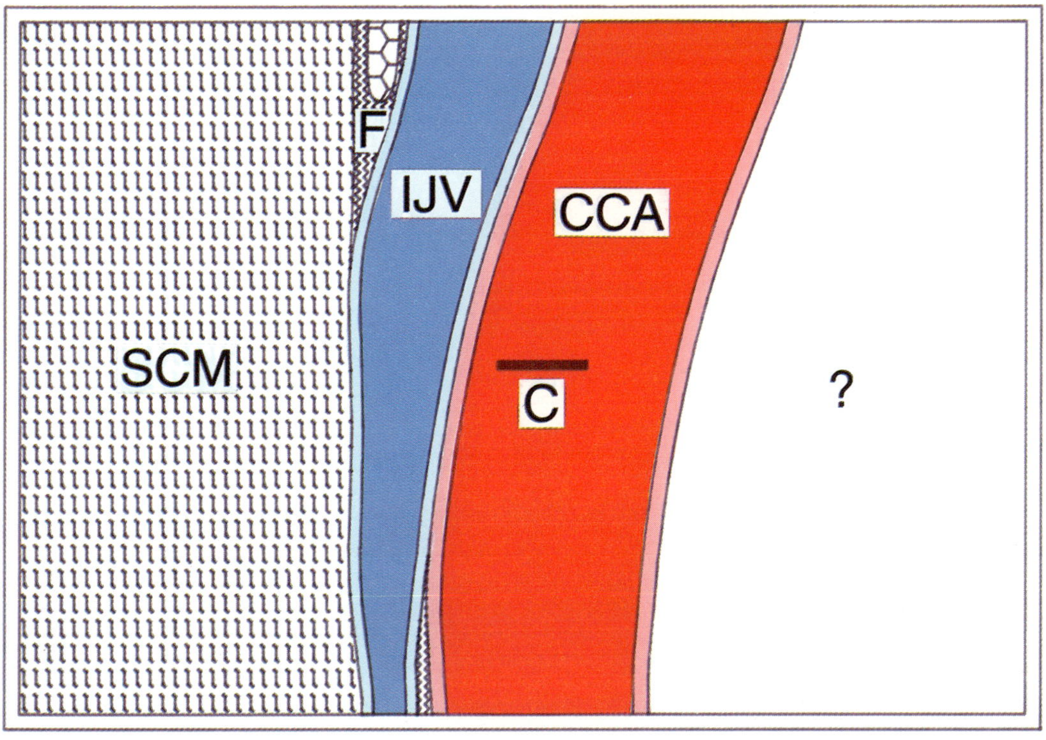
F
IJV
CCA
SCM
C
?

Figure 149. SPARK DISCHARGE ARTIFACT

Some beautiful electrical interference patterns can be obtained under certain circumstances. This is what results during the instant in which an electrocardiogram monitor is turned on. The artifact (AF) resulting from the spark discharge from closing the switch has a complicated moiré pattern of interlacing parabolas. SCM = sternocleidomastoid muscle, SQ = subcutaneous tissue, IJV = internal jugular vein, C = Doppler cursor, CCA = common carotid artery, ? = tissue of uncertain composition.

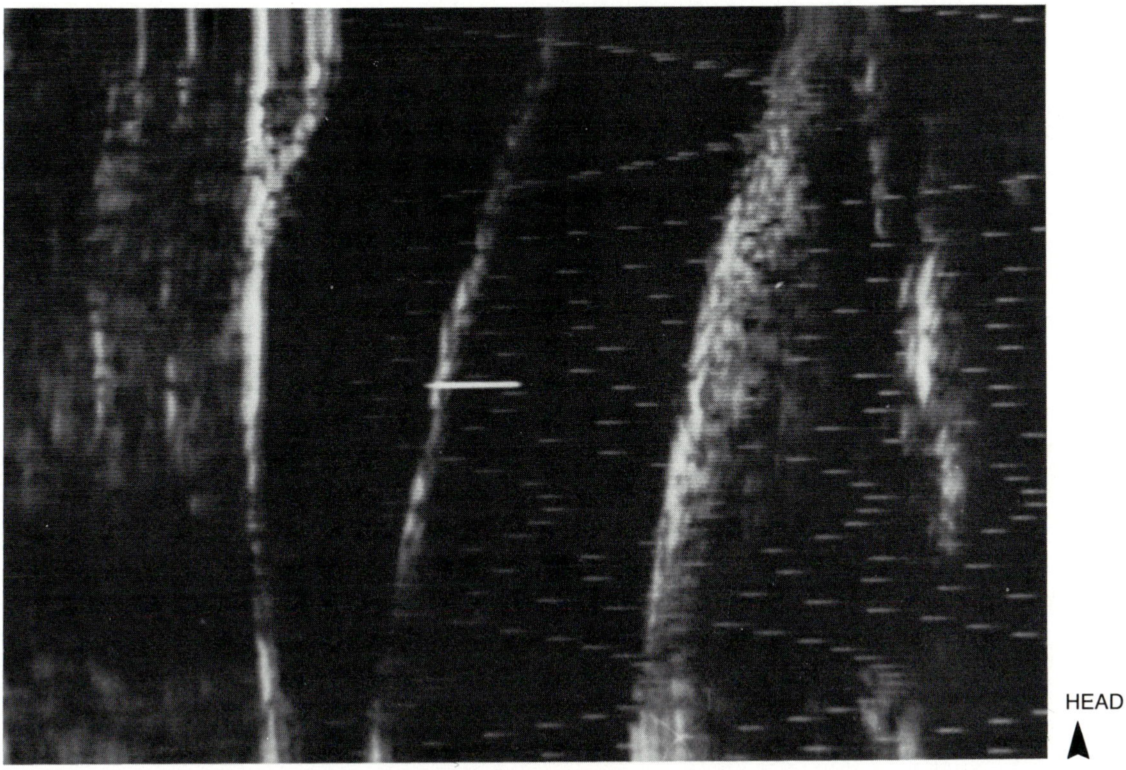
HEAD

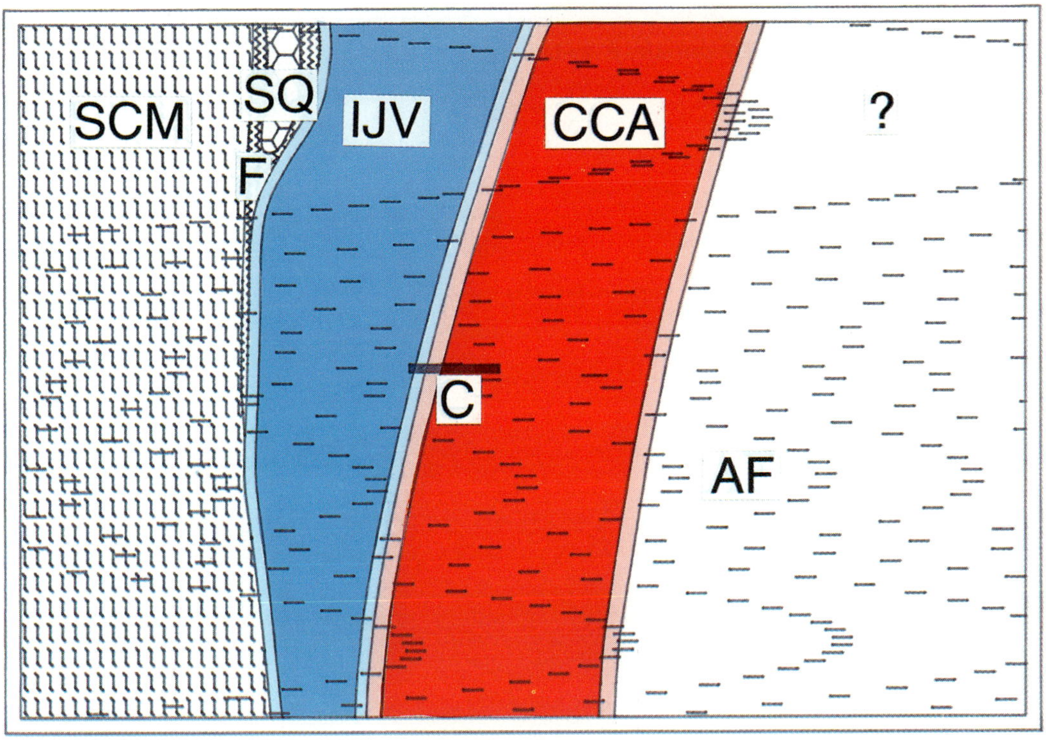
SCM
SQ
F
IJV
CCA
?
C
AF

Figure 150. BUBBLE ARTIFACT

The probes used with this machine are constructed with a fixed transducer that radiates a beam directed against an elliptically shaped concave oscillating mirror, which redirects the ultrasound beam out through the portion of the transducer head covered by an acoustically transparent membrane. The echoes returning from the tissue come back through the membrane, strike the mirror, and are redirected back to the transducer where the signal is received and converted back into an electrical waveform to be processed. The Plexiglas transducer head is filled with water in order to provide a transparent medium for sound conduction between these components. A problem that can arise with this design is the development of bubbles in the water. These tend to form at a slow rate over days to weeks as a result of "out gassing" of the water itself. The other mechanism by which bubbles can form more quickly is a crack in the Plexiglas housing.

The bubbles have two types of appearances in the ultrasound image. The first is what we have termed "large bubble artifact" (LB), which appears as large semicircular arcs usually most prominent in the far field (right half) of the image. It is believed that the semicircular shape is caused by refraction of the beam, as it passes through the bubble into a large wave front. The actual bubble itself is not visualized. The second type of bubble artifact is what we term "small bubble artifact" (SB). It has the appearance of an actual bubble often distorted into a somewhat elliptical shape. One sees a collection of vertical stripes within this circular or elliptical contour rather than the actual surface of the bubble. It is believed that this SB arises when a somewhat larger bubble enters the path of the beam in a more focused region near the surface membrane. SCM = sternocleidomastoid muscle, V = internal jugular vein, CCA = left common carotid artery, C = Doppler cursor, F = fascia, T = thyroid.

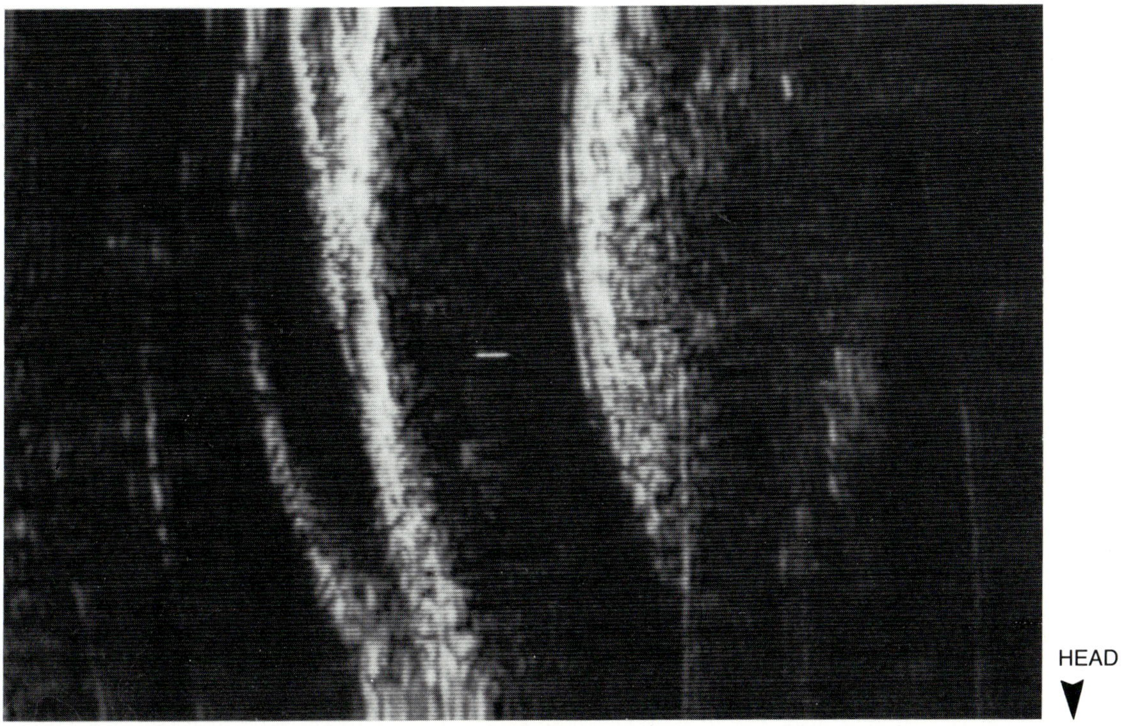
HEAD

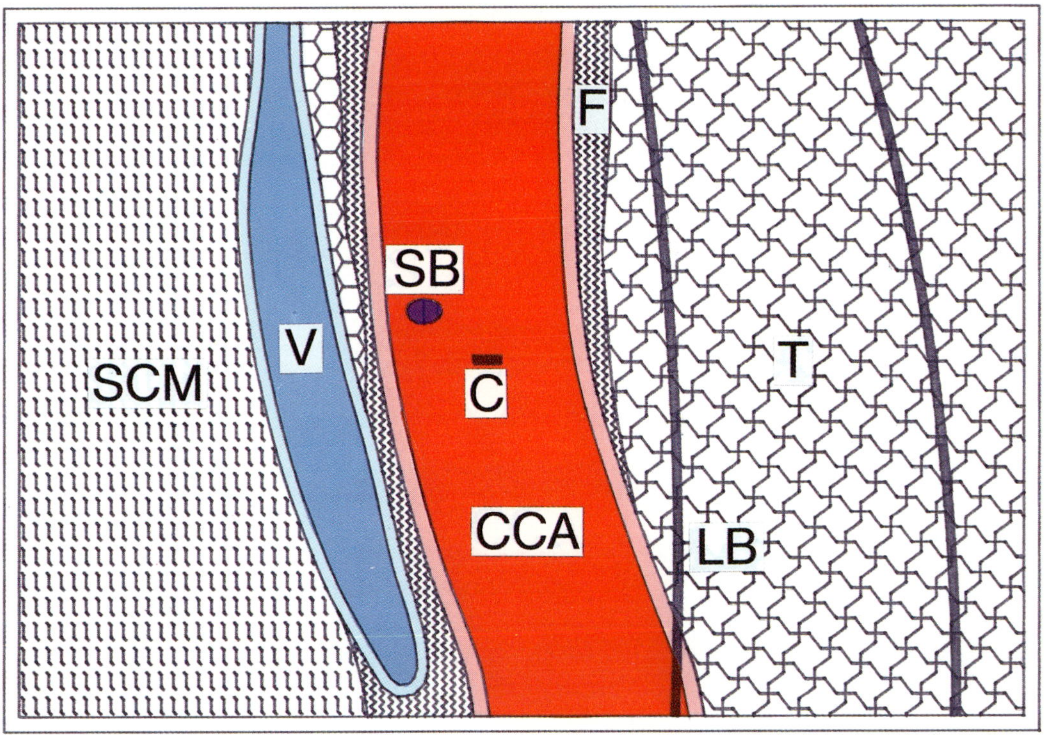
F
SB
V
C
SCM
T
CCA
LB

Figure 151. BUBBLE ARTIFACT

Note the movement of the small bubble artifact (SB) as the probe is held motionless. The bubble has moved from a previous position of 10 o'clock relative to the Doppler cursor (C) to a position almost directly overhead. By looking at the previous view alone, one could not be sure this was indeed small bubble artifact. However, the bubble is now seen much more distinctly. Note also the very slight movement of the large bubble artifact (LB) away from the deep wall of the common carotid artery (CCA). SCM = sternocleidomastoid muscle, V = internal jugular vein, F = fascia, T = thyroid.

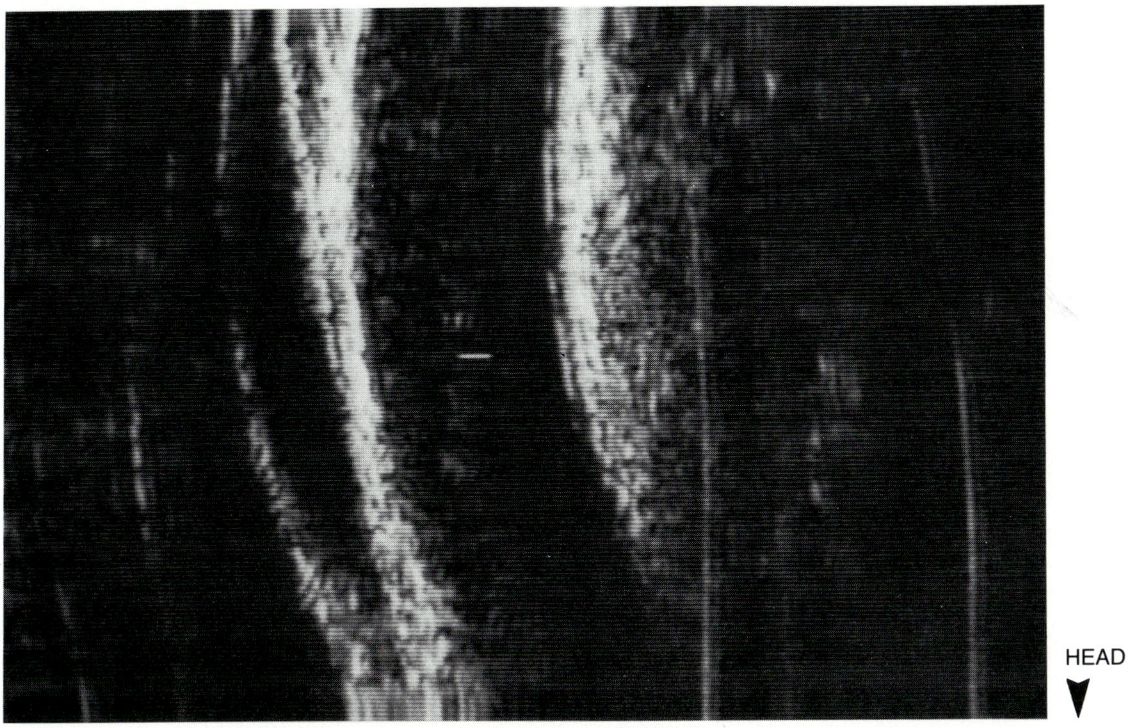
HEAD

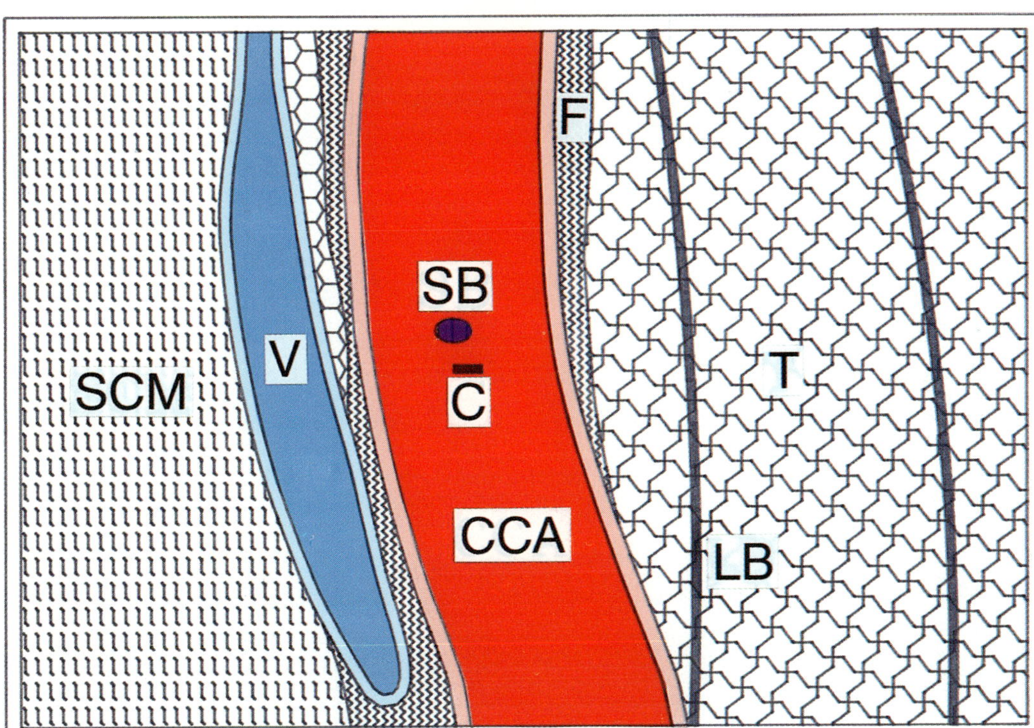
F
SB
V
SCM
C
T
CCA
LB

Figure 152. BUBBLE ARTIFACT

A few frames later, the small bubble artifact (SB) has now moved to the right of the Doppler cursor (C) at the 2-o'clock position. The large bubble artifact (LB) has also moved deeper, to the right of the common carotid artery (CCA). SCM = sternocleidomastoid muscle, V = internal jugular vein, F = fascia, T = thyroid.

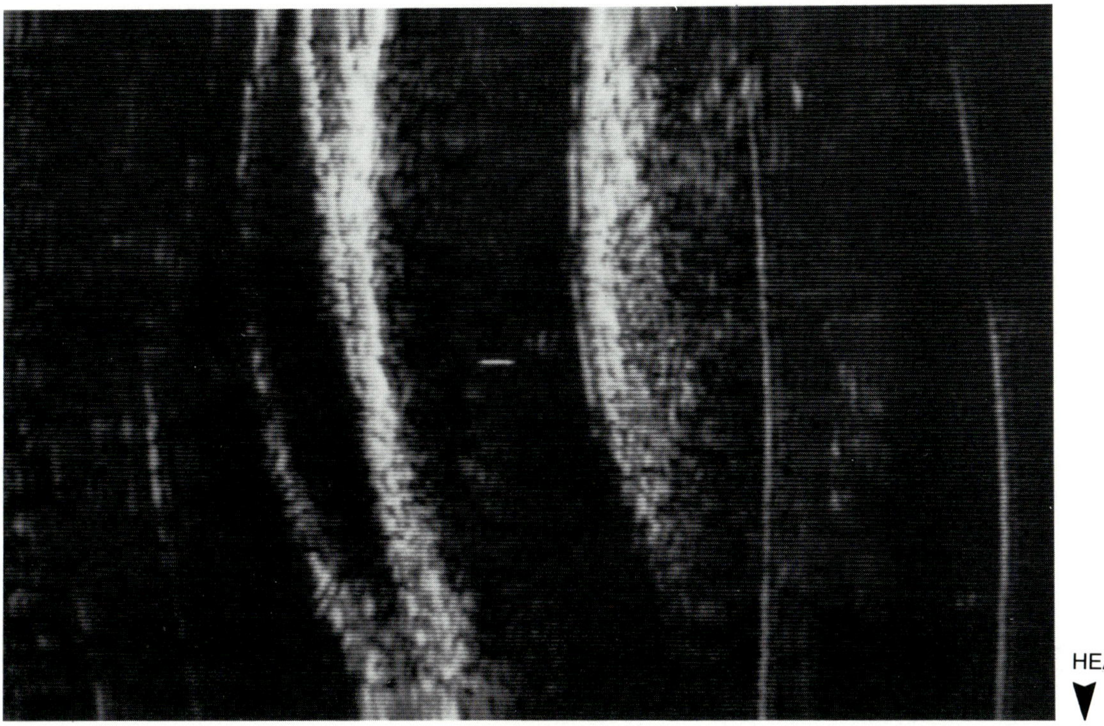
HEAD

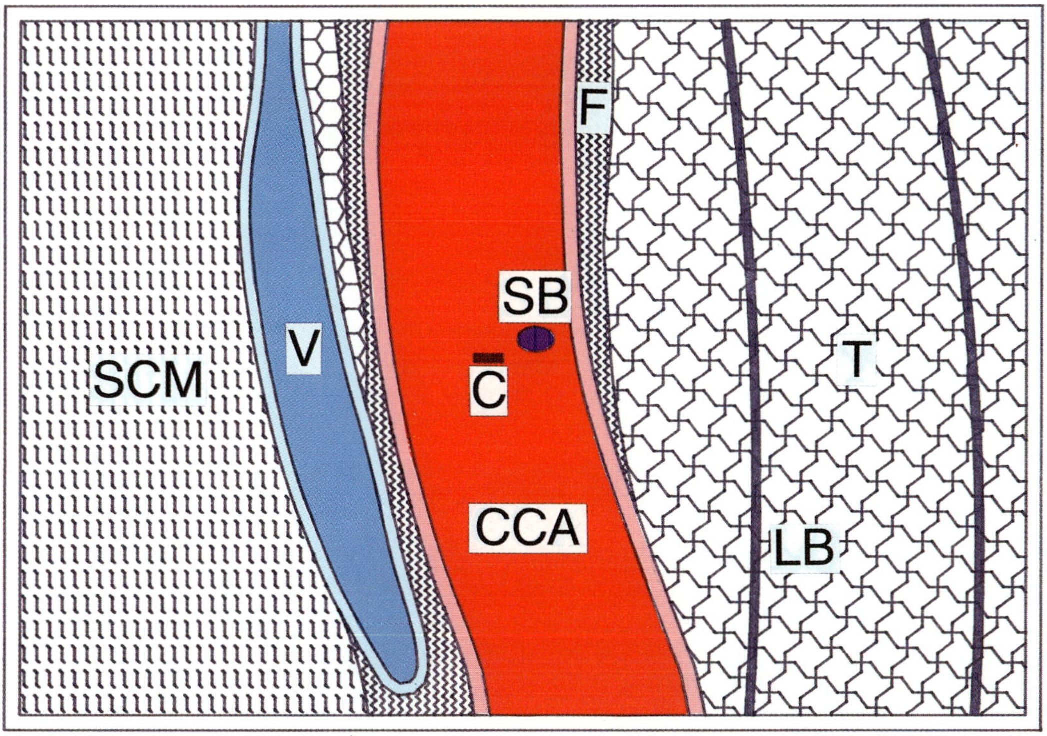
F
SB
V
C
SCM
T
CCA
LB

Figure 153. VARIOUS ARTIFACTS

This is a transverse view of a normal right carotid bifurcation, showing extensive large bubble artifact (LB). The degree of bubble artifact is related to the size and number of bubbles and also to the velocity of convection currents within the water. It is recommended that the probes not be shaken or jarred in order to avoid detachment of bubbles from the headblock into more central areas. This artifact was intentionally produced by just such a maneuver. The fascia-like zones of bright echoes in the near field (to the left) are produced by reverberation artifact (RV). In addition, a zone of artifact that we have termed "near-field artifact" (NFA) is seen as a horn-shaped zone of brightening within the sternocleidomastoid muscle (SCM). This scan has been taken in far-field focus. We believe this NFA is produced by increased ultrasound beam strength along the midline of the beam because of focusing effects. NFA is seen as an artifactually increased brightness across the middle of the near fields with less illumination of the tissues above and below. The artifact is faint and is totally obscured by the brightness of the superficial tissue layers unless they are very dark. IJV = internal jugular vein, ECA = external carotid artery, ICA = internal carotid artery, F = fascia, SQ = subcutaneous tissues (including thyroid gland where the letters SQ are located).

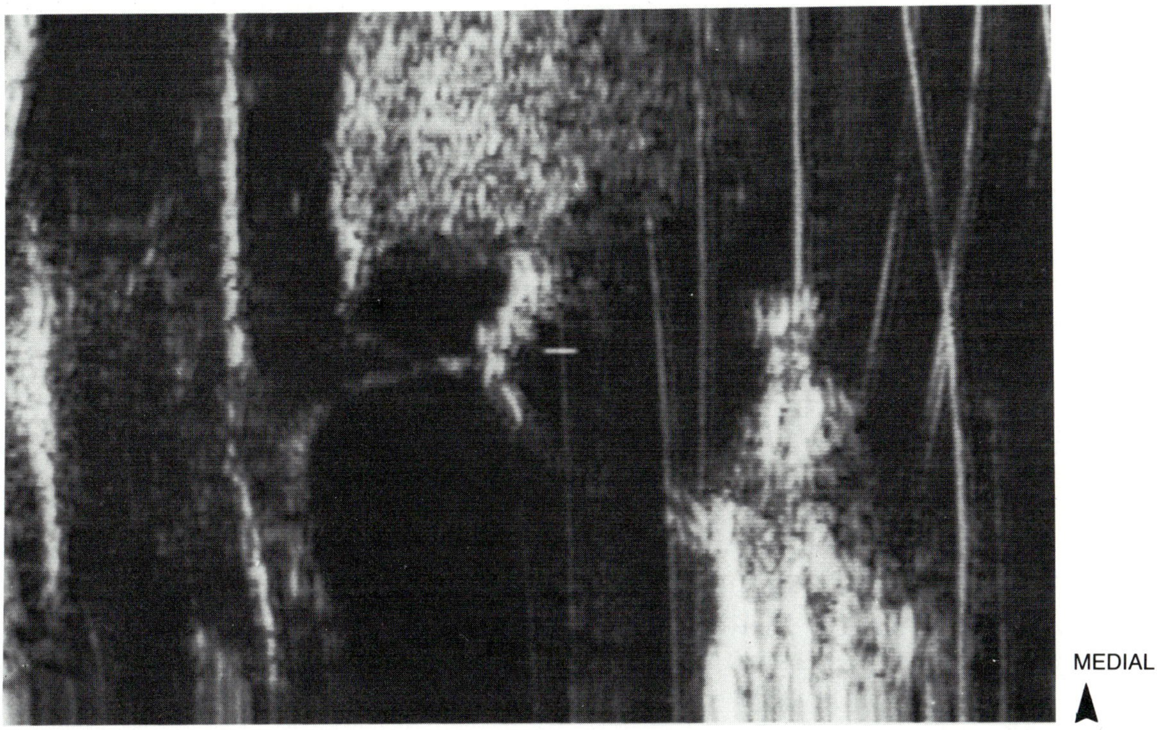
MEDIAL

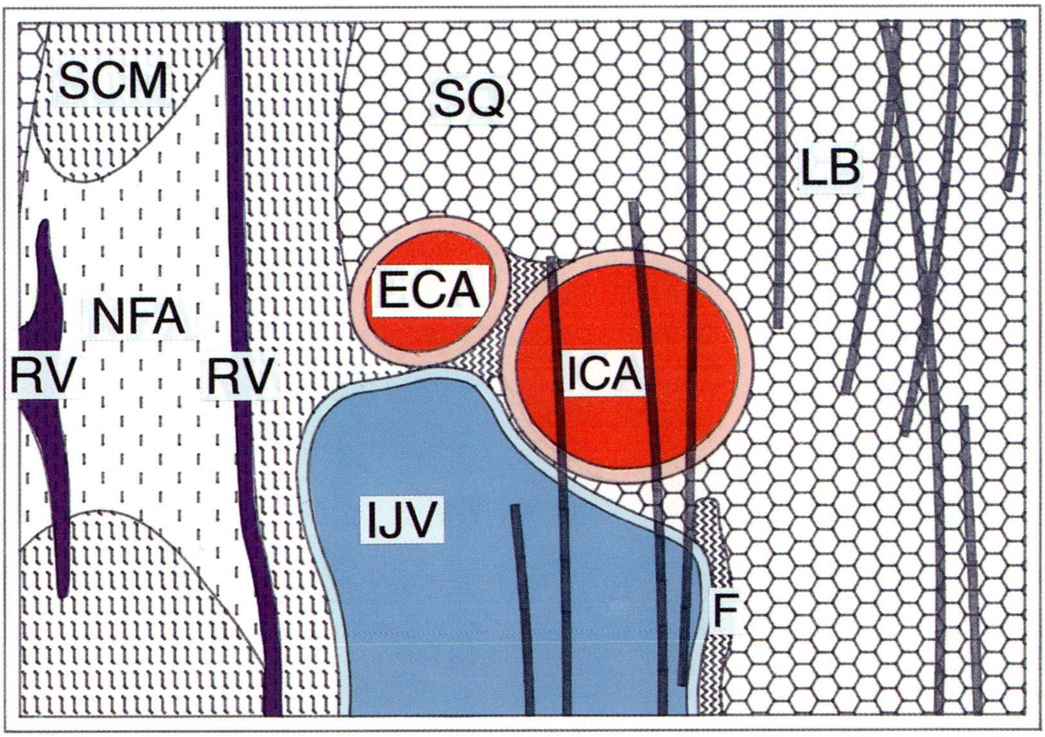
SCM
SQ
LB
ECA
NFA
RV
RV
ICA
IJV
F

Figure 154. VARIOUS ARTIFACTS

As the probe is moved down the neck to the upper common carotid artery (A) seen here in transverse view, one notices lessening of the large bubble artifact (LB) as the water settles down. Fairly well seen in this transverse view are two small bubbles (SB). The reverberation artifact (RV) and near-field artifact (NFA) remain quite prominent within the sternocleidomastoid muscle (SCM). SQ = subcutaneous tissue, IJV = internal jugular vein, FV = facial vein, F = fascia, C = Doppler cursor.

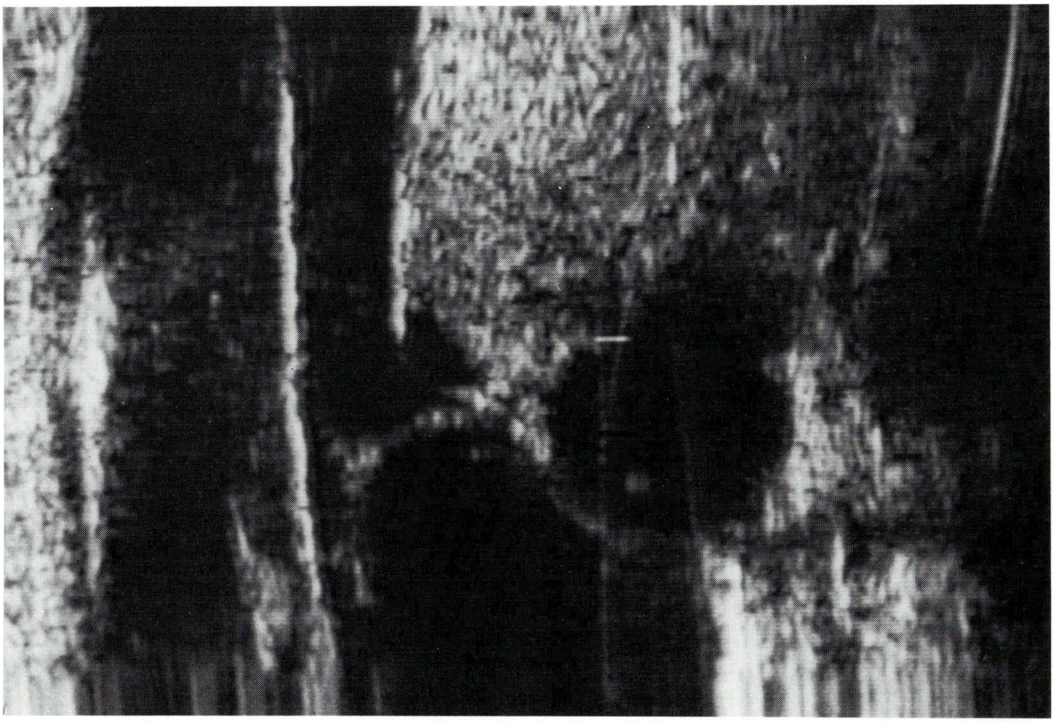
MEDIAL

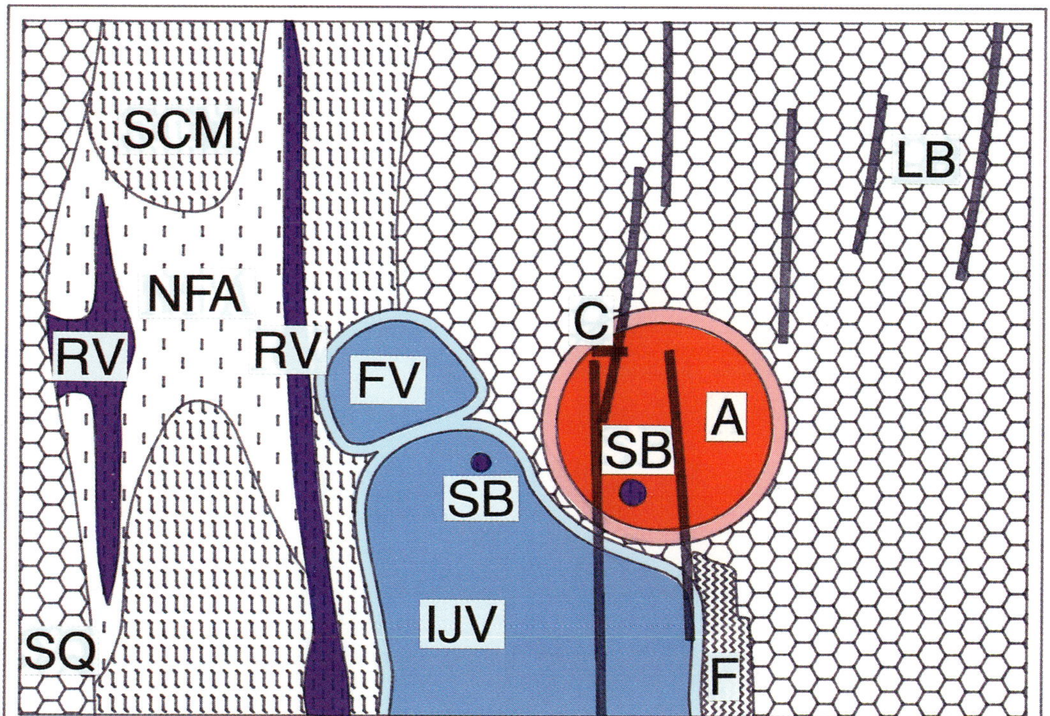
SCM
LB
NFA
C
RV
RV
FV
A
SB
SB
IJV
SQ
F

Figure 155. VARIOUS ARTIFACTS

Holding the probe motionless, one can again observe movement of the small bubble (SB) and large bubble (LB) artifacts. The reverberation artifact (RV) from the superficial tissues and near-field artifact (NFA) persist. Note the crisscross appearance of large bubble artifact within the center of the common carotid artery (CCA). Large bubble artifact that has a stationary location usually associated with a crisscross pattern of arcs is due to a bubble adherent to the oscillating mirror. SCM = sternocleidomastoid muscle, SQ = subcutaneous tissues (including thyroid gland), FV = facial vein, IJV = internal jugular vein, C = Doppler cursor, F = fascia.

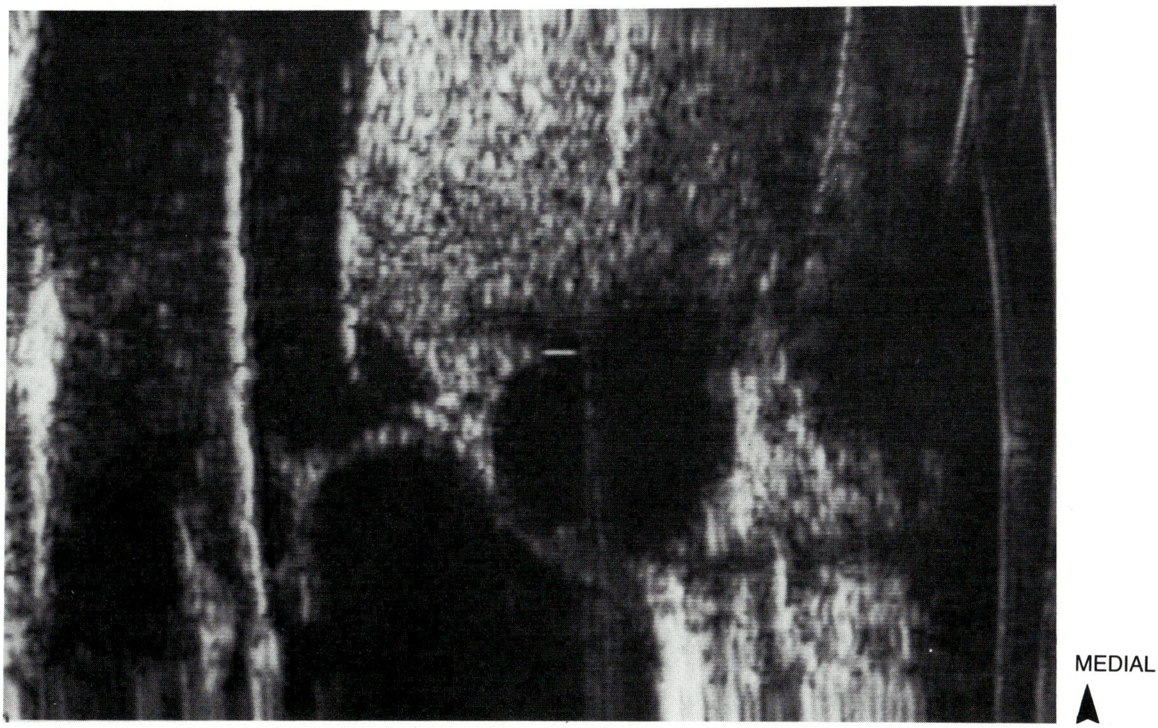
MEDIAL

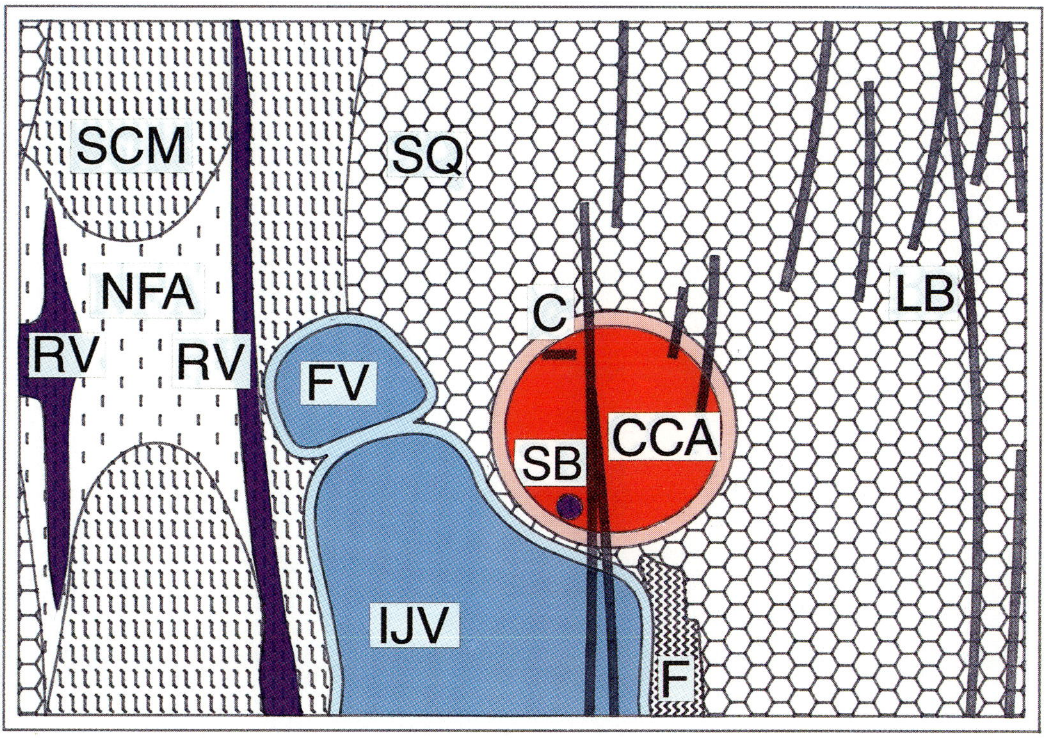
SCM
SQ
NFA
RV
RV
FV
C
CCA
SB
IJV
F
LB

Figure 156. VARIOUS ARTIFACTS

This scan has been prepared so that the subcutaneous tissues superficial to the sternocleidomastoid muscle (SCM) are no longer apparent. The near-field artifact (NFA) and tissue reverberation artifact (RV) persist. Actually, there is a second RV extending into the top of the facial vein (FV), which is not drawn on the diagram. There are two small bubble artifacts (SB) visible within the internal jugular vein (IJV) and the common carotid artery (CCA), which are more faint than the previous example (see Figure 155). C = Doppler cursor, F = fascia, LB = large bubble artifact.

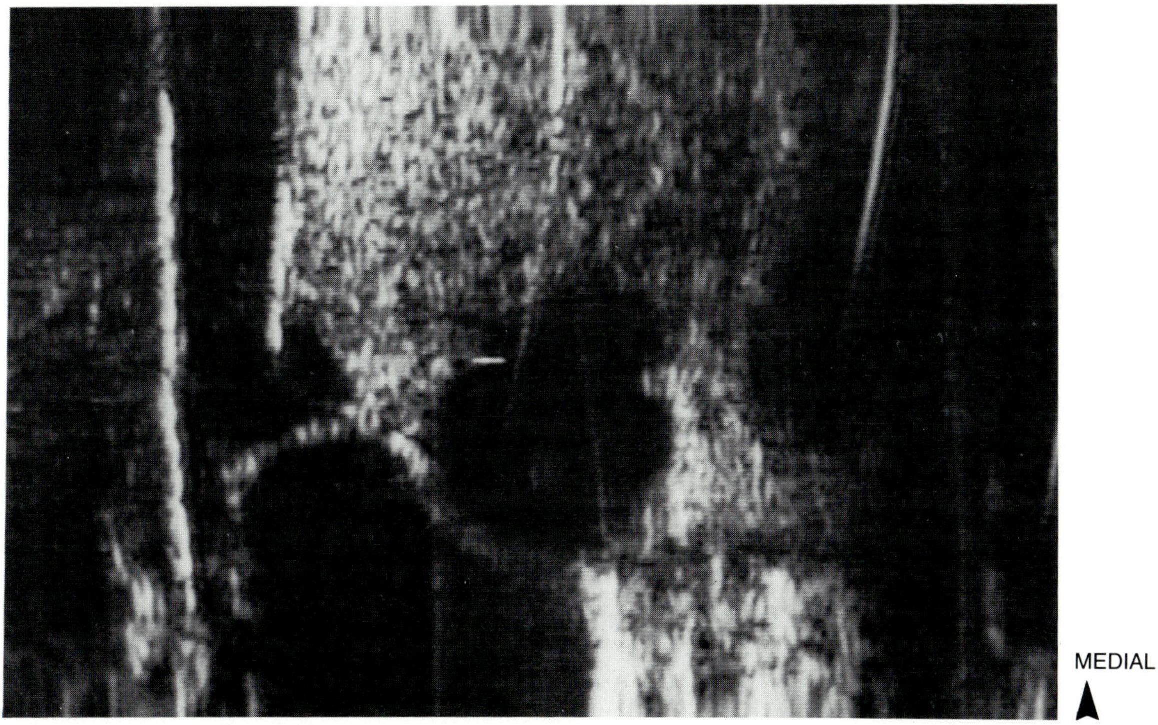
MEDIAL

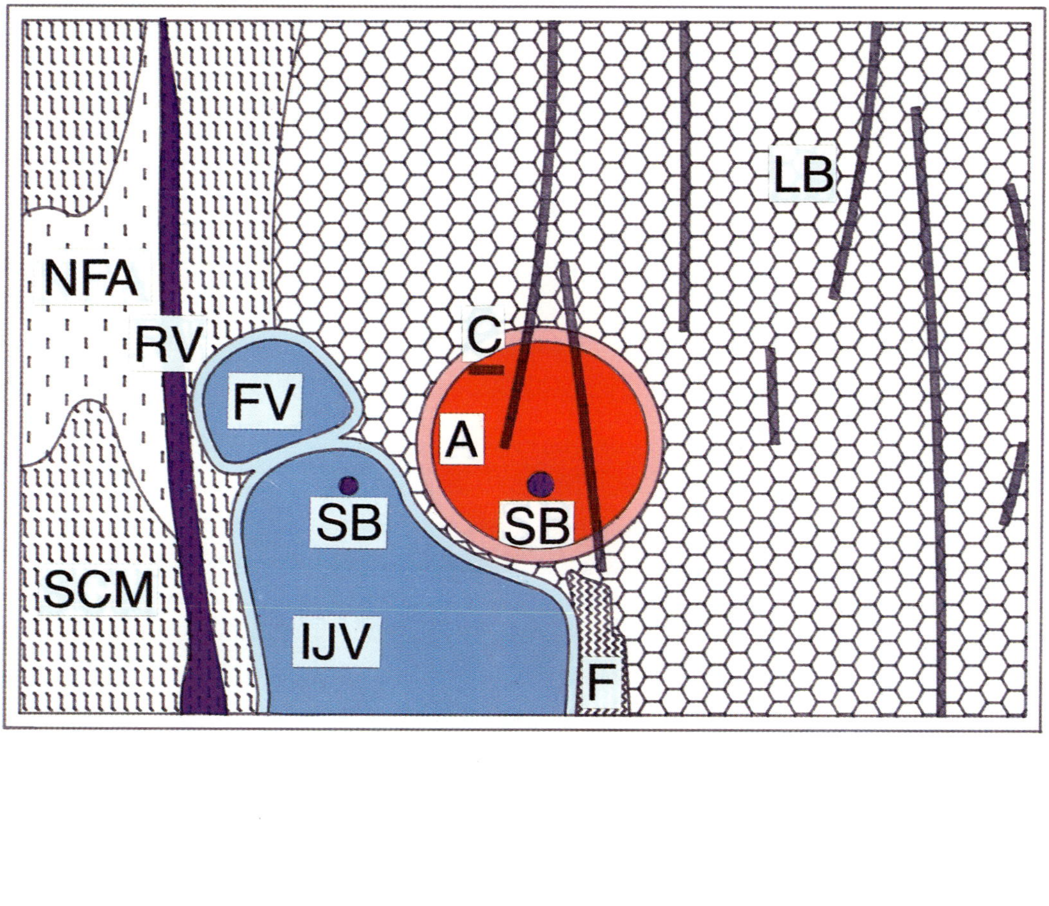
NFA
RV
FV
SB
SCM
IJV
C
A
SB
F
LB

Figure 157. VARIOUS ARTIFACTS

Two other types of artifact are illustrated in this example. The first is "hard-line" artifact (HL) that appears as a stationary group of vertical linear bands located three quarters of the distance from the left edge to the right edge of the screen. This HL is thought to be due to internal echoing of stray ultrasound beams emanating from the transducer and missing the mirror. The second artifact is seen as a constellation of semicircular arcs in the far field, which we term mirror artifact (MA). This artifact is present even when no contact with tissue is made. The artifact has a very slight flutter in real time and is thought to be due to material adherent to the surface of the mirror, such as bubbles, dirt, or algae. M = sternocleidomastoid muscle, F = fascia, V = internal jugular vein, CCA = common carotid artery (with an elliptical shape because the view is not perfectly transverse).

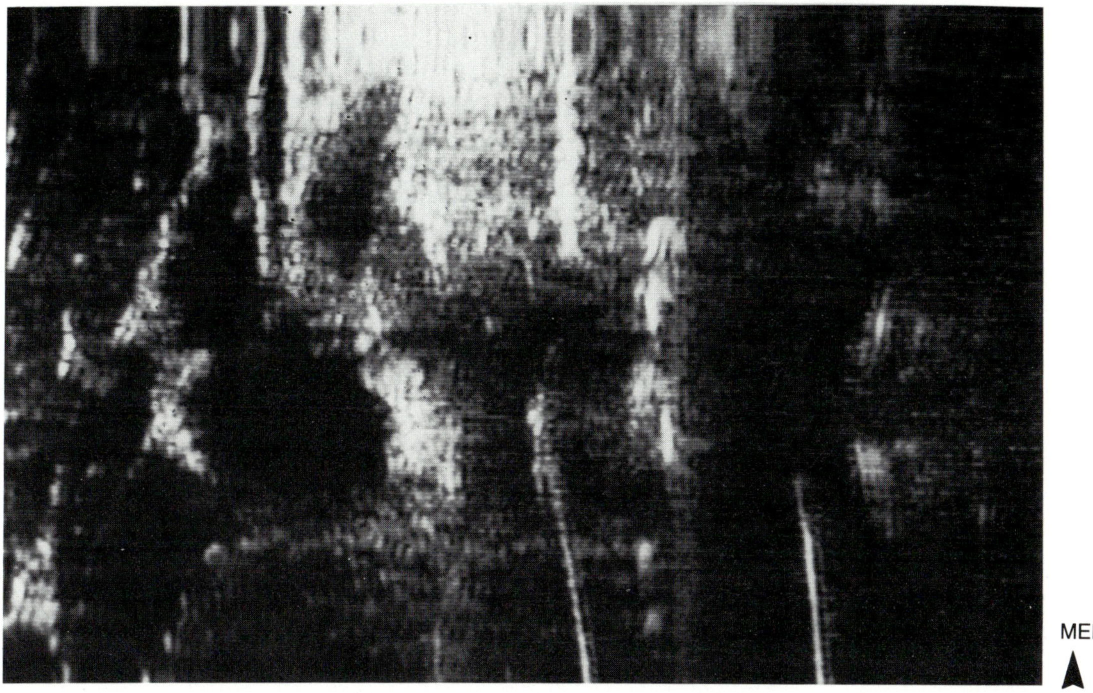
MEDIAL

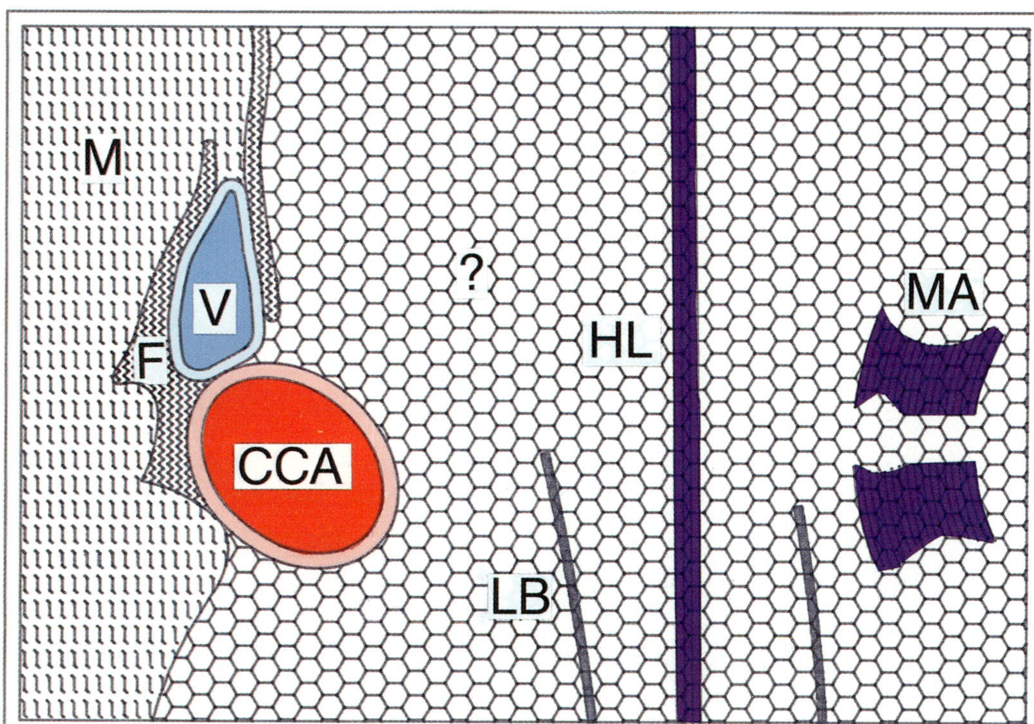
M
V
F
CCA
?
HL
LB
MA

Figure 158. "HARD-LINE" ARTIFACT

This is a prominent example of "hard-line" artifact (HL). This artifact is more prominent when the 8 MHz probe is adjusted to mid field focus. HL usually dramatically improves or disappears when the probe is switched to far-field focus. The brightness of this artifact varies from probe to probe. This manufacturer is working on a sound-absorbing insert that will line the inside of the headblock in hope of eliminating this artifact. Overall, this scan has a very blotchy, high contrast appearance with loss of gray scale and fine detail that is an artifact of the photographic settings and was not present in the original. The settings, however, did bring out the thrombus (T) present within this native aneurysm (AN) of this right common carotid artery (CCA) at the bifurcation. Compare this illustration with the other illustrations of this patient shown in Figures 134 and 135. SQ = subcutaneous tissue, SCM = sternocleidomastoid muscle, F = fascia, IJV = internal jugular vein, P = plaque, ICA = internal carotid artery, ? = tissues of uncertain composition.

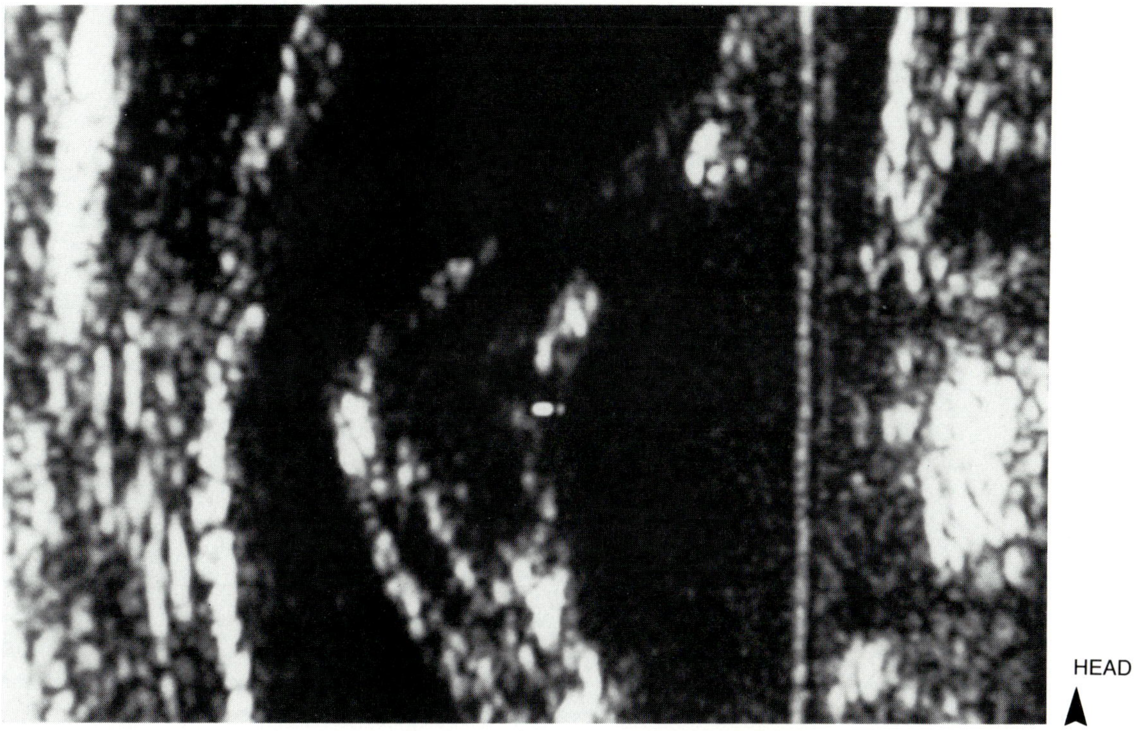
HEAD

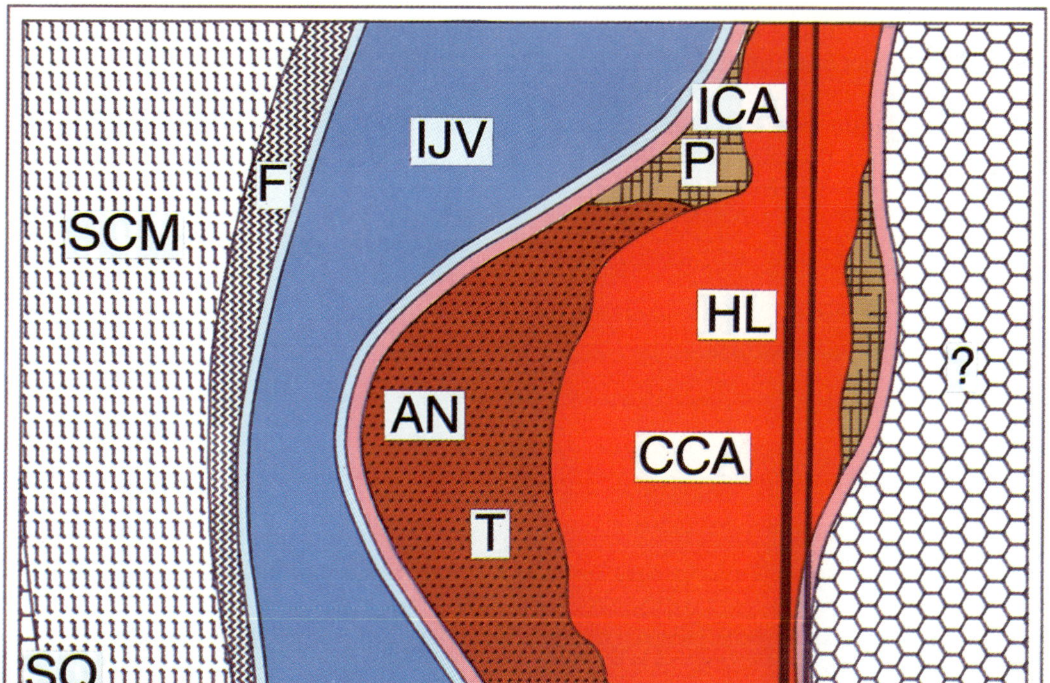
IJV
ICA
P
F
SCM
HL
?
AN
CCA
T
SQ

Figure 159. REVERBERATION ARTIFACT

This is a particularly good example of a type of reverberation artifact we call tissue artifact. It is thought to be caused by reflection of a particularly strong echo returning from the tissue. The sonic ping that is reflected from the bright tissue boundary does not make it all the way back into the probe. The ping is re-reflected off the probe face or a more superficial tissue layer, travels back out to strike the deeper tissue boundary a second time, and is reflected back once more before it finally makes a complete path back to the transducer. This results in an M-shaped path of the original ping with respect to time before part of the original echo is received. The resulting time delay caused by the extra path length of the rebounding echo causes the ultrasound circuitry to display a weaker "ghost" in the deep field.

In this case, the "ghost" of the original fascial boundary (F), which is particularly bright within Circle 1, is seen at a deeper distance from the transducer and appears as artifact (AF) within Circle 2. The artifact caused by this double echo is slightly expanded from the original echo (F) because of diffusion of the ultrasound beam. Artifact can be distinguished from plaque by the fact that as one bears down on the probe and causes foreshortening of the superficial layers by compression against the probe (small arrow), one sees this artifact move toward and away from the probe at an accelerated speed (large arrow) in concert with the superficial tissues. It thus appears to be moving back and forth within the vessel rather than attached to a wall of an artery, which in this case is the common carotid artery (CCA). The relative speed as well as the relative size of the "ghost" is proportional to the ratio between the distances of the "ghost" and original echoes from the transducer crystal. Note the similarity in appearance between the artifact and the superficial fascia. Relative motion of echogenic "tissue" within an artery is an extremely important criterion in distinguishing the presence of true plaque from re-echoing of overlying tissue. Also note the small thyroid cyst (C) within the gland. M = sternocleidomastoid muscle, SQ = subcutaneous tissue, V = internal jugular vein.

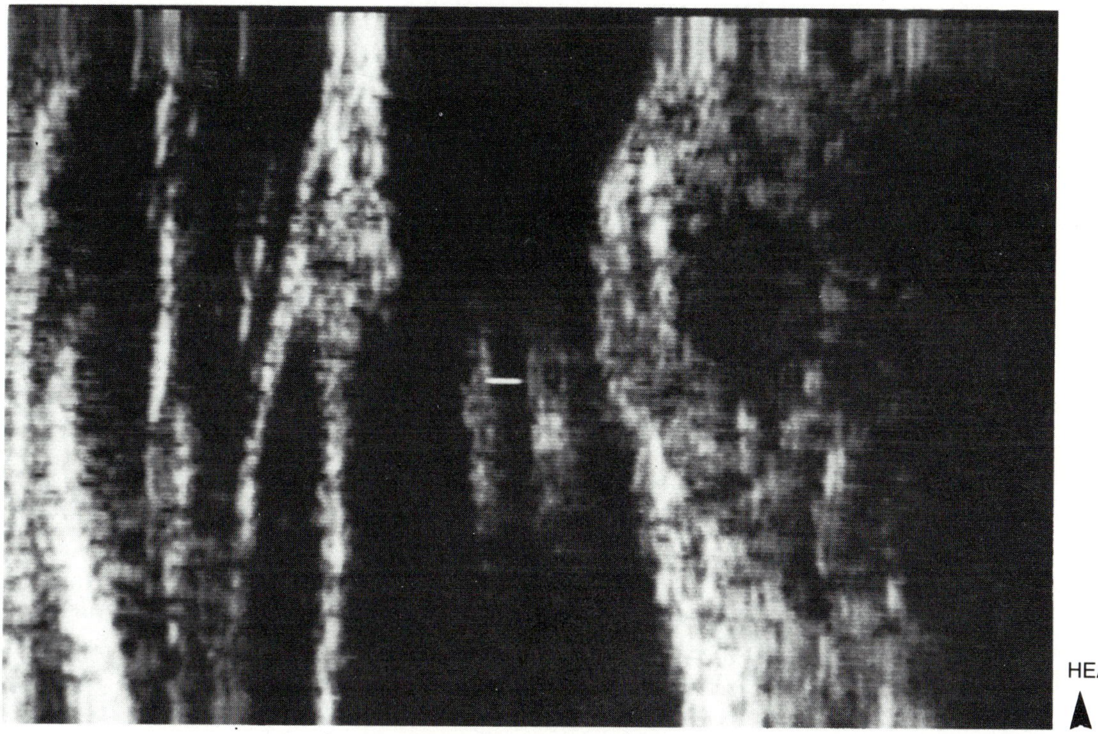
HEAD

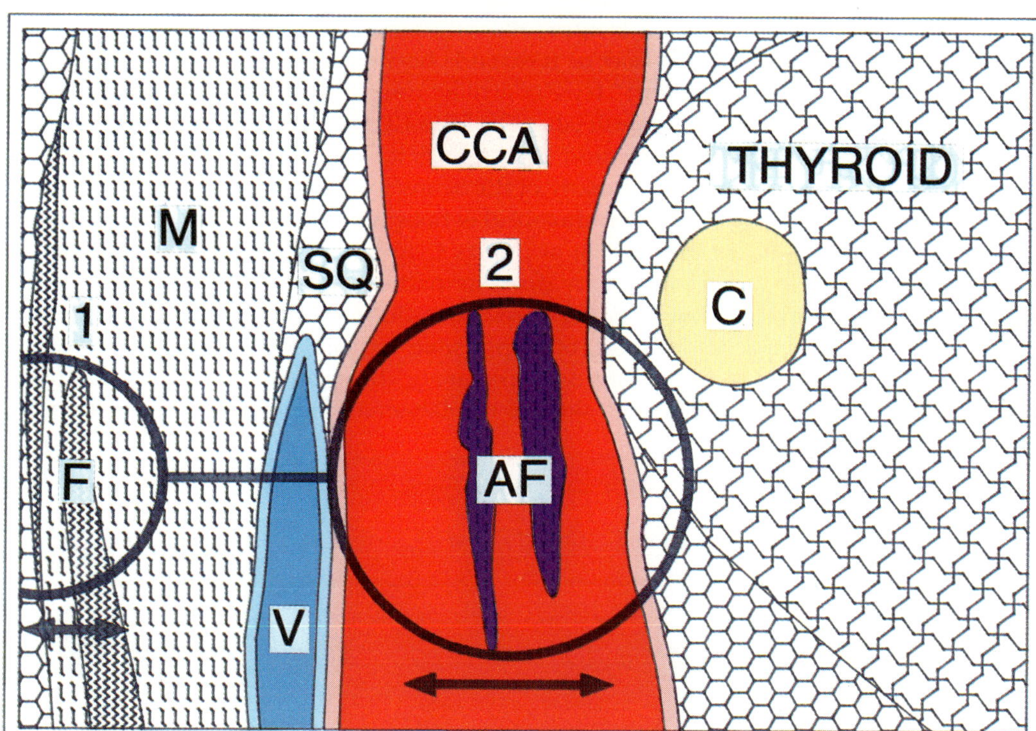
CCA
THYROID
M
SQ
2
1
C
F
AF
V

Figure 160. INTRA-ARTERIAL ARTIFACT

This and the following scan of a right common carotid artery (CCA) demonstrate the presence of tissue artifact (AF) within an otherwise normal CCA. The first criterion by which this artifact can be distinguished from plaque is the presence of a normal "intimal stripe" particularly along the deep wall of the artery that continues up through the middle of the apparent "plaque." The second criterion indicating that this is artifact and not plaque is the lack of a discrete boundary along the inner surface of the artifact, particularly along the superficial wall of the artery. The lack of discrete echoes suggesting a well-defined surface should make one suspicious of the presence of artifact rather than plaque. Faint white vertical bars overlying the artery and internal jugular vein (IJV) to the left represent the 2-mm separations between lines of the gradicule on a machine used to measure arterial diameter.

In this case, the artifact is due to reverberation of the ultrasound beam alternately striking the highly reflective boundaries of the deep, then the superficial, then the deep walls of the IJV. The vein is surrounded by brightly echogenic fascia (F), consisting mostly of arterial adventitia along its deep wall. There is also a bright zone of subcutaneous tissue in front of the superficial wall of the IJV. This re-echoing of the ultrasound beam back to points A and B is perceived as coming from points A′ and B′, respectively, as the image is processed. The net effect is that the tissue artifact (AF) in front of the deep wall of the CCA is a mirror reflection of the superficial wall of the IJV as reflected from the intervening fascia (F). Note the corresponding concavity of the artifact that matches the concavity of the superficial wall of the IJV. Also note that the artifact at point A′ is much thicker than at B′ because it is apparent only against the dark background of the arterial lumen and is obscured, as it extends beyond the arterial "intimal stripe."

There is also a "fade-out" type of artifact (not drawn) behind the superficial walls of the IJV and the superficial wall of the CCA (C′ to D′). This "fade-out" or smearing effect extending behind the superficial wall of a vessel is a common artifact, as one will note from many of the scans in this atlas. This type of artifact is also due to reverberation of ultrasound echoes within the tissue. Possible paths for this echo to occur are shown at points C and D and perceived as artifact at points C′ and D′. There are many possible paths by which the beam can reverberate, including double and triple reverberations within the fascia (F). Many times it is not clear which path is responsible for this "fade-out." Nevertheless, it is important not to interpret this as plaque or thrombus behind the superficial walls of arteries and veins. S = skin, M = platysma muscle, SQ = subcutaneous tissue.

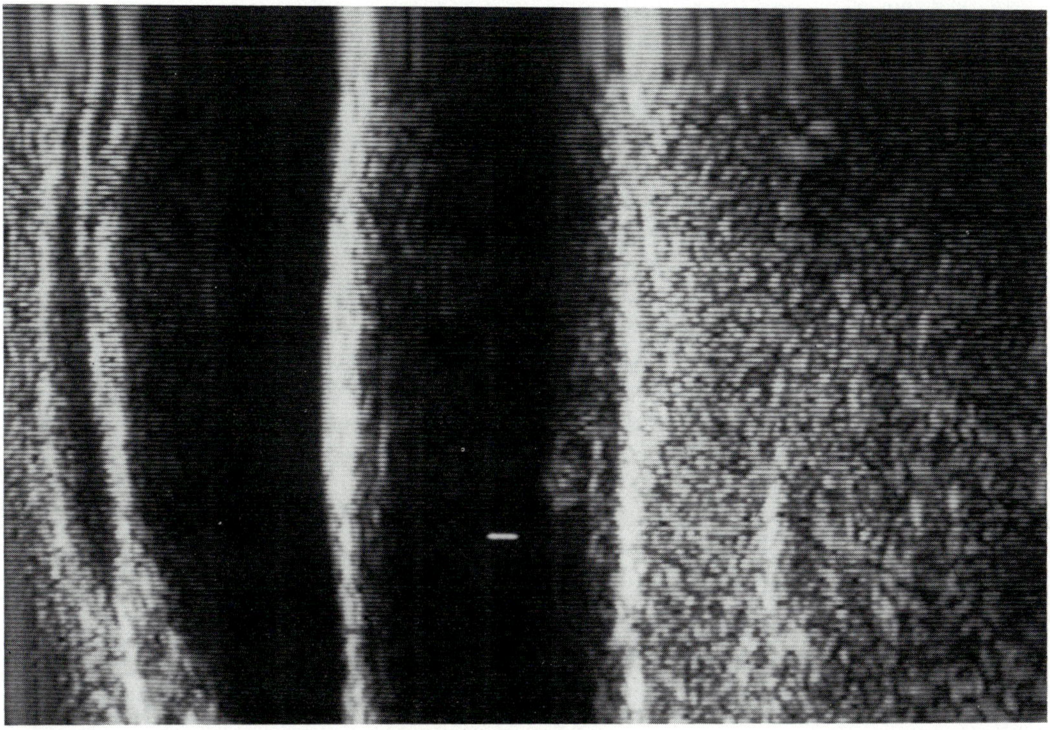

HEAD

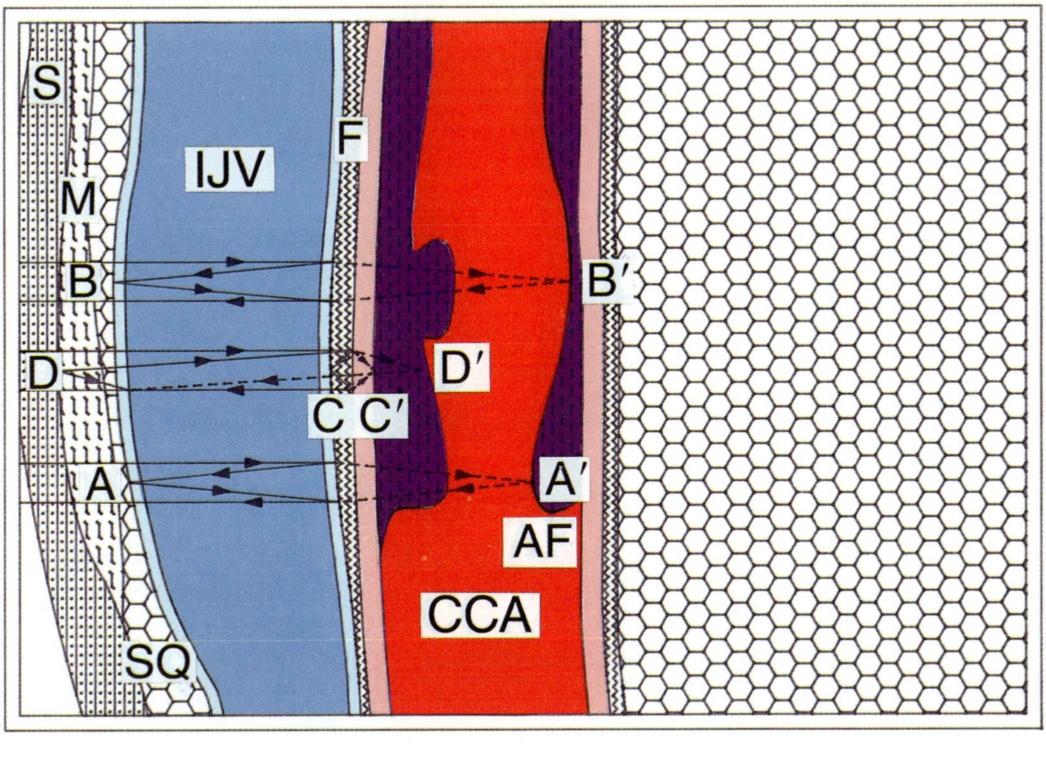

Figure 161. INTRA-ARTERIAL ARTIFACT

As the probe is held absolutely steady, one notes that this artifact (AF) disappears with each cardiac pulsation, resulting in greater prominence of the normal "intimal stripe." The common carotid artery (CCA) is much more normal in appearance in comparison with the previous scan, although some internal echoes within the artery remain. Note the movement of the AF in front of the deep arterial wall, which in comparison with the previous scan has moved out more into the center of the lumen. The cause of this movement is apparent, since with arterial systole there has been a simultaneous narrowing of the internal jugular vein (IJV). The AF, therefore, is moved correspondingly closer to its mirror image, which is the superficial wall of the internal jugular vein (IJV). Such tissue AF is usually and most easily distinguished by pressing with the probe to obtain a relative shift of the echogenic material in comparison with the arterial walls. At times, close observation of normal pulsation is all that is necessary to distinguish artifact from plaque. S = skin, M = platysma muscle, SQ = subcutaneous tissue, F = fascia (including arterial adventitia).

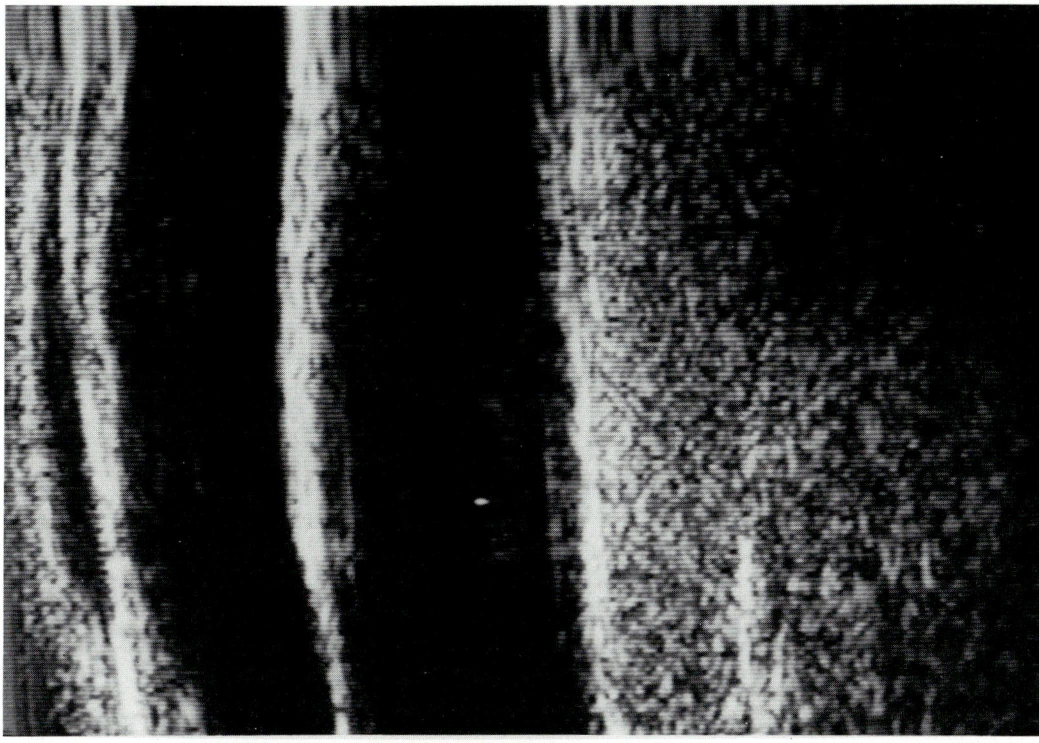

HEAD

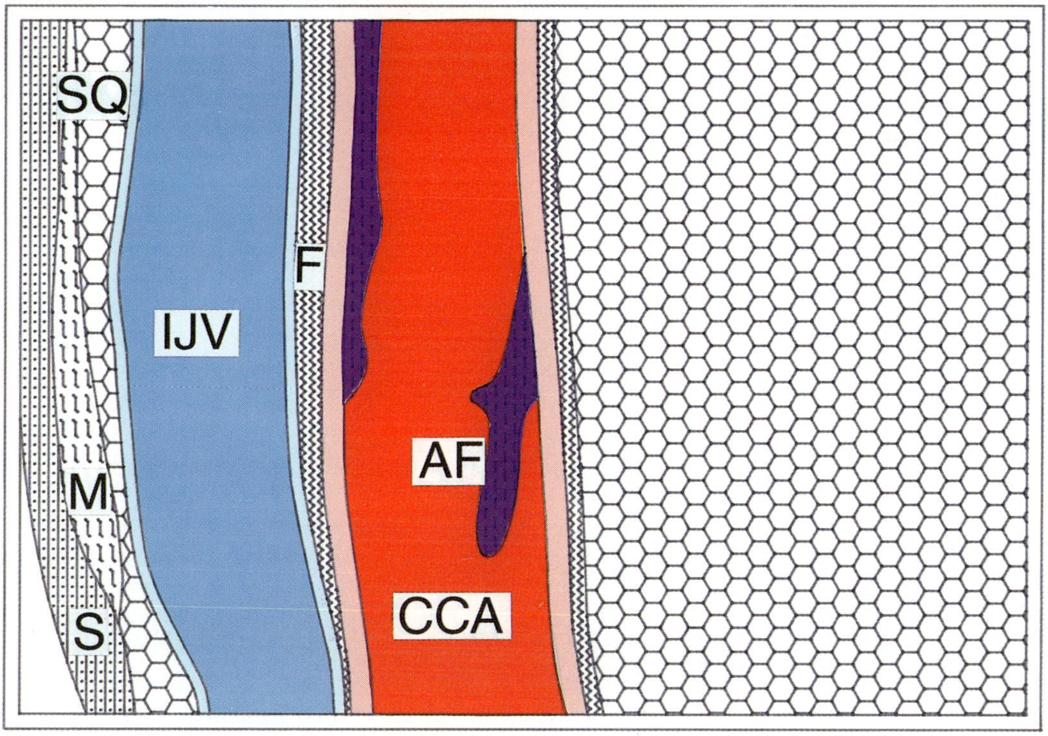

Figure 162. REVERBERATION ARTIFACT

Note the presence of moderately echogenic artifact (AF), particularly along the deep wall of this common carotid artery (CCA) but also in the center of the scan to a much fainter degree along the superficial wall. This AF can be distinguished from the plaque (P) behind it by six criteria. The first and most important is that it is not consistently the same in location relative to the artery as seen in real time (see Figures 46 and 163). The second criterion is that it fluctuates in intensity, depending upon the position of the overlying tissues as seen in multiple views and in relation to overall gain settings. The third criterion is that AF can be made to move across the artery by compression of the probe. The fourth criterion is that the borders of the AF tend to be fuzzy, fading into the background as opposed to the borders of the normal artery and plaque, which tend to have sharper contours. The appearance of the AF itself in many cases bears a resemblance to some layer of the overlying tissue or to a peculiar electronic or mechanical artifactual shape, which is easily recognized and is the fifth criterion. The sixth criterion is the extension of the echoes outside the borders of the artery. In this case, the AF is probably arising from reverberation between the bright band of fascia (F) superficial to the artery and the bright plane of subcutaneous tissue (SQ) superficial to the sternocleidomastoid muscle (M) in a manner similar to that shown in Figures 160 and 161. S = skin, AS = acoustic shadowing from the brightly echogenic plaque, ? = tissue of uncertain origin.

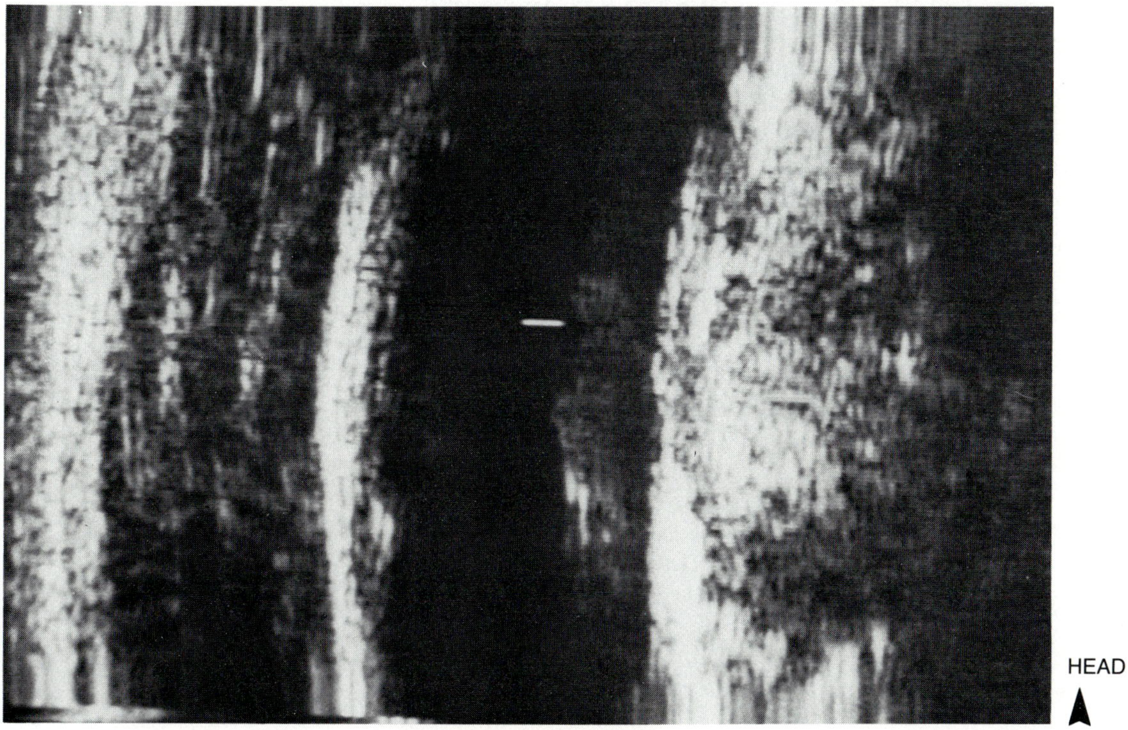
HEAD

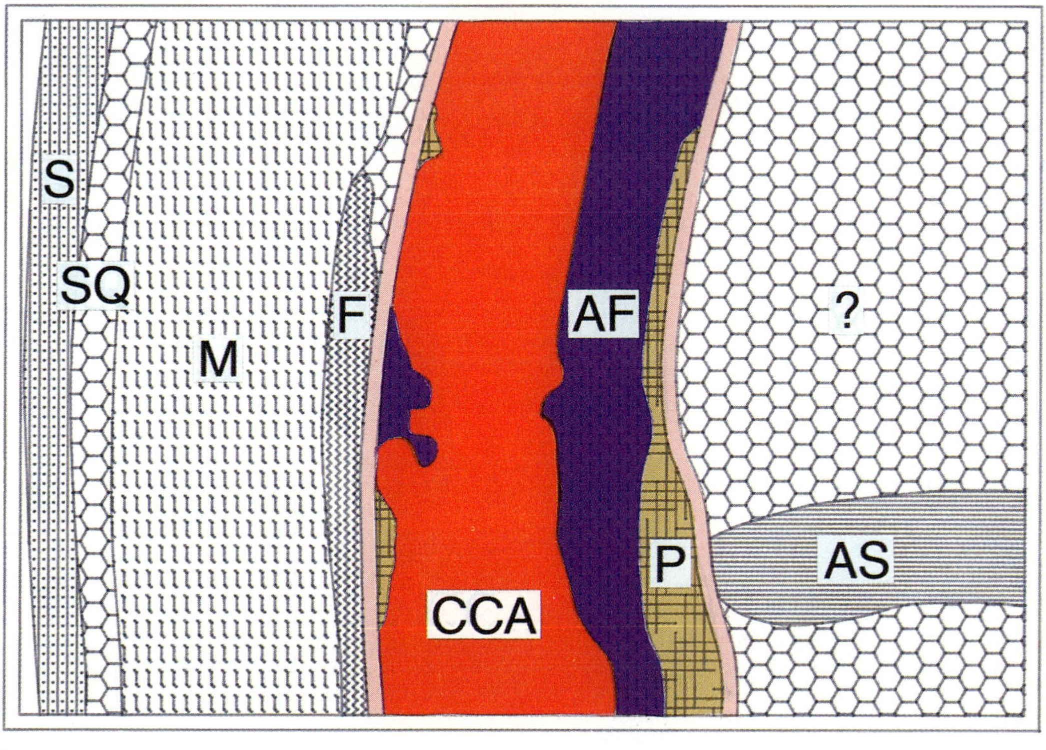
S
SQ
M
F
CCA
AF
P
?
AS

Figure 163. REVERBERATION ARTIFACT

Note the change in appearance of the same artifact (AF) as Figure 162 as the probe is held motionless over the common carotid artery (CCA). The AF is now faded generally; specifically, it is considerably less visible directly superficial to the brightest area of plaque (P) (on the left) associated with acoustic shadowing (AS). Note also the artifactual shape of the faint double lines in the small portion of AF next to the superficial wall. This parallel "railroad-track" shape is not caused by plaque. G = gel, S = skin, SQ = subcutaneous tissue (including platysma muscle), M = sternocleidomastoid muscle, F = fascia.

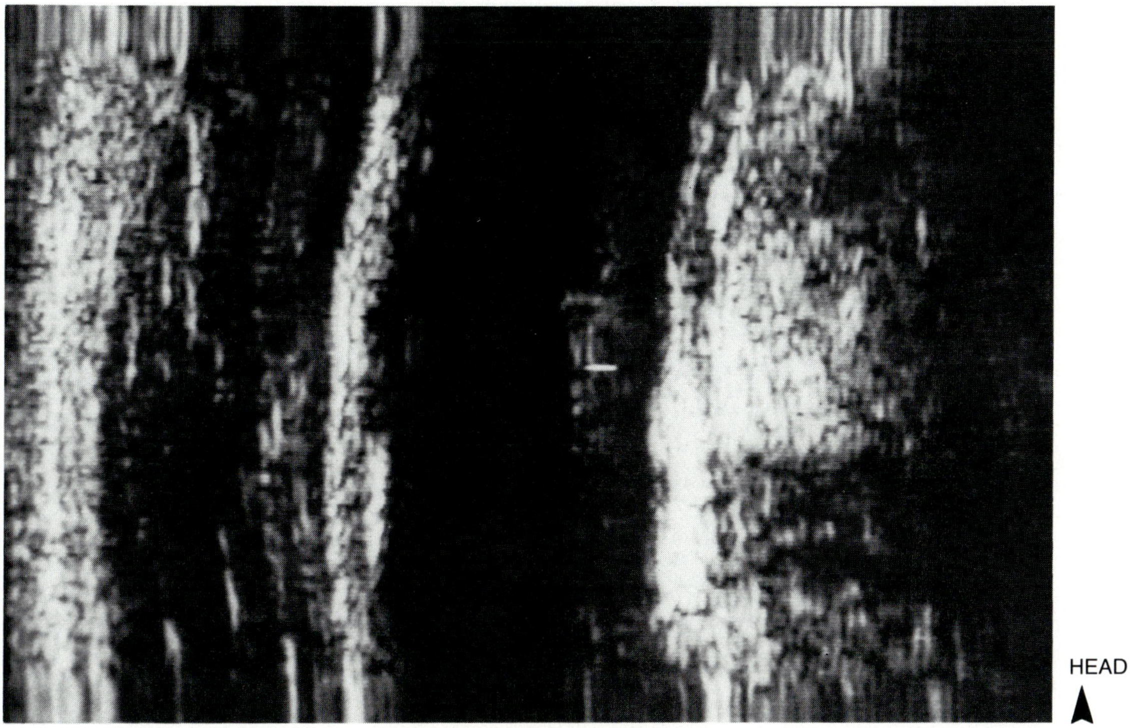
HEAD

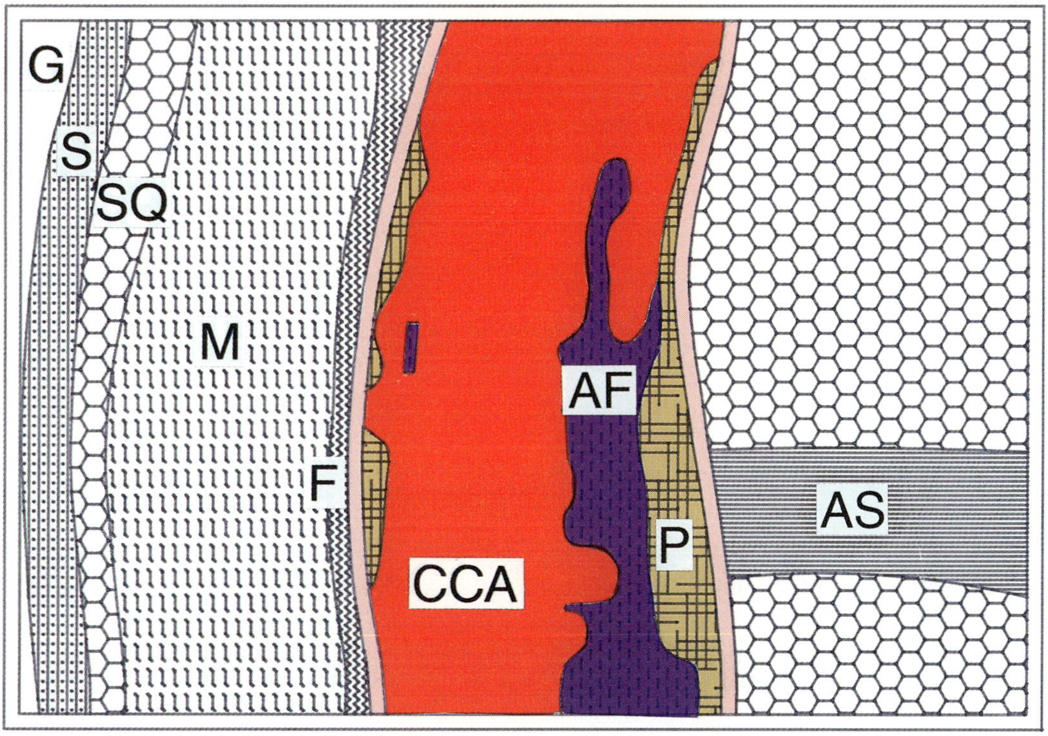
G
S
SQ
M
F
CCA
AF
P
AS

Figure 164. VARIABLE TISSUE ARTIFACT

This is an example of a left common carotid artery (CCA) showing tissue artifact as seen in transverse view. The artifact (AF) is of the same brightness as the plaque (P) on the superficial and deep walls of the artery and might even be thought to be a free-floating clot within the arterial lumen. S = skin, SQ = subcutaneous tissue, M = muscle, VN = vagus nerve, AS = acoustical shadowing, ? = tissue of uncertain composition.

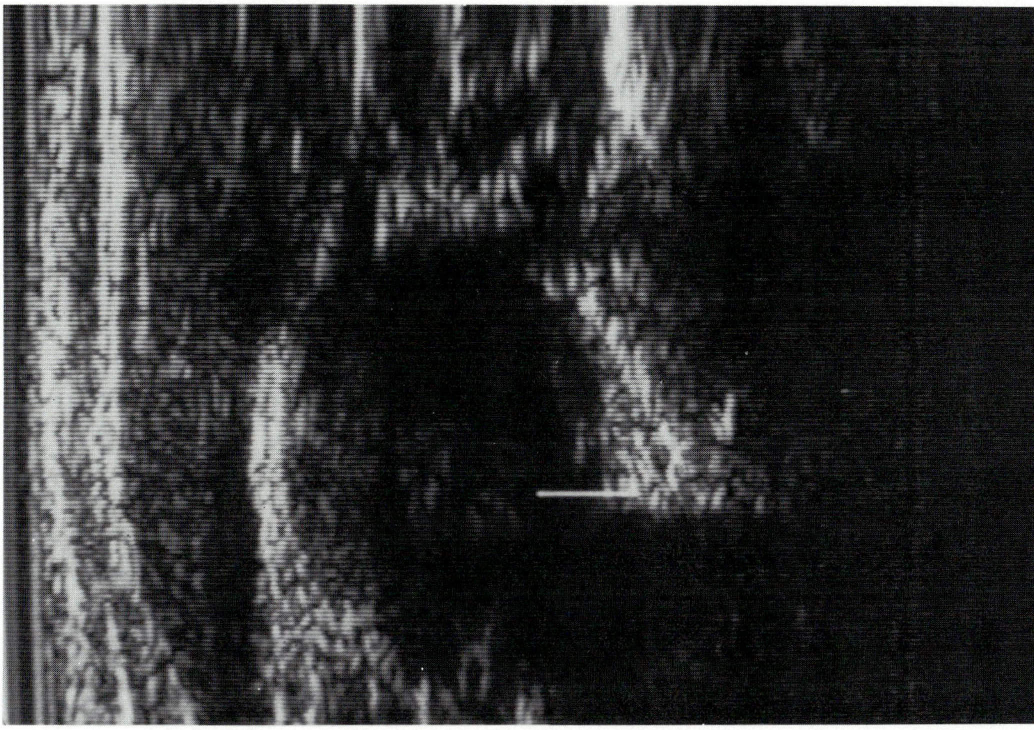

MEDIAL

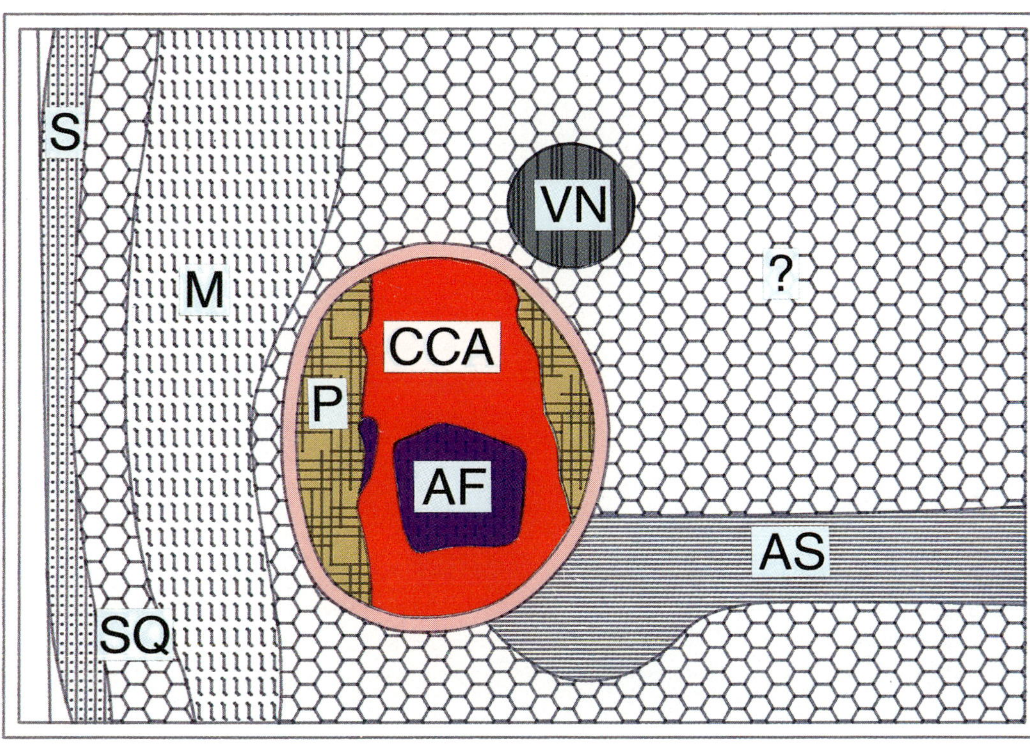

Figure 165. VARIABLE TISSUE ARTIFACT

As one keeps the artery under observation, this artifact (AF) both fades and changes position within the artery. The plaque (P), particularly along the superficial wall, becomes more distinct. S = skin, SQ = subcutaneous tissue, M = sternocleidomastoid muscle, VN = vagus nerve, CCA = common carotid artery, AS = acoustic shadowing (from the vessel wall), ? = tissue of uncertain composition.

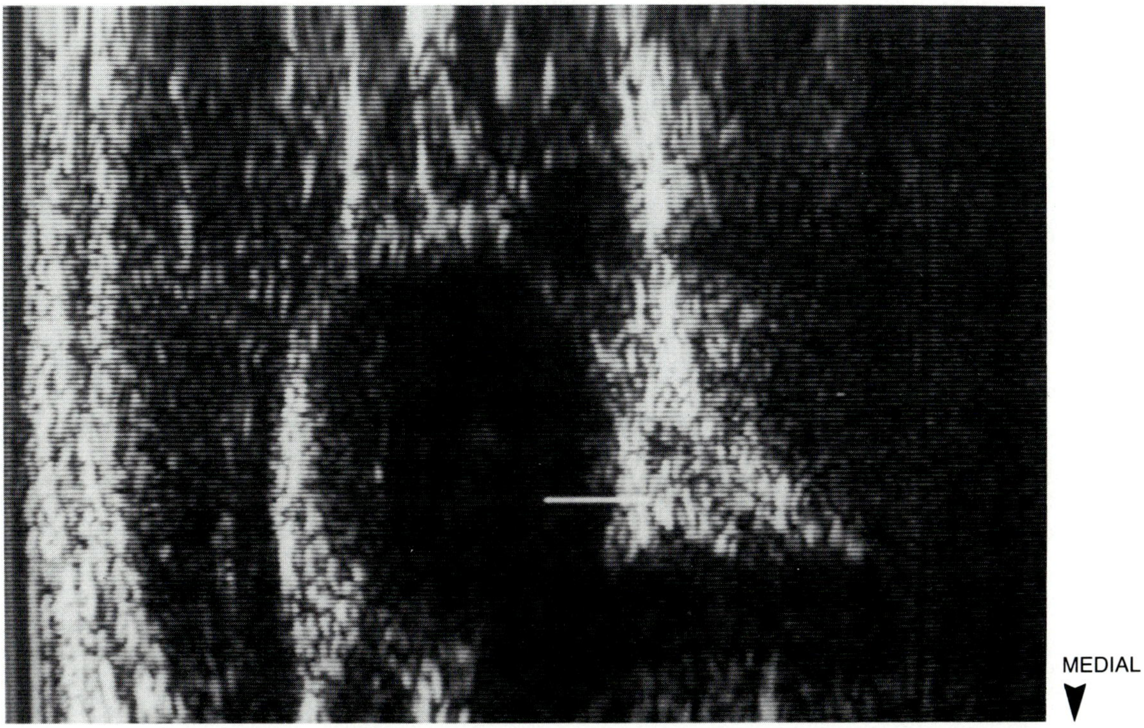
MEDIAL

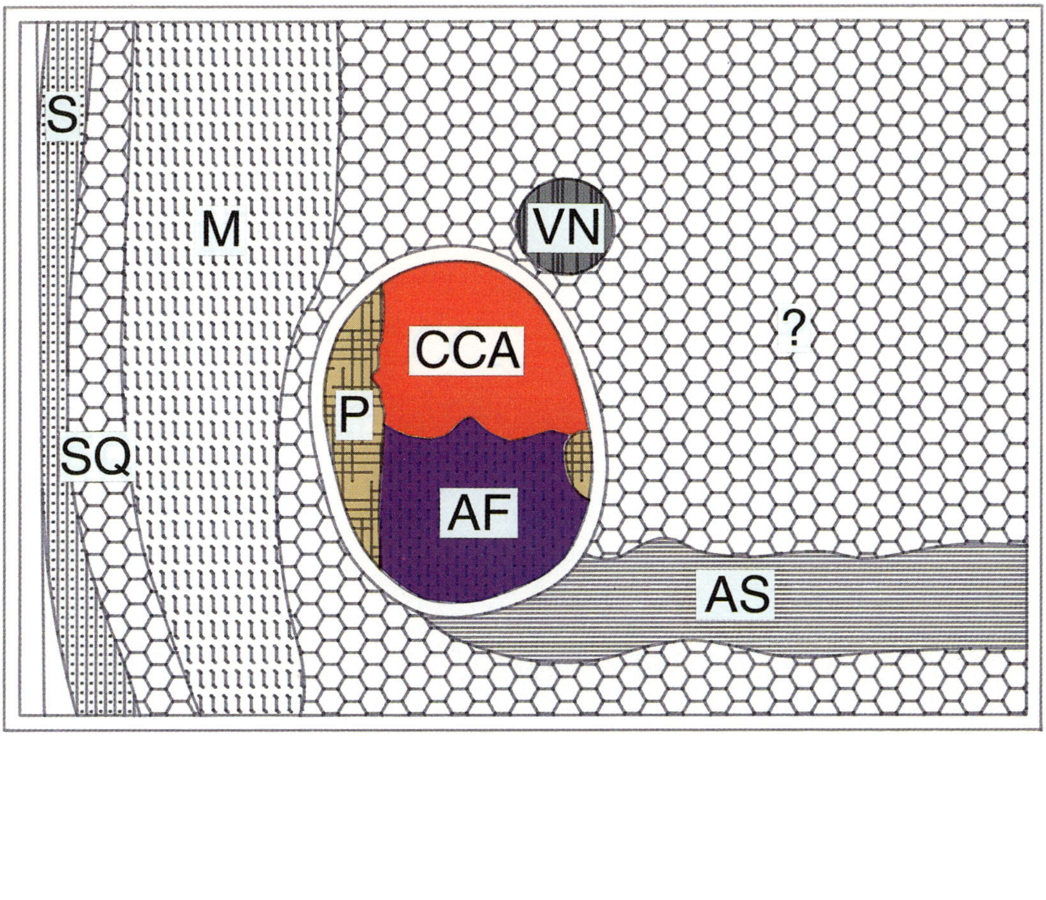
S
M
VN
?
CCA
P
SQ
AF
AS

Figure 166. REVERBERATION ARTIFACT

In this longitudinal view of the mid section of a left common carotid artery (CCA), one sees several linear echoes, owing to artifact (AF). This is another example of tissue AF caused by reverberation of the ultrasound beam within superficial tissue boundaries. The result is the production of virtual images of the superficial layers that appear as "ghosts" within the widely patent CCA that has no plaque. There is a relative shift of these echoes within the artery upon compression of the superficial tissues. In addition, the linear contours and peculiar "double-bar" shape are clues that the echoes are AF. "Double-bar" echoes, as seen here, are almost always produced by reverberation. S = skin, M = platysma muscle, F = fascia, SCM = sternocleidomastoid muscle, ? = tissue of uncertain composition.

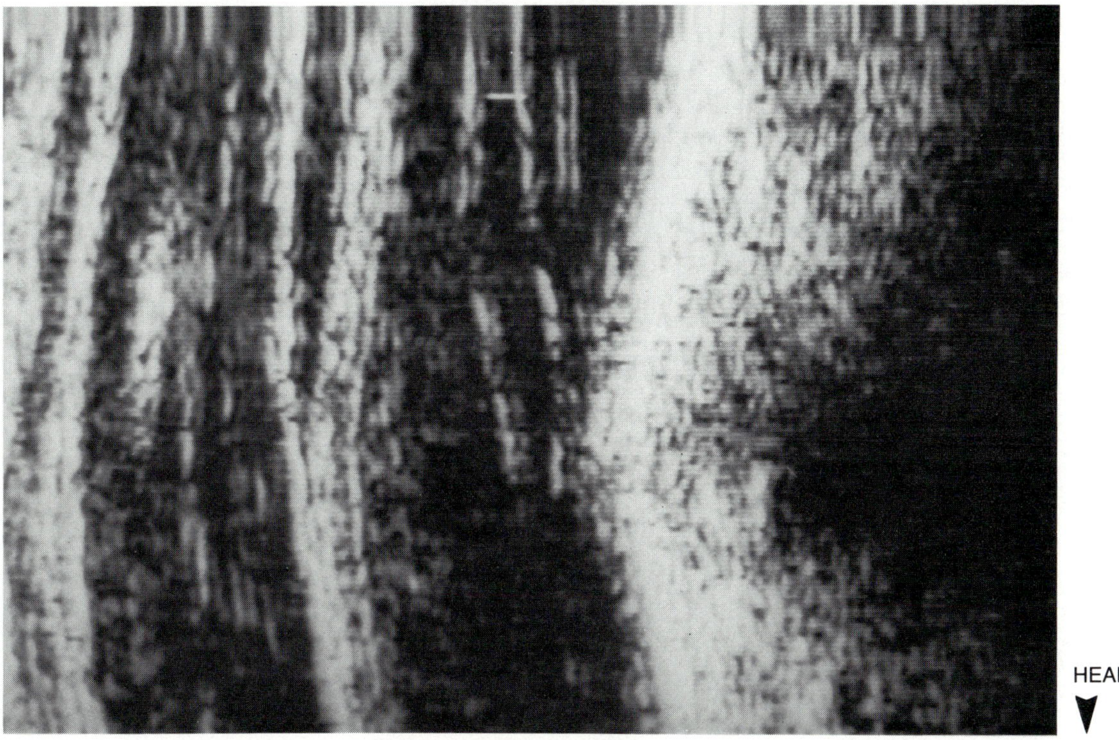
HEAD

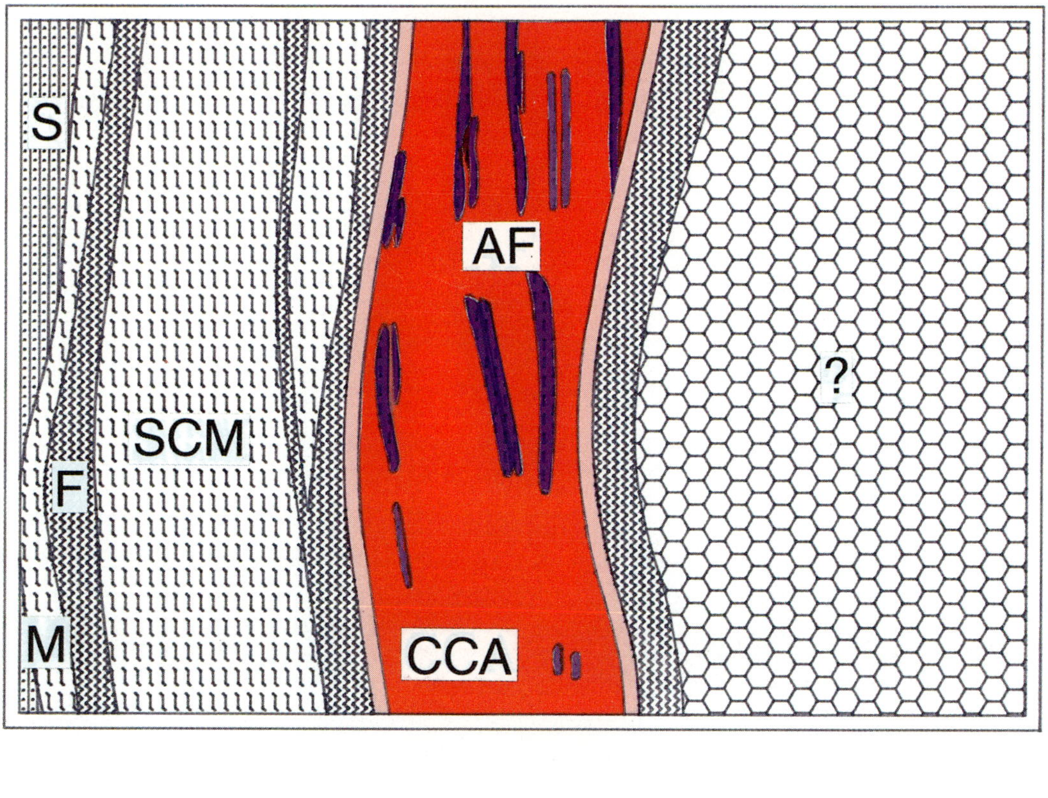
S
AF
?
SCM
F
M
CCA

APPENDIX

GOOD SAMARITAN HOSPITAL VASCULAR LABORATORY
CAROTID ULTRASOUND EXAMINATION

Patient ______________________ Date ______________
Age/Sex ______________________ Hospital # ______________
Physician ______________________ Room # ______________

Right	Resid. Lumen	% Stenosis
ICA		
ECA		
CCA		

Left	Resid. Lumen	% Stenosis
ICA		
ECA		
CCA		

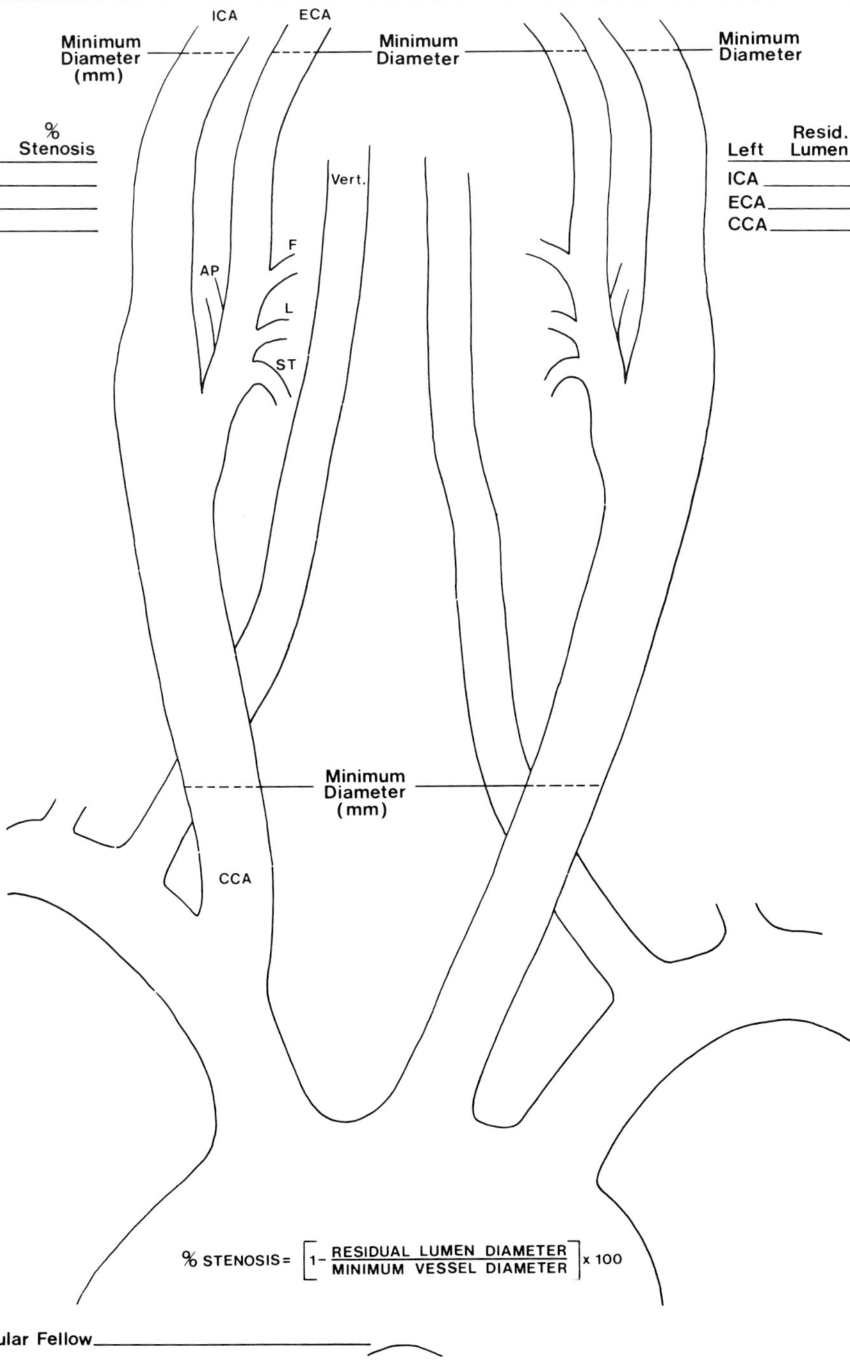

Peripheral Vascular Fellow ______________________

The first diagram is used for reporting the results of carotid ultrasound scans. Note the inclusion of the formula for the percent stenosis at the bottom of the page. Note also the blank columns and lines for inserting arterial and normal lumen diameters.

GOOD SAMARITAN HOSPITAL VASCULAR LABORATORY
CAROTID ULTRASOUND EXAMINATION

Patient M.W. **Date** 4/24/87
Age/Sex F/69 **Hospital #** 592919-5
Physician J. Cranley **Room #** 1215-2

Right	Resid. Lumen	% Stenosis
ICA	3.0	40%
ECA	1.5	50%
CCA	6.6	10%

The B-mode scan on the right is of good quality and reveals lightly echogenic, heterogeneous atherosclerotic plaque, which begins in the area of the common carotid artery and extends into the external and internal carotid arteries. There is a very unusual protuberance of the wall of the common carotid artery just prior to the internal carotid origin. This protuberance presses against the jugular vein and appears to be an aneurysm, which contains moderately echogenic, heterogeneous material consistent with thrombus within the aneurysm. There is no significant stenosis of the common carotid artery. There is 40% stenosis of the internal carotid artery and 50% stenosis of the external carotid artery. The plaque is highly irregular, but no distinct ulceration can be identified.

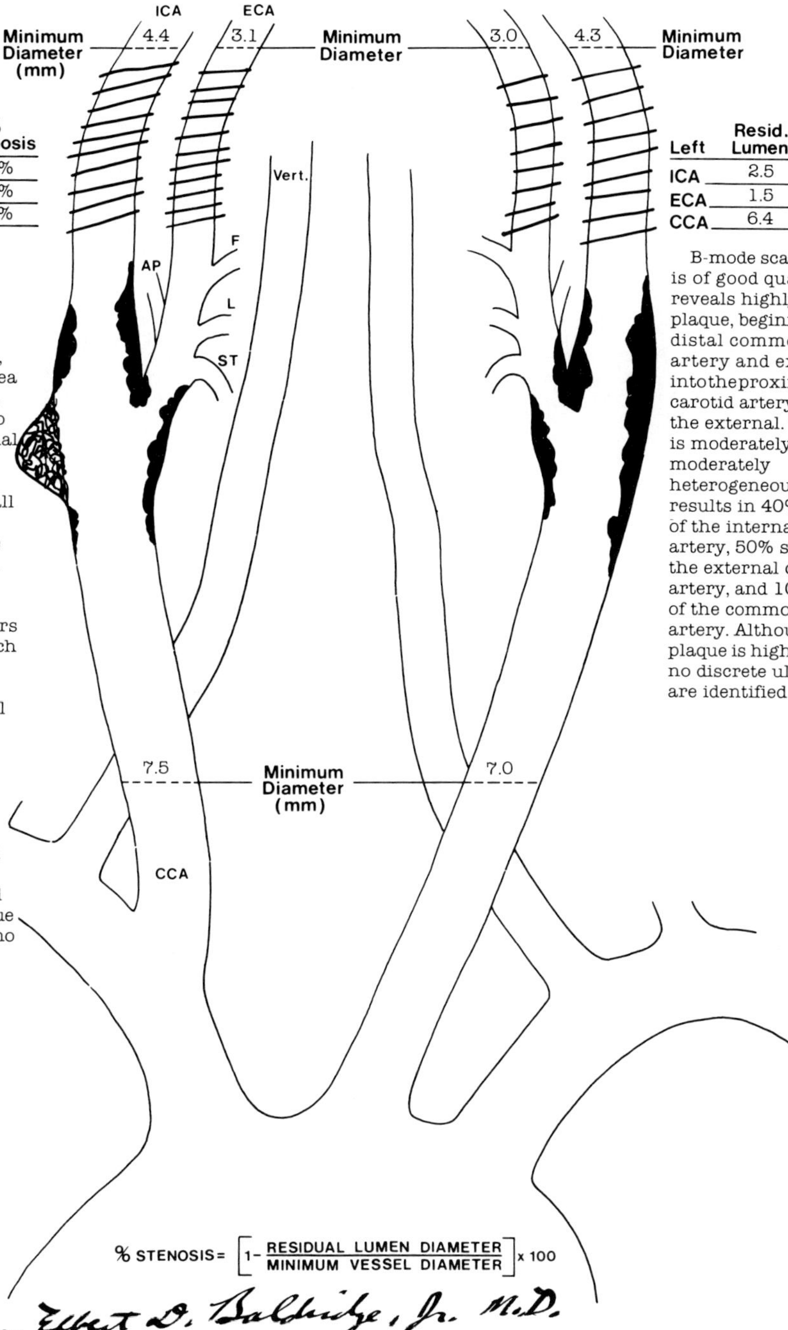

Left	Resid. Lumen	% Stenosis
ICA	2.5	40%
ECA	1.5	50%
CCA	6.4	10%

B-mode scan on the left is of good quality and reveals highly irregular plaque, beginning in the distal common carotid artery and extending intotheproximalinternal carotid artery as well as the external. The plaque is moderately echogenic, moderately heterogeneous, and results in 40% stenosis of the internal carotid artery, 50% stenosis of the external carotid artery, and 10% stenosis of the common carotid artery. Although the plaque is highly irregular no discrete ulcerations are identified.

$$\% \text{ STENOSIS} = \left[1 - \frac{\text{RESIDUAL LUMEN DIAMETER}}{\text{MINIMUM VESSEL DIAMETER}}\right] \times 100$$

Peripheral Vascular Fellow Elbert D. Baldridge, Jr. M.D.

The second diagram has been completed for the patient whose right carotid aneurysm was shown in Figures 134, 135, 158. Although the left internal carotid artery contains considerable plaque, there is only a 40% stenosis relative to the distal artery. This is the value of illustrating plaque with a drawing. Otherwise the physician might think a 0% stenosis means an absence of plaque. Note also the cross hatching that indicates nonvisualized parts of the distal arteries. Any drawing showing the arteries in only one plane must be a composite and not an identical likeness to any single ultrasound scan. The purpose is to communicate an overall impression of the extent of disease.

INDEX